ACUTE CARE NURSE
PRACTITIONER CERTIFICATION
EXAMINATION:
Review Questions and Strategies

Barbara A. Todd, RN-C, MSN, FNP, ACNP
Director Clinical Services, Cardiac Surgery
Temple University Hospital
Philadelphia, Pennsylvania

 F. A. Davis Company • Philadelphia

F. A. Davis Company
1915 Arch Street
Philadelphia, PA 19103
www.fadavis.com

Printed in the United States of America

Last digit indicates print number: 10 9 8 7 6 5 4

Acquisitions Editor: Joanne P. DaCunha, RN, MSN
Developmental Editor: Diane Schweisguth, RN, BSN
Cover Designer: Louis J. Forgione

As new scientific information becomes available through basic and clinical research, recommended treatments and drug therapies undergo changes. The author and publisher have done everything possible to make this book accurate, up to date, and in accordance with accepted standards at the time of publication. The author, editors, and publisher are not responsible for errors or omissions or for consequences from application of the book, and make no warranty, expressed or implied, in regard to the contents of the book. Any practice described in this book should be applied by the reader in accordance with professional standards of care used in regard to the unique circumstances that may apply in each situation. The reader is advised always to check product information (package inserts) for changes and new information regarding dose and contraindications before administering any drug. Caution is especially urged when using new or infrequently ordered drugs.

Library of Congress Cataloging-in-Publication Data

Todd, Barbara, A.
  Acute care nurse practitioner certification examination : review questions and strategies/ Barbara A. Todd.
    p. cm.
  ISBN10:0-8036-0957-4   ISBN13: 978-0-8036-0957-0
  1. Intensive care nursing—Examinations, questions, etc.
RT120.I5 T64 2001
610.73′61—dc21

2001047102

This book is dedicated to my mother, Mattie Todd, and the memory of my father, Julius Todd, Sr., for their guidance and support in shaping my nursing career.

Preface

In my 23 years as a clinician practicing in acute care and serving as clinical preceptor to numerous nurse practitioner, nursing, and medical students, I have come to appreciate the value of using sample examinations as pedagogical tools. This book was written as a guide for nurse practitioner students who are preparing for the acute care nurse practitioner (ACNP) certification examination. To that end, I have provided numerous questions that reflect both the content of the ACNP exam and the constant evolution of the fields of nursing and medicine. I have made every attempt to ensure that the information presented is current and relevant.

This book is organized into six units. Unit I, which comprises Chapters 1 and 2, includes test-taking strategies. Unit II, Chapters 3 to 12, covers system-specific health problems. Unit III, Chapters 13 to 29, communicates common problems in acute care. Unit IV encompasses issues in acute care, covered in Chapter 30. Unit V covers health promotion and risk assessment, covered in Chapter 31. Unit VI consists of two practice examinations, each containing 175 questions. A CD, intended to simulate the test environment, also accompanies the book. It includes two practice examinations, each containing 225 questions.

I sincerely wish you luck on the certification examination. I hope that this book provides an invaluable tool to help you assess your readiness to take the ACNP certification examination.

Barbara A. Todd

Acknowledgments

I would like to acknowledge my countless patients and colleagues who have contributed to this book and to my professional development. I would especially like to thank my colleague and mentor, V. Paul Addonizio, MD, for his ongoing support of my professional endeavors.

I would also like to thank my family and friends for their constant encouragement during this project.

A special thanks to the F. A. Davis team, Joanne DaCunha and Diane Schweisguth, for their assistance.

Most of all, I would like to thank God for the gift of life and the vision for this professional mission.

Contributors

Karen Stuart Champion, RN, BSN, MS
Instructor
Indian River Community College
Fort Pierce, Florida
(Coauthor, Chapter 2: Test-Taking Skills and Designing Your Study Plan)

Lynne M. Dunphy, RN, PhD, FNP, CNS
Associate Professor
College of Nursing
Florida Atlantic University
Boca Raton, Florida
(Author, Chapter 1: Achieving Success on a Certification Examination;
Coauthor, Chapter 2: Test-Taking Skills and Designing Your Study Plan)

Consultants

Rosanne Iacono, RNCS, MSN, ARNP
Nurse Practitioner
Thomas Jefferson University Hospital
Philadelphia, Pennsylvania

Otilia A. Loya, RN, MS, MBA
Consultant
Castro Valley, California

Pamela McDonald, RNC, RNFA, WHCNP, APCNP
Nurse Practitioner
Blackhawk Medical Center
Danville, California

Alice S. Poyss, RN, PhD, CRNP
Associate Professor
MCP Hahnemann University
Philadelphia, Pennsylvania

Contents

INTRODUCTION

1

● LYNNE M. DUNPHY

Achieving Success on a Certification Examination

Congratulations! With the purchase of this book, you have taken your first step along the road to becoming a certified advanced practice nurse! The earlier in your educational process you begin preparing for the certification examination (we will be using the term "exam" from now on for the rest of this book), the greater your chance of success will be. However, if you are a practitioner who has been "out there" for a number of years, this book will also help you understand the certification process and the steps to take to be successful on the certification exam of your choice. Regardless of your situation, the important point is that you have begun! Remember: The longest journey begins with but a single step.

Adapted from Winland-Brown, JE, and Dunphy, LM: Adult and Family Nurse Practitioner Certification Examination: Review Questions and Strategies. FA Davis, Philadelphia, 2000.

Certification and Why It Is Important

There are basic differences between becoming licensed (something you achieved at the completion of your basic nursing program by sitting for the state board or National Council Licensure Examination [NCLEX]) and becoming certified. A good understanding of the difference between the two is important to your ultimate success on the certification exam. Becoming "test savvy" demands a thorough understanding of the underlying premises and purposes of the exam for which you are sitting.

Licensure

Licensure is mandated for practice and is a legal delineation. Its purpose is to protect the public from unsafe practitioners. Legal regulation of nursing practice is the joint responsibility of state legislators and the state boards of nursing. Minimum competency is assessed on a licensure exam: Have you met the basic criteria for safe and effective nursing practice? The test questions on the licensure exam are from frequently updated job analyses conducted about entry-level nursing practice. They reflect those functions a registered nurse (RN) needs to know and perform for safe entry-level practice. Currently, the licensure exam is prepared and administered by the National Council of State Boards of Nursing. Composed of representatives from every state board across the United States including its territories, this body assumes responsibility for setting a national standard for safe and effective entry-level nursing practice and assessing it through administration of a national licensing exam, the National Council Licensing Examination for Registered Nurses (NCLEX-RN). Passing this exam is mandatory for state licensure as a registered nurse in every state.

Certification

In contrast, *certification* is the process by which a nongovernmental agency or association grants recognition to an individual who has met predetermined standards for specialty practice. Certification validates superior knowledge of a nursing specialty, and through the process of recertification, implies continued high achievement in that specialty. In 1974, the American Nurses Association (ANA) initiated a national voluntary certification process to recognize excellence in nursing practice. By 1978, the purpose had broadened and included the assurance of quality beyond basic nursing practice. This was partly to recognize professional achievement but also to identify nurses potentially eligible for third-party reimbursement.

The purpose of certification (Table 1–1) is quite different from that of licensure. Certification is a voluntary process, although currently many states require passage of the appropriate certification exam for licensure to perform advanced practice nursing functions.

Purpose of Certification

Debate remains heated on the continuation of voluntary certification administered through professional associations such as the ANA and its subsidiary, the American Nurses Credentialing Center (ANCC) versus a mandatory second-level licensure exam specifically for advanced practice nursing functions. At present, however, certification is the only means available to validate

TABLE 1–1. **PURPOSE OF CERTIFICATION**

- Required for practice in some states
- Indicates specialized and advanced knowledge base
- Provides greater career opportunities
- Increasingly required for third-party reimbursement

your advanced practice nursing knowledge nationally. (Table 1–2 lists associations and organizations offering advanced-practice nursing certification.)

Associations and Organizations Offering Advance-Practice Nursing Certification

National certification and specialty designation play an increasingly central role in both state licensure at an advanced practice level and in reimbursement for advanced nursing services, as well as prescriptive priv-

TABLE 1–2. **ASSOCIATIONS AND ORGANIZATIONS OFFERING ADVANCE-PRACTICE NURSING CERTIFICATION**

Association or Organization	Advance Practice Nursing Certification
American Academy of Nurse Practitioners	Nurse Practitioner • Adult • Family
American Nurses Credentialing Center	Nurse Practitioner • Acute care (jointly with American Association of Critical-Care Nurses) • Adult • Family • Gerontologic • Pediatric • School Clinical Nurse Specialist • Community health • Gerontologic • Home health • Medical-surgical • Psychiatric and mental health (adult); psychiatric and mental health (child and adolescent)
American Association of Nurse Anesthetists	Certified Registered Nurse Anesthetist
American College of Nurse-Midwives	Certified Nurse Midwife
National Certification Board of Pediatric Nurse Practitioners and Nurses	Nurse Practitioner • Pediatric
National Certification Corporation for the Obstetric, Gynecologic, and Neonatal Nurse Practitioner Nursing Specialties	Nurse Practitioner • Neonatal • Woman's health
Oncology Nursing Certification Corporation	Advanced Oncology Nursing for Nurse Practitioners and Clinical Nurse Specialists

ileges in certain states. Some forms of reimbursement are contingent on national certification. As of 1998, certification became necessary to receive Medicare reimbursement, and the Veterans Affairs Medical Systems mandate national certification for advanced practice nurses. Likewise, certain managed-care organizations, as well as hospitals, require national certification as a criterion for credentialing of the provider.

Certification of advanced practice nurses (APNs) serves to ensure that individuals titled at an advanced practice level have mastered a specific body of knowledge and acquired a particular set of specialized skills unique to their areas of practice. APNs are expected to have expert competence, knowledge, and skills. Consensus has increasingly emerged regarding the competencies and specialty skills of APNs. The skills and abilities of APNs as outlined by the National Council of State Boards of Nursing in 1992 include:

- Advanced ability to synthesize and analyze data
- Advanced ability to apply nursing principles
- Ability to provide expert guidance and teaching
- Ability to work with clients, their families, and other health-care workers
- Ability to manage clients' health or illness status
- Ability to recognize practice limits
- Ability to use abstract thinking and conceptualization
- Ability to make decisions independently
- Ability to diagnose and prescribe
- Ability to consult with or refer clients to other health-care workers[1]

YOUR ROLE

You are making an important, timely, and professionally astute decision by deciding to become certified. Margretta Madden Styles, President, American Nurses Credentialing Center, noted in a recent edition of *Credentialing News*, ". . . as the global tide turns from governmental regulation and public protectionism toward competitive quality improvement of services and informed consumer choice, voluntary credentialing is a movement whose time has come."[2] We concur.

CERTIFICATION EXAMS

Certification exams from ANCC are designed to assess your abilities as an APN in the delivery of acute care services. Table 1–3 lists the requirements for nurse practitioner certification.

Requirements for Nurse Practitioner Certification

AMERICAN NURSES CREDENTIALING CENTER

In 1973, the ANA established its certification program to recognize professional achievement in a defined clinical or functional area of nursing. This was in response to a proliferation of specialties in nursing, as

TABLE 1–3. REQUIREMENTS FOR NURSE PRACTITIONER CERTIFICATION

American Nurses Credentialing Center (ANCC)

SPECIALTY AREAS
- Acute Care Nurse Practitioner
- Adult Nurse Practitioner
- Family Nurse Practitioner
- Gerontological Nurse Practitioner
- Pediatric Nurse Practitioner
- School Health Nurse Practitioner (recertification only)

REQUIREMENTS
- Master's degree level Nurse Practitioner program from an accredited institution of higher learning
- Meet practice requirements specific to certification type

EXAMINATIONS
- Computer-based
- Administered at Sylvan Learning Centers on request
- Year 2000 exam costs: $230 for member, $370 for nonmembers

CONTACT
ANCC
600 Maryland Ave, SW
Suite 100 West
Washington, DC 20024-2571
800-284-2378
http://www.ana.org/ancc/index.htm

well as the increasing emphasis in graduate nursing education on an area of clinical specialization. The exams were first offered in 1974. It was a voluntary process, and 691 nurses were initially certified, including psychiatric mental health clinical nurse specialists, the first APNs to promote certification and use it as a basis for reimbursement. A master's degree was required to sit for this advanced practice certification. In 1978, 10 generalist and specialty level certification examinations were available; by 2000, the number of exams available had expanded to 30. Currently, more than 130,000 nurses have achieved certification at both the generalist and advanced practice levels. Exams are published in 15 generalist categories, 12 in advanced practice categories (including clinical nurse specialist certifications and nurse practitioner certification), 4 in the nursing systems and administration category, and 1 modular certification in case management. In 1991, the ANCC was established as a separate subsidiary of the ANA. Nationally accepted standards for certification require that credentialing bodies be separate from their parent organizations to prevent conflicts of interest.

To qualify to take an exam and become certified at either the generalist or advanced level, a nurse must (1) meet requirements for clinical or functional practice in a specialized field; (2) show evidence of having pursued education beyond basic nursing preparation, and in the case of nurse practitioner exams, provide evidence of successful completion of a master's level approved curriculum; and (3) in some cases, have received the endorsement of his or her peers. After meeting these criteria, the nurse must also take and pass the certification exam to be certified in that specialty.

After you have sent in your application for the ANCC exam, you will receive a copy of the *Candidate's Handbook,* a valuable source of help in preparing for the exam. The handbook contains a test content outline (TCO) that describes the domains of practice and content areas, topics, and subtopics that will be covered on the exam. It also includes information about how that content is weighted, that is, the number of test questions in each of the major content areas. For example, the June 1998 TCO for the Family Nurse Practitioner Certification Exam indicated that there would be 37 questions (24.7%) on the evaluation and promotion of client wellness, 105 questions (70%) on the assessment and management of client illness, and 8 questions (5.3%) on issues in primary care. The domain content of issues in primary care consists of the nurse-client relationship, ethical and legal considerations, and access to care. Additionally, questions were further classified along a second dimension, that of life span, which included non–age-specific content, aging adult, adult, adolescent, child, infant, and childbearing woman. A third dimension identified as problem areas, organized content by body systems, such as respiratory and cardiovascular. What this means is that each test question is characterized by all three dimensions. For example, a test question that asks about the treatment of a 70-year-old man with a diagnosis of benign prostatic hypertrophy would be categorized as an assessment and management of client illness test question, requesting content about the aging adult, specifically to do with the genitourinary system. Be aware that the TCO may be changed from exam to exam, so you need to carefully examine your handbook for the most current one.

The computer-based exam for the year 2000 had 150 test questions. The number of items on the test may vary from 75 to 150, depending on your pattern of testing. The passing scores for the Acute Care Nurse Practitioners exams taken from August 1999 to February 2000 were 97 out of 150 questions. During that time, 239 persons sat for the exam; 209 passed, or 87.5%. A criterion-referenced standard is used to reflect a level of specialty knowledge independent of the group taking the exam. In this approach, each examinee's score is compared with an absolute number determined by the content experts who develop the exam. The passing score is determined by the test development committee after careful consideration of the content of the test questions, as well as statistical examinations of the reliability and validity of the "piloted" test questions. *The passing score is always expressed in terms of the number of questions you must answer correctly on the total test.* Your score report will provide you with detailed information regarding how many test questions you got correct in each of the major content domains; however, it is your performance on the total test that determines your success or failure. These reports are mailed to you within 6 to 8 weeks after the

exam. You will need to recertify every 5 years. This may be accomplished by retaking the exam or by keeping your practice current; at present 1000 hours of clinical practice in your specialty area are mandated for recertification, along with 75 continuing education credits.

ACHIEVING SUCCESS

Much of the focus in your various practitioner programs has been on assessment, management, and evaluation of disease. In addition, this is the role most of you readers perform in your respective work settings. The ability to diagnose and treat disease is paramount to your safe and effective functioning as an APN and the certification exams increasingly reflect this reality. However, it is important never to lose sight of the fact that these exams are certifying your abilities as an APN, and as such have an underlying bias *toward health, health promotion, and human responses to health and illness.* As a nurse, your reaction to the various manifestations of health and illness phenomena is instinctively different than that of another primary-health-care provider. This is manifested in different ways on each exam, but it is an important distinction to keep in mind as you sit and ponder various distracters and wonder what answer the examiner wants. Similarly, the test blueprints and type of questions asked reflect a continued commitment to concepts of health promotion and disease prevention, as well as underlying principles of therapeutic communication skills so essential to forging meaningful nurse-client relationships. Nursing-based elements of growth and development, nutrition, and therapeutic communication, as well as content on cultural differences and cross-cultural communication, will be integrated with the more specific content of diagnosis, pharmacology, and disease management.

Physical assessment and history-taking skills, as well as content from advanced physical assessment courses, remain prominent. Although a certain amount of basic pharmacologic content is included, the latest drugs and pharmacologic interventions may not always appear because the exam questions are prepared and tested in advance. Questions about your knowledge of prescribing safely for the pregnant woman almost always appear on the FNP exams.

If you have been in active practice for some time, care must be exercised as you take the exam. Distractors (see Chap. 2) will not necessarily correlate with what you currently see and do. Remember, the exam reflects the *ideal* answer according to the certifying body and not always the realities of your practice! Answers rely on national guidelines and standards of practice from a variety of bodies. Your practice is often actualized in specialty areas, across different geographic regions, and at sites with different practice patterns and priorities. The questions on the exam are looking for much more generalized responses and might well reflect phenomena you have very seldom experienced. Allowing yourself to become frustrated with the distracters offered will not help, but rather will hinder, your ability to succeed. This is why it is essential that your study consist of taking large numbers of sample test items (more about this in Chap. 2).

Being familiar with testing and succeeding on a multiple-choice exam are far different abilities than the expert skills you bring to your professional practice. But these skills are not mutually exclusive. It is a matter of the correct "mind set." This mind set is predicated on an awareness of the *nursing* base of the certification exam coupled with an understanding of the test blueprint. Determine not to select an anecdotal answer based on experience from your own practice, but rather on nationally recognized, clinically based guidelines rooted in the literature.

You have taken the first and hardest step: You have purchased this book! Mentally review the important reasons to become nationally certified. Fix the end goal vividly in your mind. Imagine how you will feel opening the envelope telling you that you have succeeded, that you are a nationally certified APN. It is a worthwhile goal.

Take the next step on the road to success. Turn to Chapter 2. It will assist you in the development of important test-taking skills as well as providing guidelines for your individualized study plan.

You can succeed!

References

1. National Council of State Boards of Nursing: National Council of State Boards of Nursing Position Paper on the Licensure of Advanced Nursing Practice. National Council of State Boards of Nursing, May, 1992.
2. Styles, M: The road ahead. ANCC Credentialing News 1:1, 1998.

Bibliography

American Nurses Certification Corporation: 1998 Certification Catalog. American Nurses Certification Corporation, Washington, DC, 1998.

Henerson, T, et al: Scope of Practice and Reimbursement for Advance Practice Registered Nurses: A State-by-State Analysis. Intergovernmental Health Policy Project, Washington, DC, 1995.

King, CS: Second licensure. Advanced Practice Nursing Quarterly 1:7, 1995.

National Certification Board of Pediatric Nurse Practitioners and Nurses: Pediatric Nurse Practitioner Certification and Certification Maintenance Programs. National Certification Board of Pediatric Nurse Practitioners, Cherry Hill, NJ, 1995.

Oncology Nursing Certification Corporation: Oncology Nursing Certification Corporation Test Bulletin, Oncology Nursing Certification Corporation, Pittsburgh, PA, 1996.

Pearson, L: Annual update of how each state stands on legislative issues affecting advanced nursing practice. Nurse Pract 23:1, 1998.

Sheehy, CM, and McCarthy, M: Advance Practice Nursing: Emphasizing Common Goals. FA Davis, Philadelphia, 1998.

Your Guide to Certification and How to Get a License: Career Guide 1998. Am J Nurs, 1998.

Resources

American Nurses Credentialing Center (ANCC)
600 Maryland Ave, SW
Suite 100 West
Washington, DC 20024-2571
800-284-2378
http://www.ana.org/ancc/index.htm.

To find out whether your state has certification requirements for advance practice nursing, use the World Wide Web to get a list of all state Boards of Nursing (BON) with web sites:
http://www.ncsbn.org/files/otherweb.html#sbon

2

● LYNNE M. DUNPHY and KAREN STUART CHAMPION

Test-Taking Skills and Designing Your Study Plan

Adapted from Winland-Brown, JE, and Dunphy, LM: Adult and Family Nurse Practitioner Certification Examination: Review Questions and Strategies. FA Davis, Philadelphia, 2000.

This chapter has several parts. The first parts deal with the specifics of answering multiple-choice test questions and the skills necessary to succeed when taking a multiple-choice examination (we will use the term exam from this point on). We specifically discuss the American Nurses Credentialing Center (ANCC) acute care nurse practitioner exam. The second part actively assists you in developing and setting up an individualized study plan that will enable you to succeed in achieving your goal: becoming a nationally certified advanced practice nurse.

Test-Taking Skills: An Acquired Art

Both certification exams consist of multiple-choice test questions. The ability to select the best response to the question posed is what determines your success on the exam. Knowledge of the content is unfortunately not enough to guarantee success. If you are not able to communicate your knowledge through the medium of a multiple-choice exam, you will not succeed in becoming certified. Achieving success on a multiple-choice test is a skill, and like any other skill, it can be learned. Think of it as playing tennis. The more you practice, the stronger the muscles in your arm become and the better you get. The same is true for test taking. To begin strengthening your test-taking "muscles," we discuss some specific test-taking strategies.

STRATEGY #1: UNDERSTANDING AND ANALYZING THE ANATOMY OF A TEST QUESTION

A multiple-choice test question consists of three parts:

- An introductory statement, which sets up the clinical situation
- A stem, which poses a question
- Options, from which you must select the correct answer

The first step in analyzing a multiple-choice test question is to separate what the question *tells* you from what it is *asking*. The *introductory statement,* which may vary considerably in length, provides information about a clinical situation, a disease process, or a nursing response. This statement includes a specific question, referred to as the *stem,* that you must answer on the basis of your advanced practice nursing knowledge. Stems may be worded in different ways. Some stems are in the form of a question; others are in the form of an incomplete statement. You must select the *option* that best answers the question posed or completes the incomplete statement from a number of potential options, referred to as *distractors.*

Recognizing these components will assist you in analyzing the information presented and focusing on the question's intent or issue. Let's look at an example that includes an introductory statement in the form of a clinical situation. The stem is in **bold print.**

EXAMPLE 1

*A 78-year-old woman with a history of hypertension but no other health history is **noted to have a systolic ejection murmur heard at the second right intercostal space.** The rest of the physical examination is normal. You would suspect:*

A. mitral stenosis.
B. aortic sclerosis.
C. aortic stenosis.
D. mitral regurgitation.

The introductory statement of Example 1 gives you information about the clinical situation (the 78-year-old woman with history of hypertension) and the stem gives you the physical assessment findings. The option that provides the most accurate response is B.

Understand what the question is asking. Test questions designed to assess nursing knowledge do so in two ways: recall (memory-based questions) and comprehension (application-based questions). This question is an example of a recall question. Nursing, however, is a practice-based discipline. Application of nursing knowledge is essential to safe, competency-based practice. Application frequently implies analysis of information. Review the following example.

EXAMPLE 2

A 68-year-old man with hypertension and diabetes should have influenza vaccination:

A. yearly.
B. every 5 years.
C. every 6 months.
D. every 10 years.

This question is asking about information related to recommendations regarding immunizations.

Additionally, a stem will request one of two types of responses: a *positive response* or a *negative response.* Remember, the stem asks you to answer a question, to solve a problem, or select a response. To select the correct *option,* you need to determine the *type of stem.* Positive-response stems request an answer that is true, appropriate, or accurate, whereas negative-response stems request the option that is incorrect, false, inaccurate, or inappropriate. Negative-response stems frequently contain words such as *except, not, false,* or *least.* Consider this example.

EXAMPLE 3

*Risk factors for osteoporosis include all of the following **EXCEPT:***

A. alcohol.
B. obesity.
C. age.
D. sedentary lifestyle.

Example 3 is a straight recall question testing your knowledge about osteoporosis and its risk factors. The key word in the stem, *except,* is a negative. Putting it another way, to select the correct response for this question, which is B, you must select the answer that is wrong or that is *not* a positively correlated risk factor for osteoporosis. Be sure to determine whether the stem is a positive-response stem or a negative-response stem in order to select the correct answer.

STRATEGY #2: IDENTIFYING THE QUESTION'S CRITICAL ELEMENTS AND KEY WORDS

The ability to identify those *critical elements* and *key words* in a test question is crucial to correct interpretation of the question. For example, they determine whether the stem is asking for a positive or negative response. Additionally, key words are important words or phrases that help focus your attention on what the question is specifically asking. Key words usually appear in the stem, whereas the critical elements, such as the key concepts and conditions, tend to appear in the introductory statement. Examples of key words include most, first response, earliest, priority, on the first visit, on a subsequent visit, common, best, least, except, not, immediately, and initial. Often, but not always, these words appear in bold or italicized print. Take a look at this example.

EXAMPLE 4

*Which of the following is an example of a **primary** preventive intervention?*

A. Tetanus prophylaxis
B. Screening sigmoidoscopy
C. Papanicolaou smear
D. Blood pressure screening

Example 4 is a recall question with a positive-response stem. Although all of the interventions are preventive, the key word is **primary,** allowing you to choose the correct answer, A.

You must also identify the *issue* the question is asking about. For example, the question might be requesting information about a disorder.

EXAMPLE 5

*Mr. Williams, age 76, is seen in the ambulatory care clinic. He is complaining about incontinence, suprapubic pain, urgency, and dysuria. Urinalysis reveals the presence of white blood cells (WBCs), red blood cells (RBCs), and bacteria. Your **assessment** is:*

A. prostatitis.
B. nephrotic syndrome.
C. benign prostatic hypertrophy (BPH).
D. cystitis.

By selecting the correct answer, D, you have demonstrated knowledge related to a disease process, the *issue* about which this question requested informa-

tion. Other examples of issues include drugs, for example, antibiotics or immunizations; a diagnostic test, such as urinalysis or serum glucose; a toxic effect of a drug, such as rash or vomiting; a problem, for example, knowledge deficit or substance abuse; a procedure, such as bone marrow aspiration or cardiac catheterization; a behavior, for example, agitation or overeating; or occasionally a combination of the above. Consider this example.

EXAMPLE 6

*Which drug is **not** used in the treatment of acute gout?*

A. A nonsteroidal anti-inflammatory drug (NSAID)
B. Colchicine
C. An antibiotic
D. An analgesic

This is a *recall* question with a negative-response stem. The *key word* is *negative* (**not**), and the issue is knowledge of drugs. The correct answer is C.

STRATEGY #3: USING THERAPEUTIC COMMUNICATIONS

In communication-type questions, you are always looking for a *therapeutic response,* the cornerstone of the nurse-client relationship. To communicate therapeutically, you need to use communication tools and avoid communication blocks. Remember your basic therapeutic nursing role. The nurse, whether at a generalist or advance-practice level, is *always* therapeutic. Your role is *not* that of an authority figure. This may cause some confusion for practitioners from other cultures in which health-care providers are conceptualized as authority figures who give directions. Remember, this is a *nursing*-based exam. Your *initial response* is *always* the therapeutic response, the acknowledgment and validation of the client's feelings.

EXAMPLE 7

Ms. Doe, age 55, is very fearful because of a breast lump you have just identified. She begins to cry and states: "I'm afraid of having a mammogram." Your initial response is:

A. "You must have the mammogram."
B. "Don't worry; I'm sure it is nothing."
C. "Wonderful advances have been made in breast cancer research."
D. "You feel scared?"

The correct answer is D. Communication skills learned in Nursing 101 are important components of successful test-taking strategies. Table 2–1 reviews communication techniques that facilitate therapeutic communication and those that block therapeutic communication.

TABLE 2–1. COMMUNICATION TECHNIQUES

Techniques	Examples
TECHNIQUES THAT FACILITATE THERAPEUTIC COMMUNICATION	
Offering self	"I'll stay with you."
Showing empathy	"I see you are upset."
Silence	Remaining present but silent
Giving information	"You need to take this drug two times a day."
Restatement	"You feel hurt?"
Clarification	"You are saying that . . ."
Reflection	"You seem to be anxious."
TECHNIQUES THAT BLOCK THERAPEUTIC COMMUNICATION	
False reassurance	"Everything will be okay."
Disapproval	"That was wrong."
Approval	"That was right."
Requesting an explanation	"Why did you do that?"
Giving advice	"I think you should . . ."
Deferring	"You need to talk with your doctor about that."
Defensiveness	"We are understaffed!"
Devaluing feelings	"That's silly, don't be upset!"

Communication Techniques

Another important component in selecting the correct answer to questions that address your ability to communicate therapeutically is prioritization of responses. More than one option may contain a therapeutic response. But which is the *first, best,* or *most therapeutic* response in that situation? Communication theory emphasizes that it is a priority to address the client's *feelings first.* Validate, validate, validate. "You seem to be very sad today, Mr. George." "I can see that you are upset." "You seem very anxious, Mrs. Smith." This should always be done *before* clarifying or presenting information. Is there a need to address these feelings? If so, this takes priority. Empathy, restatement, reflection, and being silent, as well as remaining with the client, are all excellent nursing strategies that can potentially validate clients' feelings. The only exception to this rule would be the presence of a pressing or interfering physical problem.

STRATEGY #4: IDENTIFYING THE PERSON WHO IS THE FOCUS OF THE QUESTION

Another critical element is your ability to identify the person who is the focus of the question. This person might be the client or the person with the health problem, whereas other questions might address a family member, or neighbor of the person with the healthcare problem, or another member of the health-care team. Take a look at this example.

EXAMPLE 8

Mr. Boyd, age 84, has dementia and is in a long-term-care facility. His daughter and son-in-law are visiting. As they get ready to leave and begin to say good-bye, Mr. Boyd grabs his daughter's arm and begins to cry, saying "Don't leave me here. I will die in this place." As she leaves the room, his daughter is visibly upset and asks you whether she ought visit again soon because it has so upset her father. The best reply for you to make is:

A. "You might try telephoning next time instead of visiting. Your father will know that you are thinking of him then."
B "I will give you the number of the social worker. She will be able to arrange a team conference and family meeting."
C. "This is a very upsetting time for all of you. However, it is important that you continue to visit regularly. For now, I will go in and sit with your father for a little while."
D. "He needs time to adjust to this new setting. Perhaps it might be easier on you all if you just didn't visit for a few days."

In this question, the person who is the focus of the question is Mr. Boyd's daughter, not Mr. Boyd. The *key word* in the stem is *best* response. It is also helpful to identify the issue the question is asking. The *issue* in this question is one of therapeutic communication. The issue is Mr. Boyd's daughter's feelings of concern about her father. C is the correct response because it validates the daughter's feelings first.

STRATEGY #5: DETERMINING THE BEST RESPONSE

There may be more than one option in a test question that is correct. Even so, which is the *best, first, or most therapeutically sound* response to the question posed? Application-based test questions often involve decision making, which is based on prioritization. To assist you in the correct selection, follow a few tips:

- Assessment always comes before diagnosis and treatment.
- The key word, *initial,* usually implies the need to assess.
- Remember Maslow's Hierarchy of Needs.
- In communication-based questions, you must address the client's feelings first.
- In teaching and learning situations, learning is contingent upon **motivation**.

According to Maslow, physiologic needs always come first. For example, you might recall the mnemonic "A, B, C" (referring to *a*irway, *b*reathing, *c*irculation) from basic cardiopulmonary life support as a way of prioritizing treatment. This is handy to remember for questions that present a sudden emergency situation or any situation that is potentially life-threatening for the client. If basic physiologic needs are met, safety is the next priority, followed by psychosocial needs. Therapeutic communication skills teach the acknowledgment of feelings first. Teaching and learning theory remind us that unless the client is motivated to learn, no client teaching will be successful. If the client is not motivated, this issue must be addressed first.

STRATEGY #6: AVOIDING COMMON PITFALLS

A very common cause of test-taking error is misreading the test question. To avoid common pitfalls, follow these tips:

- Ask yourself, "What is this question *really* asking?"
- Look for the key words.
- Restate the question in your own words. Eliminate any options that require you to make assumptions about information that was not presented in the case scenario and any options that contain information not presented in the scenario. *Do not read into and overanalyze the test question!* Go with your first, most straightforward response. It is usually your best bet for answering the test question correctly.
- Carefully review the question using the systematic format and strategies suggested in this book.
- Make a decision about each option as you read it; this is an efficient approach to test taking. Do *not* go back to that option once you have eliminated it; do *not* overcomplicate the case scenario presented; and do *not* rely on anecdotal data from your own practice! These are national exams with testing content based on national standards of practice.

STRATEGY #7: SELECTING THE BEST ANSWER WHEN YOU DO NOT KNOW THE ANSWER

We now discuss more specific strategies for selecting the best answer. Okay. You are beginning your exam. You have answered a few questions easily, but now you have come to a test question to which you do not know the answer. You have identified the introductory statement and the stem (whether it is a positive-response stem or a negative-response stem) and read through the distractors. You have identified the issue and the person who is the focus of the question. You are still uncertain about the correct answer. If this happens, follow these tips:

- Eliminate incorrect options. This is very important. Frequently, you will be able to eliminate two choices easily. This gives you a 50% chance of guessing the correct answer, even on a test question that you do not know!
- Select the most global response option. The option that is the most comprehensive or general statement is often a better answer than an option that is

more specific and thus limited. A global response, by definition, means a more general statement.
- Eliminate similar options or those that contain words like "always" or "never." If options say essentially the same thing, neither can be correct. Absolute options containing the words "always" or "never" are seldom correct.
- Look for similar words or phrases in the introductory statement or stem and in the options.

Try this strategy if you need to guess.

- Be alert to relevant information from earlier questions.
- Watch for grammatical inconsistencies between the stem and the options. If three of the four options sound similar, the "odd" one should win out.
- Look for the longest option. It is often the correct response.

Key test-taking tips are given in Table 2–2.

Key Test-Taking Tips

TEST-TAKING SKILLS: KNOW YOURSELF

Which Test-Taking Type Are You?

A fun part of this exercise can be to diagnose your own studying and test-taking style. Are you a tortoise or a hare? Are you a peacock? Or are you more like a pig? Knowing this can assist you in both designing your study plan for the exam and answering test questions on the exam. For example, are you a tortoise, moving slowly and laboriously through each question, taking far too long, and then having to rush at the end, thus increasing your chance of error? Or are you a hare, racing through the exam questions as fast as you can, often misreading information and likely to make quick guesses as opposed to carefully thought out responses.

TABLE 2–2. KEY TEST-TAKING TIPS

- Eliminate options you know are incorrect. If you can eliminate two options, even a guess has a 50% chance of being correct.
- Answer all questions as if the situations were ideal.
- Read the test question carefully.
- Separate what the question tells you from what it is asking.
- Identify all false-response stems.
- Select the most global response.
- Eliminate options that are incorrect or similar, or that contain words such as "always" or "never."
- Look for grammatical inconsistencies between the stem and the options, words in the options that have appeared in the stem, and the longest option.
- Be alert to information relevant to answering the question in the stem or in earlier questions.

Are you preoccupied with grades and personal achievement, viewing the certification exam as a threat? Do you procrastinate about studying rather than developing and sticking to a well-designed study plan, thus increasing your anxiety? Do you argue with some test questions and their options? None is right, you think, according to your practice! Then you may be a peacock. Remember, exam questions are *not* perfect, but they still require that you choose the *best* available option. Do *not* waste time and energy arguing mentally with a test question. Select what you feel is the best option and *move on!* Or are you a pig? Pigs frequently doubt their own knowledge and may change initial correct responses. Usually pigs are smart, but lack confidence. They are often academically successful, but experience anxiety when information is presented in a different format. Table 2–3 will assist you in identifying your test-taking personality as well as providing concrete suggestions for maximizing your study efforts.

TABLE 2–3. **IDENTIFYING YOUR TEST-TAKING TYPE***

Hare	*Tortoise*	*Peacock*	*Pig*
STUDY STYLE			
Crams Feels anxious during study sessions	Obsessive Focuses on details; misses the bigger picture	Procrastinates Puts off studying; does not think there is a need to study	Diligent Smart, has good study habits, but lacks self-confidence
TEST-TAKING STYLE			
Often first to finish Rushes; does not thoroughly read questions and answers Makes quick guesses Feels anxious when answer is not readily apparent	Often last to finish Spends too much time examining the details and rereading questions and answers May have to rush at end to complete exam in allotted time	Reads own ideas into questions Changes initial responses often because expected answer is not present Selects answer based on anecdotal experience	Questions own knowledge Changes initial responses Feels anxious when faced with information that is presented differently from expected way Voices self-doubt during testing
TEST-TAKING STRATEGIES			
Develop and stick to a study plan; avoid last-minute cramming. Focus on decreasing test-taking speed. Read questions as though speaking them aloud in your head to avoid scanning. Read all options. Time yourself in practice tests; allow no less than 1 min per question.	Focus on concepts and not details during study periods. Use concept maps. Focus on increasing testing speed. Do not linger too long over one question. Time yourself in practice tests; allow 45–60 seconds for each question. Keep a watch in front of you while taking the test; determine the halfway point and mark it on the exam.	Develop and stick to a study plan. Practice with sample tests. Maintain objectivity; avoid adding your own interpretation. Avoid changing answers.	Continue usual study activities. Work of self-confidence. Develop a self-confidence mantra to recite if you find yourself doubting your knowledge. Use practice tests to increase confidence. Avoid changing answers.
RELAXATION TECHNIQUES			
Breathe deeply. Practice positive visualization. Avoid caffeine. Develop a test-taking mantra to recite if you find yourself losing focus.	Breathe deeply. Practice positive visualization. Avoid caffeine.	Breathe deeply. Practice positive visualization. Avoid caffeine.	Breathe deeply. Practice positive visualization. Avoid caffeine.

Source: Adapted from Sides, MB, and Korchek, N: Successful Test-Taking Strategies, ed. 3, Lippincott. Philadelphia, 1998, p. 77; and Dickenson-Hazard, N: Test-taking strategies and techniques, in Kopec, CA and Millonig, VL (eds.): Gerontological Nursing Certification Review Guide, revised ed. Health Leadership Associates, Potomac, MD, 1996, pp. 3–5.

Identifying Your Test-Taking Type

WHAT IS YOUR PREFERRED LEARNING STYLE?

Awareness of your learning style can also guide you in selecting study strategies. Learning styles are related to the pathways or channels through which you prefer to absorb information. The three types of learners usually identified are visual, auditory, and tactile or kinesthetic.

Visual Learners

Visual learners learn better from reading and writing than from hearing and talking about information. They usually find that background noises, such as those from music or television, are more distracting than helpful while studying. Strategies for visual learners include:

- Reading the text in a quiet area or setting
- Watching appropriate videos
- Using concept maps, flash cards, or charts of materials
- Using highlighting markers or colored paper to take notes

Auditory Learners

Auditory learners grasp the information better by listening and talking. Combining the information with music often works well for auditory learners. Strategies for auditory learners include:

- Reading the text aloud
- Listening to audio tapes of the learning material
- Making up a song and singing about the tape content (especially helpful if you are having difficulties in a particular area)
- Listening to background music or other noise
- Talking about the content with a study partner

Tactile or Kinesthetic Learners

Tactile or kinesthetic learners prefer to learn "hands-on." They may have difficulty sitting to study for long periods. During study sessions, it might help to stand and move around or take frequent stretch breaks. Combining physical activity with the study session works well for kinesthetic learners. Strategies for tactile learners include:

- Moving around while studying
- Reading while exercising on a stationary bicycle
- Listening to tapes of learning material while walking or biking
- Rewriting or typing notes

Although most everyone is capable of learning through all their sensory pathways, most have a preferred channel. Think about which of the three learning styles discussed works best for you. Time is often at a premium for nurses studying for certification, and capitalizing on your preferred learning style will help you study in the most efficient way. Keep strategies for your preferred learning style in mind as you develop your study plan.

No matter what your personal style, your test-taking skills *can* be improved! Remember how you improve other skills, such as your tennis skills: practice. The same holds true for test-taking skills. The more you practice answering sample test questions, the better you will become at it. The best way to accomplish this is through practice, practice, and more practice. That is why we have written this book for you. This book will provide you with 2000 sample test questions. Research has shown that two-thirds of study time should be spent taking sample tests, with only one-third of the time spent reviewing content. Various books are available to you; however, very few contain nearly the number of test questions you need to develop and flex your test-taking muscles. This book provides enough questions to enable you to do that.

Getting Started

Studying, like regular exercise, is good for the brain. As a health-care professional, you will find that it will always be your job to keep abreast of the professional literature and spend some time studying. To recertify, you are mandated to keep your practice current through a combination of a number of clinical hours and continuing education options. The earlier you begin to plan for certification, the better it will be.

The principles of effective study are actually simple but often ignored. There is one central law about study: the law of mass effect. Any worthwhile studying takes time. And in today's world, time is a precious commodity. There is no way around the hours involved. Therefore, if you want to study, you need to set aside adequate time and plan accordingly. There are no shortcuts! But you need to make it easy to begin.

Tips for Studying

Just as a cold engine will run a little rough, settling down to study when one is out of the habit can be difficult. The following suggestions can make it easier to begin studying and to return to it on a regular and consistent basis:

- *Create a pleasurable personal environment.* This is a very basic but frequently overlooked requirement for successful study. Organize all your study materials in one area. Try to create a pleasant and regular workspace for yourself—perhaps just a part of a room, but an inviting part. Decorate it with flowers, pictures, or whatever makes the area appealing to you. Decide whether background music is helpful to you or distracting. Background music may be helpful for an auditory learner, whereas a visual learner may find it a distraction. For the kinesthetic learner, an open area that allows free movement may be better than a small office.

- *Plan your activities in advance and be realistic.* Plan in advance what you are going to work on and do not be overly ambitious. Blocks of 1-1/2 hours at most are recommended, with a 10-minute break every 45 minutes. List the tasks beforehand; otherwise you might spend valuable time trying to decide what material to review today. Set specific targets for the time available.
- *Keep focused on the goal: becoming certified!* Keep the benefits of the study clearly in mind, in this case the joy of receiving your passing score in the mail, followed by your embossed certificate. Imagine how the envelope feels when it comes in the mail. Feel your relief and joy when you open the envelope and read your passing score! Picture the certificate framed, hanging in your office. Write down a list of all the things that you stand to gain from passing the exam and read it over when you are ready to begin to study. Maybe it is a raise, an advanced level of licensure, a new job, or prescription-writing privileges. Focus on these results and how they make you feel. Close your eyes and allow the feelings to flood through you!
- *Leave the environment in readiness for your next session.* Leave your work environment inviting for the next time. Put your materials away so that they are easily accessible. Do not leave the area cluttered, but rather make it more pleasing. Spend the last few minutes of your study time tidying up so that your environment is all set for your next session. This is also an excellent time to plan what you will do the next time you sit down to study. Believe it or not, these small, concrete habits can make a big dent in your natural tendency to procrastinate.
- *Reward yourself.* Last but not least, reward yourself! This must be done for each study period. You might decide that if you spend 3 hours studying on Saturday, you will see a movie that you want to see on Saturday evening, or go to the mall, or treat yourself to a long, leisurely bubble bath! Be good to yourself.

There are many ways you can make studying more fun. Make use of your best time of day. For some, this might mean arising early while the rest of the household sleeps and stealing time alone, undisturbed, with a hot cup of tea or coffee. For others, evening is preferable. Study for short periods with frequent breaks. Remember to integrate whichever learning modalities work best for you. For example, if you are an auditory learner, use audiotapes while you are walking (especially good for tactile or kinesthetic learners). Think in terms of "bite-size" pieces and structure your study plan accordingly; otherwise you might become overwhelmed and defeated before you begin. Variety is also essential. For example, break up the time between test question review and content review or break up the study period into different tasks—perhaps studying with a study group for a part of the time. Discussing the materials with others is a good strategy for auditory learners. Take notes part of the time and read for a part of the time. Do not keep at any one activity for longer than 45 minutes—even your practice exams.

Study with the purpose in mind, in this case passing the certification exam. As suggested earlier, research has shown that two thirds of the study time is most effectively spent taking sample test questions. Do not lose sight of this! Studying does not necessarily mean sitting and reading textbooks. For example, reading books in a linear fashion is often not the most effective way to master information. Always keep the purpose and the end result in mind.

Use the "salami" principle—cut large tasks into smaller ones and digest one at a time! You will avoid indigestion! Also, be prepared to delay the start of new projects until this one is complete and you have successfully taken the exam!

Designing Your Study Plan

ASSESS

Review the phases of the nursing process in creating your study plan: assess, plan, implement, and evaluate. Begin by taking some sample test exams: you might try an integrated content exam first and score yourself. This will give you an idea of your baseline and how intensive your study plan needs to be. Reflect, as part of your assessment, on your test-taking type, preferred learning style, and personality.

Use the analysis of scoring in Table 2–4 to help you make an accurate assessment of *why* you missed the questions you did. Did you miss the correct answer because you did not know or remember the content? Or did you miss a key word, read into the test question, or change the answer? This indicates a need for continued work on test-taking skills, best achieved through continued testing of oneself with sample test questions, such as the ones provided for you in this book. Evalu-

---

**TABLE 2–4. ANALYSIS OF SCORING
QUESTION NUMBER**

TEST-TAKING ERROR

- Missed key word
- Did not read all of the distractors carefully
- Read into the question
- Misread or misunderstood the question
- Changed the answer

CONTENT WEAKNESS

- Forgot or did not recognize or understand the content
- Applied wrong concept or rationale

ate the percentage of questions you missed because of lack of knowledge of content and how many you answered incorrectly because of test-taking error. Design your study plan accordingly. Use the analysis of scoring to continue to track your progress.

Analysis of Scoring

You need to answer anywhere from 75 to 150 test questions on the computerized exam. That is a passing score of approximately 66%. Aim for 85% on your practice exams to demonstrate some level of mastery of content. Assess your passing score on an integrated content exam. Any test score below 80% indicates a need to initiate a more aggressive and intensive exam review. A score of 80% or above, however, does not mean that you should not prepare! You should still aim to review approximately 2000 to 3000 sample test questions before sitting for the exam, and do some basic content review. An initial score below 80% means you should aim for a minimum of 5000 sample test questions before the exam, as well as a more intensive content review. Attending a certification review class is an additional way to shore up your knowledge base.

PLAN AND IMPLEMENT

The certification exam timeline and study calendar (Table 2–5) offer out a suggested 6-week timeline, a countdown to exam time from the time of registration for your respective exam. Use the "salami technique." Study a little everyday. Improve your self-image! Believe you are a good student and behave like one! Stick to your study plan! Setting clear-cut goals and objectives is always helpful.

Certification Exam Timeline and Study Calendar

Spend some time taking approximately 100 test questions in a specific content area. Assess your score. If it is between 85 and 95%, move on! Feel confident! Continue to review through sample test questions. If your score is lower, however, use the diagnostic grid.

As noted in Chapter 1, the ANCC exam covers pathophysiologic content organized by body system. This is how you should organize your study time: by body system as well as associated content areas. We suggest following the table of contents of this book, modeled on the practice domains spelled out by both certifying bodies. After assessing your baseline knowledge through use of the integrated exams provided in this book, move on to the content areas in which you scored the lowest. For some people, this might be the neurologic content; for others, it might be the endocrine content or perhaps the psychiatric content.

To review disorders and help you prioritize, use the following tips:

- Organize content by body system.
- Begin with the system you find the most difficult.
- Review the pathophysiology of that system, if necessary.
- List pertinent disorders of that system.
- Review incidence and contributing factors.
- Review early and late disease manifestations.
- Review the sequelae, prognosis, and life-threatening complications.
- Determine treatment; adjust for age.
- Review associated teaching and learning needs.
- Review coping techniques, prevention, and health promotion.

Using content maps is another approach to mastering content. Figure 2–1 is an example of a content map approach to reviewing disease processes. A content map is a picture or pattern of information. It also shows relationships between pieces of information. Developing content maps can help you to find content areas in which you are weak and avoid studying content you already know. People are drawn to study what they already know. They feel comfortable with that information, whereas new information can produce anxiety. In the long run, however, this is not a good strategy. Few people can read a book and visualize the exact page, word for word, in their minds. A content map helps you find the information in your memory, where it is usually stored in patterns related to other memories. Using this structure, you can find out which areas you may not completely understand. Content maps start with general information and move to specifics. They can be helpful for persons who spend so much time studying the details that they miss the bigger picture.

EVALUATE

To help you evaluate your progress, consider these tips:

- *Take a sample test and use the test-taking analysis of scoring.* Review one of your sample content area tests. Why did you answer the questions that you got wrong incorrectly?
- If content is forgotten, use a content review. Did you not recognize or remember the content? This would indicate a need to review content using a book of condensed information, for example, Dunphy's *Management Guidelines for Adult Nurse Practitioners,* an outline-review book, or attending a certification review. It does not mean that you should return to your textbook or class notes.
- *If a rationale is misunderstood, go back to textbooks.* Did you not comprehend the content? For example, perhaps your basic understanding of the cardiac cycle was not thorough enough to include the severity and implications of various murmurs (i.e., which ones are relatively normal physiologic events and which ones are indicative of more severe pathology). This would indicate a need to go back to one of your textbooks; perhaps audiotapes or

TABLE 2–5. **CERTIFICATION EXAM TIMELINE AND STUDY CALENDAR***

Sunday	*Monday*	*Tuesday*	*Wednesday*	*Thursday*	*Friday*	*Saturday*
COMMITMENT						

- Register for the examination.
- Evaluate your test-taking type and preferred learning style.
- Take assessment examination.
- Evaluate exam with analysis of scoring.
- Develop study plan and gather study materials.
- Fill out study calendar and begin.
- Make arrangements for going to the exam.

(Dates)						
Week 1	Content: Score:	Content: Score:	Content: Score:	Content: Score:	Content: Score:	Content: Score:
(Dates)						
Week 2	Content: Score:	Content: Score:	Content: Score:	Content: Score:	Content: Score:	Content: Score:
PERSEVERANCE						

- Continue studying.
- Take a week off from studying.

(Dates)						
Week 3	Content: Score:	Content: Score:	Content: Score:	Content: Score:	Content: Score:	Content: Score:
(Dates)						
Week 4	Content: Score:	Content: Score:	Content: Score:	Content: Score:	Content: Score:	Content: Score:
FOCUS AND REWARD						

- Focus on content areas in which you scored less than 80% on sample questions.
- Make final arrangements for going to the exam.

(Dates)						
Week 5	Content: Score:	Content: Score:	Content: Score:	Content: Score:	Content: Score:	Content: Score:
(Dates)						
Week 6	Content: Score:	Content: Score:	Content: Score:	Content: Score:	Content: Score:	Content: Score:

Source: Adapted from Hoefler, P: Successful Problem Solving and Test-Taking for Nursing and NCLEX-RN exams, ed. 4, MEDS, Silver Spring, MD, 1997, p. 111.

videotapes, or both, with more detailed content; and a review of basic pathophysiologic processes.

- *If the error is in test taking, continue to take the sample exams.* Did you answer a question incorrectly because you missed a key word? Did you not read all the distractors carefully enough? Did you read something into the question? Did you change an answer? All these are indications of test-taking error. This indicates a need to continue taking sample exams.

- *Practice, practice, practice sample test questions.*

Using the analysis of scoring as you score yourself on an integrated exam followed by exams for specific body-system content will enable you to design an individualized study plan that has specificity and relevance for you. For example, you may need to spend 1 week on neurologic content but only 1 day on cardiac content. You can succeed in becoming certified!

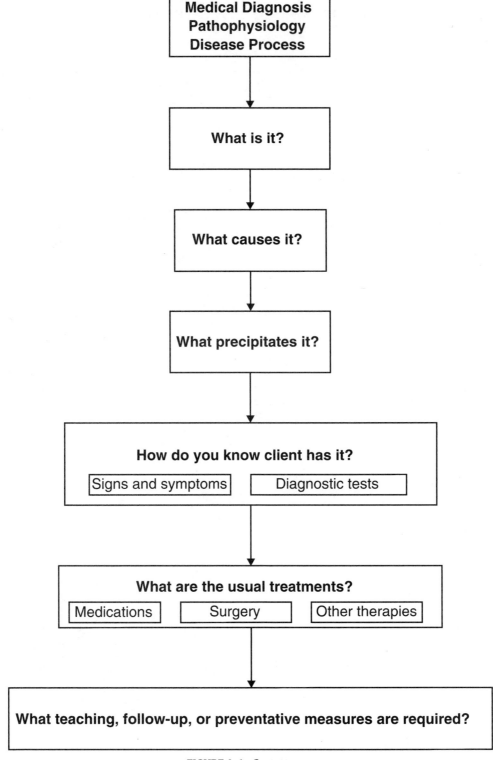

FIGURE 2–1. Content map.

LAST-MINUTE PREPARATIONS: RELAXED AND READY

Well, you are finally there! The day of the exam! Several tried-and-true techniques can also help you get through this day with success and confidence. The night before the exam, get a good night's sleep. Try relaxation techniques to assist you. Do *not* cram the night before, although you may want to review a few notes. It might be better to do something relaxing and enjoyable like going to a movie. Find the exam site the night before to ease your anxiety on the morning of the exam. Know where to park and how long it will take you to get there.

The morning of the exam, do a few exercises to get your blood pumping to your brain. Eat lightly, but *do* have breakfast. Bring identification, your registration for the exam, at least two sharpened pencils if you are taking a paper-and-pencil exam, and a watch. Dress in layers. Avoid stimulants and depressants. Go light on the caffeine. Find the rest rooms. Use the bathroom before the exam begins.

Listen carefully to the instructions. Do deep breathing and positive relaxation exercises to calm yourself as the exam is being passed out. Stay focused! Pace yourself, do not spend too long on any one test question. Go with your first choice. Move on. Try to avoid changing answers. On the computerized exam, you will not be able to go back. Use test-taking strategies when you do not know the answer. Identify distractions, such as backache or neck ache, noise, reading the same questions over and over, feeling tired, or thinking of your vacation. If these occur, *stop,* take a few minutes to take a few deep breaths, refocus, then get back on track! Do not panic if someone finishes before you! Stretch as nec-essary. Practice positive visualization if your mind begins to drift and you find it difficult to concentrate. Do not overcomplicate the test questions! Do not overanalyze the test questions! Move on! Think positively about your success. Stay focused on your goal: becoming a nationally certified advanced practice nurse!

Begin now by using this book as suggested. After all, the longest journey begins with a single step. Take that step now. Turn the page and begin.

Bibliography

American Nurses Credentialing Center: Credentialing News 1:1, 1998.

Dickenson-Hazard, N: Test-taking strategies and techniques. In Kopac, CA, and Millonig, VL (eds): Gerontological Nursing Certification Review Guide, revised ed. Health Leadership Associates, Potomac, MD, 1996.

Hoefler, P: Successful Problem Solving and Test-Taking for Beginning Nursing Students, 2nd ed. MEDS, Silver Spring, MD, 1997.

Hoefler, P: Successful Problem Solving and Test-Taking for Nursing and NCLEX-RN Exams, 4th ed. MEDS, Silver Spring, MD, 1997.

Sides, MB and Korchek, N: Successful Test-Taking, 3rd ed. Lippincott-Raven, Philadelphia, 1998.

Stein, A and Mariano, D: Test Smart: How to pass NCLEX-RN. In NCLEX Excel! Course. Allegheny University of Health Sciences, Philadelphia, 1997.

UNIT TWO

SYSTEM-SPECIFIC HEALTH PROBLEMS

3

Cardiovascular Problems

1 *A 45-year-old man is being referred to your clinic for cardiac rehabilitation. As you discuss disease prevention with him, you state that cardiac rehabilitation is which form of prevention?*

a Primary
b Secondary
c Restorative
d Tertiary

2 *A 60-year-old man has been referred to your cardiac surgery practice for aortic valve replacement due to aortic stenosis. Cardiac catheterization revealed severe aortic stenosis with normal coronary anatomy. While you take the history and do the physical exam, the patient states that he has had multiple episodes of angina. What is the most likely physiologic explanation for his anginal symptoms?*

a Coronary vasospasm
b Coronary embolization
c Excessive metabolic demand
d Hypoxia

3 *When examining this patient you would expect to hear a:*

a late systolic murmur, heard at the left sternal border (LSB).
b holosystolic murmur; heard at the LSB and radiating to the axilla.
c late diastolic murmur; heard at the LSB.
d diamond-shaped systolic murmur; heard at the second right intercostal space and radiating to the neck.

4 *Mitral valve prolapse is most frequently associated with:*

a aortic stenosis.
b female athletes.

c a diastolic click.
d a late systolic murmur.

5 *A 50-year-old female patient is 4 days post coronary artery bypass graft (CABG) surgery. You are called to see her secondary to new onset of atrial fibrillation with a ventricular response to 140 beats/min. The patient's blood pressure is 120/70 mm Hg and spot pulse oximetry is 95% on room air. Appropriate medications for rate control would include all of the following **EXCEPT**:*

a digoxin (Lanoxin).
b verapamil (Calan, Isoptin, Verelan).
c nifedipine (Procardia).
d metoprolol (Lopressor).

6 *The most common cause of primary right ventricular infarction is:*

a pulmonary hypertension.
b pulmonary embolus.
c pericardial effusion.
d an inferior myocardial infarction.

7 *A 69-year-old male patient is 4 hours post coronary artery bypass graft (CABG) surgery. Four grafts were done: the left internal mammary artery—left anterior descending (LIMA-LAD), left internal mammary artery—radial (LIMA-RADIAL) composite to obtuse marginal 1 and 2, and right internal mammary artery—right coronary artery (RIMA-RCA). As the acute care nurse practitioner, you are called to see the patient because of ST segment elevations in leads II, III, and AVF. The CABG you would be most concerned about is the:*

a LAD graft.
b obtuse marginal 1 graft.

c RCA graft.
d obtuse marginal 2 graft.

8 *A 30-year-old female patient is admitted to the hospital with an 8-week history of fever, chills, and malaise. Past medical history is unremarkable except for a heart murmur noted at age 20. Physical exam reveals a thin woman who appears ill with temperature 100°F, pulse 110, and blood pressure 110/40 mm Hg. Cardiac exam reveals a diastolic murmur II/VI heard at the LSB with a normal first heart sound and no extra heart tones. Lung fields revealed fine basilar crackles. The liver and spleen were not enlarged. Skin revealed petechiae on the arms. What is the most likely diagnosis?*

a Congestive heart failure
b Pneumonia
c Endocarditis
d Pericarditis

9 *The symptoms classically associated with aortic stenosis include all of the following* **EXCEPT:**

a edema.
b syncope.
c angina.
d dyspnea.

10 *The most common cause of mitral stenosis is:*

a endocarditis.
b congenital absence of leaflets.
c rheumatic fever.
d scarlet fever.

11 *Causes of respiratory muscle weakness after cardiac surgery include all of the following* **EXCEPT:**

a sepsis.
b phrenic nerve injury.
c hypercalcemia.
d poor nutritional status.

12 *A favorable high-density lipoprotein (HDL) to total cholesterol ratio is:*

a 2.5:1.
b 6.0:1.
c 10.0:1.
d 4.5:1.

13 *A 55-year-old man with angina is currently taking beta blockers and has moderate left ventricular dysfunction with an ejection fraction of 30%. You plan to supplement his medication regime. Which drugs should be used cautiously in this patient?*

a Transdermal nitrates
b Calcium channel blockers

c Angiotensin-converting enzyme (ACE) inhibitors
d ACE blockers

14 *Risk factors for coronary disease in women include all of the following* **EXCEPT:**

a a family history of coronary disease.
b diabetes.
c obesity.
d hypothyroidism.

15 *A 19-year-old female college student was found to be hypertensive (blood pressure 160/100 mm Hg) at a school screening. She denies earlier blood pressure elevations. As the nurse practitioner, what would be your initial treatment plan?*

a Obtain an echocardiogram.
b Order a 24-hour urine test for metanephrines.
c Obtain a complete history and physical examination.
d Have her return in 24 hours for a blood pressure check.

16 *Causes of secondary hypertension include all of the following* **EXCEPT:**

a renal artery stenosis.
b aortic aneurysm.
c Cushing's syndrome.
d pheochromocytoma.

17 *A 45-year-old woman diagnosed with postpartum cardiomyopathy is awaiting heart transplantation as an outpatient. You see her in the transplant clinic. She states that over the past week she has had several episodes of syncope and palpitations. What would be your treatment plan?*

a Check the patient's electrolyte and magnesium levels.
b Place the patient on a 24-hour cardiac monitor.
c Admit the patient to the hospital for further evaluation.
d Have the patient monitor episodes and report back in a week.

18 *Vasodilators that may be used in the treatment of heart failure include all of the following* **EXCEPT:**

a enalapril (Vasotec).
b isosorbide (Isordil).
c metoprolol (Lopressor).
d hydralazine.

19 *A 40-year-old male patient was admitted to the hospital with new onset of atrial fibrillation with a ventricular response of 150. He has no known medical history. What is your differential diagnosis?*

a Hyperthyroidism
b Congenital heart disease
c Hypercalcemia
d Hypermagnesemia

20 *A 72-year-old female patient is 5 hours post aortic valve replacement with a pericardial valve. The intraoperative course was reported as being uneventful. Her past medical history is significant for obesity, hypertension, and a knee replacement complicated by a hematoma. The patient had been receiving aspirin preoperatively but stopped 5 days before the surgery. As the acute care nurse practitioner, you are asked to evaluate her because of increased chest tube bleeding. The chest tube output has been 300 to 400 mL/h for the past 3 hours. The patient has received eight units of packed red blood cells (PRBCs), six units of fresh frozen plasma (FFP), and two pools of platelets. The patient is hemodynamically stable, but her blood pressure drops unless she is given blood products. What is the most appropriate next step?*

a Administer cryoprecipitate.
b Increase the positive end expiratory pressure (PEEP) on the ventilator to try to decrease the bleeding.
c Obtain a repeat chest radiograph.
d Notify the cardiac surgeon of the need to return the patient to the operating room.

Questions 21–22 refer to the following scenario:

A 55-year-old female patient was admitted to the coronary care unit 5 days previously with a transmural myocardial infarction. Her past medical history was significant for having hypertension since age 45, smoking, and asthma. The staff nurse notifies you that the patient is complaining of chest pain and pain with inspiration, and has a loud friction rub.

21 *What is the most likely diagnosis?*

a Extension of the infarction
b Pneumonia
c Aortic dissection
d Pericarditis

22 *The most appropriate pharmacologic treatment for this 55-year-old female patient is the administration of:*

a beta blockers.
b intravenous nitrates.
c nonsteroidal anti-inflammatory drugs.
d bronchodilators.

23 *Which antiarrhythmic drug mediates its effect by interfering with the movement of calcium through the "slow channel?"*

a Metoprolol (Lopressor)
b Amiodarone

c Diltiazem (Cardizem)
d Atropine

24 *Mitral stenosis may be associated with all of the clinical findings* **EXCEPT:**

a angina.
b right ventricular failure.
c hoarseness.
d dysphagia.

25 *A 70-year-old man was admitted to the coronary care unit (CCU) 4 days earlier with an anterior myocardial infarction. You are called to the CCU to see the patient because the patient is experiencing shortness of breath, has a pulse oximetry 85% on room air, is hypotensive with a blood pressure of 80/60 mm Hg, and has a heart rate of 120. The physical exam reveals a loud holosystolic murmur at the LSB with radiation to the axilla. What is your most likely diagnosis?*

a Extension of the myocardial infarction
b Pulmonary embolus
c Adult respiratory distress syndrome
d Acute ventricular septal defect

26 *Which of the following classes of antihypertensive agents would be the best choice for a diabetic patient with hypertension?*

a Calcium channel blockers
b Diuretics
c Beta blockers
d ACE inhibitors

27 *Differential diagnoses in a 65-year-old woman who presents with chest pain include all of the following* **EXCEPT:**

a pericarditis.
b cholecystitis.
c acute myocardial infarction.
d renal calculi.

28 *A 30-year-old man presents to your office for a routine work physical exam. He has no known medical problems, but has a family history of hyperlipidemia. He smokes a pack of cigarettes a day. A cholesterol test is performed, and the result is 260 mg/dL. What would be appropriate counseling for this patient?*

a Tell him that this is a normal cholesterol level for his age.
b Tell him that this is a high cholesterol level and that he should be further assessed by having fasting low-density lipoprotein (LDL) and high-density lipoprotein (HDL) cholesterol levels drawn.
c Tell him that he should be started on lipid-lowering agents immediately.
d Tell him to have his cholesterol level rechecked in 2 years.

29 *Common causes of pericarditis include all of the following* **EXCEPT:**

a renal failure.
b metastatic tumors.
c viral illness.
d mediastinitis.

30 *One cause of secondary hypertension is:*

a coronary artery disease.
b coarctation of the aorta.
c abdominal aneurysm.
d valvular heart disease.

31 *Which of the following statements is true concerning coarctation of the aorta?*

a The right carotid artery lies distal to the coarctation.
b Ventricular septal defects are always present.
c Both systolic and diastolic pressures are elevated proximal to the coarctation.
d Surgical correction should be performed early in life.

Questions 32–34 refer to the following scenario:

A 55-year-old man with a 15-year history of hypertension, type 2 diabetes, and hyperlipidemia was seen in the emergency department with complaints of stabbing upper back pain for the past 3 days unrelieved by acetaminophen (Tylenol) and heat applications. The patient is also complaining of shortness of breath with exertion, and fatigue. A physical exam reveals blood pressure of 180/110 mm Hg in both arms, and a heart rate of 92. A cardiac exam revealed a 3/6 diastolic blowing murmur heard at the LSB and an S4 heart sound.

32 *What diagnostic test should be done to confirm the diagnosis?*

a Magnetic resonance imaging (MRI)
b Chest radiograph
c Transthoracic echocardiogram
d Contrast computed tomography (CT) scan

33 *What would be the best pharmacologic agent to control the blood pressure in this patient?*

a Esmolol (Brevibloc)
b Sodium nitroprusside (Nipride)
c Dilitiazem (Cardizem)
d Intravenous nitroglycerin

34 *What is the most likely diagnosis for this patient?*

a Myocardial infarction
b Aortic dissection
c Pulmonary embolus
d Aortic stenosis

35 *A 50-year-old woman with no known medical history is seen in the emergency department with complaints of shortness of breath and severe midsternal chest pain associated with nausea that she has had for the last 2 hours. She took 2 tablespoons of Maalox with no relief. She is 2 years postmenopause, takes no medications, and has no allergies. As the acute care nurse practitioner, you are asked to evaluate this patient. The electrocardiogram (ECG) reveals ST depression in leads I and II, and AVF. What is your initial plan of care?*

a Obtain an arterial blood gas measurement.
b Obtain an immediate chest radiograph.
c Administer sublingual nitroglycerin until the patient is pain free.
d Administer heparin.

36 *The patient has an inferior wall infarction, but remains hemodynamically stable. An echocardiogram is obtained and reveals an ejection fraction of 25%. As the acute care nurse practitioner, you have been asked to review the medication regime for the patient before she is discharged. The patient should be placed on which of the following medication regimes?*

a Aspirin, a beta blocker, and warfarin (Coumadin)
b Coumadin, an ACE inhibitor, and a beta blocker
c A diuretic, aspirin, and a beta blocker
d Digoxin (Lanoxin), a calcium channel blocker, and aspirin

37 *Ischemic episodes in patients with known coronary disease may be caused by all of the following mechanisms* **EXCEPT:**

a adequate vasodilatory reserve.
b increased myocardial oxygen demands.
c coronary artery spasm.
d platelet aggregation.

38 *A 25-year-old man is admitted to the coronary care unit with complaints of fatigue, shortness of breath, and chest pain for the last 2 weeks. He has no prior health problems. An echocardiogram is done which reveals biventricular dilatation and left ventricular ejection of 10%. A pulmonary artery catheter was inserted and measurements indicate a cardiac index of 1.4, mixed venous oxygenation of 40%, pulmonary artery pressures of 60/38, and a right atrial pressure of 25. The patient was placed on inotropic agents without much improvement. What are the immediate treatment options for this patient?*

a Intra-aortic balloon counterpulsation
b Cardiac transplantation
c Cardiac muscle stimulation
d Ventricular assist device

39 *A 45-year-old woman is admitted to your service for pacemaker generator failure. She had an initial* pacemaker placed at age 37 secondary to complete heart block resulting from Lyme disease. What are the causes of complete heart block?

a Myocardial infarction
b Coronary artery disease
c Calcific valvular heart disease
d All of the above

40 *A 55-year-old woman presents to you for a routine physical exam. A routine chest radiograph was taken and revealed cardiomegaly. What would be your next step in evaluating this finding?*

a Obtain a chest CT scan.
b Obtain a detailed history and perform a complete physical exam.
c Obtain a cardiac echocardiogram.
d Repeat the chest radiograph.

41 *A 70-year-old man is being seen for a follow-up appointment after a recent hospitalization for congestive heart failure (CHF). On physical exam, his lungs have fine basilar crackles, and his heart rate is 80 and regular with normal first and second heart sounds. The patient also has a S3 audible at the LSB, and his blood pressure is 170/90 mm Hg. The clinical significance of the S3 include all of the following* **EXCEPT:**

a ventricular failure.
b normal variant.
c ischemic heart disease.
d systemic hypertension.

42 *A 58-year-old postmenopausal woman presents to your office with complaints of fatigue and vague midsternal chest discomfort that awakens her at night; this is sometimes relieved by taking Tums. The episodes of chest discomfort have been occurring nightly over the last week. The patient's past medical history includes diabetes, hypertension, and obesity. Her current medications include glyburide (Micronase) 5 mg daily and enalapril (Vasotec) 5 mg BID. What is your initial plan of care?*

a Refer the patient to a cardiologist for evaluation.
b Have the patient keep a diary of subsequent episodes of chest discomfort.
c Obtain a baseline ECG.
d Start the patient on nitrates.

43 *A 65-year-old man presents to your office complaining of fatigue and shortness of breath when climbing stairs that has occurred over the past 2 weeks. The patient has no prior medical history. He smokes 1.5 packs of cigarettes per day, and works as a truck driver. His family history is positive for myocardial infarction in a brother at age 50, and his father has hyperlipidemia. The patient was referred for a stress test and it was negative. Laboratory data re-*vealed normal electrolyte levels, a normal thyroid function test result, and an elevated homocysteine level. What is your plan of care for this patient?

a Start folate in an attempt to decrease the homocysteine level.
b Encourage smoking cessation.
c Counsel the patient on risk factor modification.
d All of the above.

Questions 44–46 refer to the following scenario:

A 35-year-old man with no previous health history presents to your office with a complaint of shortness of breath over the past 3 days. The physical exam is unrevealing. The patient is a thin man in no acute distress. The lungs are clear, and the cardiac exam reveals an apical impulse at the fifth intercostal space at the midclavicular line with regular rate and rhythm and no murmurs, gallops, or rubs. He has no past medical history, except that he smokes two packs of cigarettes a day and does not exercise. An ECG was done in the office which revealed Q waves in the leads II, III, and AVF, and ST depression in leads V1–3.

44 *What is the most likely diagnosis?*

a Posterior myocardial infarction
b Inferior posterior myocardial infarction
c Right ventricular infarction
d Anterior myocardial infarction

45 *As the acute nurse practitioner, what is your next plan of care for this patient?*

a Admit the patient to the hospital immediately.
b Start the patient on aspirin and nitrates.
c Send the patient for a stress test.
d Repeat the ECG and give the patient nitroglycerin.

46 *The patient stabilizes, and the peak troponin level is 35 with creatine kinase (CK) levels of 900 with 75% MB. He is referred for a catheterization that reveals a 90% circumflex lesion and he undergoes a successful angioplasty. The patient is placed on IV nitroglycerin at 60 mg/min and heparin at 900 U/h with activated clotting time of 180. In the CCU, the staff nurse notifies you that the patient is having chest discomfort radiating to the arm and nausea. The ECG reveals ST segment elevation in leads V1 to V4. Vital signs reveal a heart rate of 88 and a blood pressure of 150/70 mm Hg. What is the most appropriate first intervention?*

a Increase the nitroglycerin drip to achieve pain relief and give a dose of a beta blocker.
b Notify the cardiologist of the need for the patient to return to the catheterization lab.
c Prepare the patient for intra-aortic balloon pump placement.
d Increase the heparin drip.

47 One of your patients underwent cardiac catheterization 18 hours earlier. You are doing your rounds in anticipation of discharging this patient. At the site of the catheterization (the left femoral artery), you note a hematoma that is painful to touch. There is an audible bruit over the site, and the patient complains of left lower quadrant abdominal pain. What is the appropriate first intervention?

a Notify the cardiologist immediately.
b Have the patient walk around to see whether the discomfort abates.
c Apply warm compresses to the left femoral area.
d Obtain a complete blood count immediately, and order an abdominal CT scan.

48 A 50-year-old man who has had an earlier myocardial infarction received thrombolytic therapy. Reperfusion after thrombolysis is demonstrated by:

a development of new Q waves.
b ST segment elevation resolving quickly and resolution of Q waves.
c new ST segment elevation and development of new Q waves.
d T wave inversion in all leads.

49 Current treatments of atrial fibrillation include all of the following EXCEPT:

a amiodarone (Cordarone).
b metoprolol (Lopressor).
c amlodipine (Norvasc).
d diltiazem (Cardizem).

50 Which one of the following hemodynamic profiles is consistent with cardiogenic shock?

a Cardiac index of 2, wedge pressure of 12, and mean arterial pressure of 70
b Cardiac index of 1.8, wedge pressure of 28, and mean arterial pressure of 60
c Cardiac index of 2.5, wedge pressure of 10, and mean arterial pressure of 80
d None of the above

51 Contraindications to thrombolytic therapy in patients with myocardial infarction include all of the following EXCEPT:

a abdominal surgery within the past month.
b heme positive stools.
c a history of cerebral bleeding.
d a history of pacemaker placement 5 years earlier.

52 Which of the following diuretics is potassium sparing?

a Furosemide (Lasix)
b Bumetanide (Bumex)

c Spironolactone (Aldactone)
d Ethacrynic acid (Edecrin)

53 Symptoms of digoxin (Lanoxin) toxicity include all of the following EXCEPT:

a bradycardia.
b diarrhea.
c severe headaches.
d nausea.

54 A middle-aged male patient has been treated for CHF with furosemide (Lasix), enalapril (Vasotec), and digoxin (Lanoxin) for the past month. He complains of persistent cough since starting the medication regime. The lungs are clear and he appears to be compensated on physical exam. What is the next plan of care?

a Discontinue enalapril and start captopril (Capoten).
b Discontinue enalapril and start hydralazine (Apresoline).
c Continue the same regime and have the patient report on the progress of the cough within the next month.
d Check for other possible causes of the cough.

55 Nonpharmacologic management of CHF includes all of the following EXCEPT:

a weight reduction if applicable.
b avoidance of alcoholic beverages.
c sodium restriction to 5 g/d.
d avoidance of cigarette smoking.

56 A 60-year-old man is scheduled for coronary artery bypass graft (CABG) surgery. While doing the preoperative history and physical exam, he is noted to have a left carotid bruit. The patient denies any history of stroke or transient ischemic attacks. As the acute care nurse practitioner, what is your next plan of care?

a Notify the cardiac surgeon of the findings.
b Inform the patient of the findings, and plan a carotid duplex for further assessment.
c Notify the patient's primary care provider and ascertain whether the patient has had a previous neurologic event.
d Obtain a neurologic consultation.

57 A 50-year-old man with hyperlipidemia has been treated with lovastatin (Mevacor) for the past 2 months. What routine testing should be done on patients taking lovastatin?

a Complete blood count
b Triglyceride levels
c Liver function test
d Prothrombin time

58 *A 60-year-old patient with diabetes who at 5 days post CABG surgery is complaining of incisional pain and has a temperature that has risen to 103°F. The patient also has been hyperglycemic with blood glucose results ranging from 250 to 300. Physical exam reveals the patient has erythema of the entire sternal incision without drainage, and a sternal click. What is the most likely diagnosis?*

a Pericarditis
b Pneumonia
c Pleurisy
d Mediastinitis

59 *A 50-year-old female patient is receiving warfarin (Coumadin) therapy for atrial fibrillation with an international normalized ratio (INR) of 3.0. Previously she had been stable with an INR of 2.4. She takes 5 mg of warfarin daily. Based on this finding, you would:*

a hold the warfarin for 1 week, then restart at 2.5 mg.
b decrease the warfarin to 2.5 mg, then recheck the INR in 3 days.
c give the patient a dose of AquaMEPHYTON (vitamin K) and decrease the warfarin to 2.5 mg, then recheck the INR in 2 weeks.
d ascertain that the patient is taking the warfarin correctly, and there have been no changes in dietary patterns. If so, continue the same warfarin dose, and recheck the INR the next day.

60 *A 40-year-old female patient is 10 days post cardiac transplantation. The staff nurse notifies you that the patient is in atrial fibrillation with a ventricular rate of 150, and has a blood pressure of 130/70 mm Hg. What is your first line of treatment?*

a Digoxin (Lanoxin) 0.25 mg stat and repeat in 2 hours
b Metoprolol (Lopressor) 5 mg stat and repeat every 10 minutes until the heart rate is less than 100 and the blood pressure stabilizes
c Diltiazem (Cardizem) 10 mg bolus, then start an infusion
d Corticosteroids

61 *A 60-year-old male patient was recently diagnosed with CHF. He has diastolic dysfunction. What is the primary symptom of diastolic dysfunction?*

a Lower extremity edema
b Hoarseness
c Shortness of breath
d Abdominal bloating

62 *The most common cause of CHF is:*

a pericarditis.
b myocardial infarction.
c ventricular aneurysm.
d valvular heart disease.

63 *Treatment of diastolic heart failure includes all of the following EXCEPT:*

a diuretics.
b digoxin (Lanoxin).
c beta blockers.
d ACE inhibitors.

64 *A 40-year-old man is seen in the emergency room complaining of malaise and temperature of 103°F. He uses intravenous drugs, with the last use 4 days ago. The patient is also complaining of pain in the palms of his hands. Physical exam reveals a patient in moderate distress with hyperpigmented areas on the palms of both hands and petechiae on the upper torso. No cardiac murmurs are noted. What is the most likely diagnosis?*

a Flu syndrome
b Acute drug overdose
c Disseminated intravascular coagulopathy
d Bacterial endocarditis

65 *For a patient who is 3 months post heart transplantation, what medication is used as prophylaxis for* Pneumocystis carinii *pneumonia (PCP)?*

a Doxycycline (Doxycin, Vibramycin)
b Metronidazole (Flagyl)
c Tetracycline (Achromycin, Sumycin)
d Co-trimoxazole (Bactrim)

66 *Symptoms of right-sided heart failure include all of the following EXCEPT:*

a abdominal bloating.
b nausea.
c orthopnea.
d peripheral edema.

67 *A 45-year-old man was recently diagnosed with hypertension. He is taking furosemide (Lasix) and diltiazem (Cardizem). His heart rate is 64 and blood pressure is 140/96 mm Hg. The patient is seen in the clinic for a routine visit and states that he has a throbbing headache, which is worse in the morning hours. What is your plan of care?*

a Refer the patient to a neurologist.
b Order a head CT scan.
c Obtain a more detailed history about the headaches.
d Increase the dose of diltiazem in an attempt to better control the blood pressure.

68 *Physical exam findings that may be found in patients with essential hypertension include:*

a an atrial gallop, hypertensive retinopathy, and a laterally displaced apical impulse.
b a diastolic murmur, carotid bruit, and diminished peripheral pulses.

c   an abdominal bruit, thyromegaly, and peripheral edema.
d   a ventricular gallop, a medially displaced apical impulse, and systolic murmur.

69   *Physiologic splitting of the second heart sound is:*

a   a normal physical finding.
b   heard during expiration.
c   caused by closure of the tricuspid and mitral valves.
d   caused by closure of the aortic valve.

70   *A patient with a wandering atrial pacemaker will usually have all of the following* **EXCEPT:**

a   an irregular heart rhythm.
b   a varying PR interval.
c   normal QRS complexes.
d   a heart rate greater than 120 beats/min.

71   *Initial treatment of torsades de pointes includes the use of:*

a   beta blockers.
b   magnesium.
c   calcium.
d   amiodarone (Cordarone).

72   *A 50-year-old man is admitted to the hospital with a new onset of atrial fibrillation with a ventricular rate of 140. He admits to palpitations, but no other symptoms. He has no prior history of atrial fibrillation or other health problems and is not taking any medications. Electrolytes and thyroid function tests were normal. The patient was treated with beta blockers to control the rate and procainamide (Pronestyl), but failed to convert in 3 days. An ECG revealed normal left ventricular ejection fraction and a dilated left atrium. What is the appropriate next step?*

a   Start heparin and cardiovert the patient.
b   Start warfarin (Coumadin), continue the beta blockers and procainamide, then discharge the patient and arrange for cardioversion in 4 weeks if not converted.
c   Discontinue the beta blockers and procainamide and start the patient on amiodarone (Cordarone).
d   Bolus with heparin and start a heparin drip, then cardiovert the next day.

73   *Hypertrophic cardiomyopathy is characterized by all of the following* **EXCEPT:**

a   increased left ventricular wall thickness.
b   may occur in aortic stenosis.
c   may occur in hypertension.
d   a dilated left ventricle.

74   *A 35-year-old woman has mitral valve prolapse with mild mitral regurgitation. She tells you that she plans to go to the dentist to have her teeth cleaned. She asked if she needs antibiotics prior to the procedure. The most appropriate response is:*

a   There is no need for antibiotics.
b   You should take the antibiotics 6 hours before the procedure.
c   You need antibiotics only if you are having an extraction.
d   You should take the antibiotics 1 hour before the dental visit.

75   *The pressure gradient between the pulmonary artery end diastolic pressure (PAED) and the pulmonary artery wedge pressure (PAWP) is normally:*

a   10 to 12 mm Hg
b   1 to 4 mm Hg
c   5 to 10 mm Hg
d   15 to 20 mm Hg

76   *The normal PAWP is:*

a   6 to 12 mm Hg
b   2 to 4 mm Hg
c   10 to 15 mm Hg
d   15 to 20 mm Hg

77   *The "a" wave of the pulmzonary artery wedge tracing represents:*

a   atrial relaxation.
b   passive filling of the left ventricle.
c   left atrial contraction.
d   mitral valve closure.

78   *A middle-aged male patient had CABG surgery done. The left radial artery was harvested and used as a conduit. What instructions should be given to the patient at the time of discharge?*

a   Avoid extreme temperatures.
b   Avoid blood pressure measurements in the left arm.
c   Keep the arm elevated at night.
d   Apply an ace bandage wrap to the arm for the next month to decrease edema.

79   *A 50-year-old man, who had a cardiac transplant 1 month earlier, is readmitted with acute rejection. He is scheduled to receive muromonab-CD3 (Orthoclone OKT3). What are the immediate adverse reactions that may be associated with this drug?*

a   Pulmonary edema, fever, and rigors
b   Diarrhea, skin malignancies, and fever
c   Arthralgias, fever, and hyperkalemia
d   Hypertension, jaundice, and fever

80   *Types of distributive shock include all of the following* **EXCEPT:**

a septic shock.
b hypovolemic shock.
c anaphylactic shock.
d neurogenic shock.

81 *The initial stage of septic shock is characterized by:*

a a hypodynamic metabolic state.
b hypotension.
c normal cardiac output.
d increased vascular tone.

82 *The murmur of aortic insufficiency is a:*

a diastolic murmur heard best at the third left intercostal space.
b systolic murmur that radiates to the neck.
c diastolic murmur heard best at the base.
d diastolic murmur heard at the base, radiating to the neck.

83 *Complications of prosthetic valve replacements include:*

a endocarditis.
b hemolysis.
c paravalvular leak.
d all of the above.

84 *A 40-year-old woman is noted on physical exam to have a fixed split second heart sound. No other health history is noted, and she is taking no medications except vitamins. What is the most likely diagnosis?*

a Congenital bicuspid aortic stenosis
b Pulmonic stenosis
c Mitral regurgitation
d Atrial septal defect

85 *The potential complications that may occur as a result of unrepaired atrial septal defect include:*

a the development of arrhythmias.
b cyanosis.
c right ventricular failure.
d all of the above.

Answers

1 Answer d
Cardiac rehabilitation is a form of tertiary prevention. The goals of cardiac rehabilitation are to improve functional capacity in persons with established heart disease and aim at halting the progression of the disease process.

2 Answer c
The most likely physiologic explanation for the patient's anginal symptoms is excessive metabolic demand. Angina in patients with aortic stenosis despite normal coronary arteries (clean coronaries) occurs because of flow impedance mismatch with excessive metabolic demands.

3 Answer d
When examining a patient with aortic stenosis, you would expect to hear a diamond-shaped systolic murmur; heard at the second right intercostal space (RICS) and radiating to the neck. The classic murmur of aortic stenosis is a crescendo/decrescendo murmur (diamond shape) heard at the second RICS and may radiate to the neck and apex.

4 Answer d
Mitral valve prolapse (MVP) is most frequently associated with a late systolic murmur. Auscultation of a patient with MVP usually reveals a systolic click and a late systolic murmur.

5 Answer c
Appropriate medications for rate control of a patient with postoperative atrial fibrillation includes digoxin (Lanoxin), verapamil (Calan, Isoptin, Verelan), and metoprolol (Lopressor). Nifedipine (Procardia) would not be used. Nifedipine is a calcium channel blocker but has little to no effect on the AV node; it may actually worsen rate control in atrial fibrillation.

6 Answer d
The most common cause of primary right ventricular infarction is an inferior myocardial infarction. Primary right ventricular infarction is most commonly associated with inferior myocardial infarction and ischemia. Pulmonary embolus and pulmonary hypertension may cause right ventricular dysfunction. The presence of a pericardial effusion may impair right ventricular filling but is not associated with infarction.

7 Answer c
The coronary artery graft you would be most concerned about in the patient is the right coronary artery (RCA). The changes in the ECG (ST segment elevations in leads II, III, and AVF) suggest inferior wall injury and the RCA graft would be in question.

8 Answer c
The most likely diagnosis for the patient is endocarditis. An 8-week history of fever, chills, and malaise point to an infectious process. The presence of a diastolic murmur and petechiae with the febrile illness makes endocarditis the best answer.

9 Answer a
The symptoms classically associated with aortic stenosis include syncope, angina, and dyspnea. Edema is not a classic symptom.

10 Answer c
The most common cause of mitral stenosis is rheumatic fever, which affects the mitral valve by fusing the commissures.

11 Answer c
Causes of respiratory muscle weakness after cardiac surgery are multifactorial and include sepsis, phrenic nerve injury, and poor nutritional status. Hypercalcemia is not a cause. Hypocalcemia, however, would cause muscle weakness.

12 Answer d
A favorable high-density lipoprotein (HDL) to total cholesterol ratio is 4.5:1.

13   Answer b

Calcium channel blockers should be used cautiously in the patient with angina who has moderate left ventricular dysfunction as they may worsen left ventricular function.

14   Answer d

Proven risk factors for coronary disease in women include a family history of coronary disease, diabetes, and obesity. Hypothyroidism is not a risk factor.

15   Answer c

The initial treatment plan for a person found to be hypertensive at a screening would be obtain a complete history and physical examination. Further evaluation may include an ECG and a 24-hour urine collection for metanephrines.

16   Answer b

Causes of secondary hypertension include renal artery stenosis, Cushing's syndrome, and pheochromocytoma. Aortic aneurysm may develop as the result of hypertension but it is not a cause of hypertension.

17   Answer c

The treatment plan for a patient with postpartum cardiomyopathy who is experiencing episodes of syncope and palpitations would be to admit the patient to the hospital for further evaluation.

The episodes may be the result of ventricular arrhythmias and need to be further evaluated. The patient should have electrolytes checked and a 24-hour monitor placed. She may require an electrophysiologic study (EPS) to further evaluate the arrhythmias.

18   Answer c

Vasodilators that may be used in the treatment of heart failure include enalapril (Vasotec), isosorbide (Isordil), and hydralazine. Metoprolol (Lopressor) is a beta blocker, not a vasodilator.

19   Answer a

The differential diagnosis of a patient with new onset atrial fibrillation includes hyperthyroidism, which is one of the leading causes of new onset atrial fibrillation.

20   Answer d

The most appropriate next step for the patient described is to notify the cardiac surgeon of the need to return the patient to the operating room.

21   Answer d

The most likely diagnosis of the patient described is acute pericarditis.

22   Answer c

The most appropriate pharmacologic treatment for the patient described is the administration of nonsteroidal anti-inflammatory drugs (NSAIDs). NSAIDs are the treatment of choice for pericarditis. If the patient is unresponsive, systemic corticosteroids may need to be used.

23   Answer c

Diltiazem (Cardizem) is an antiarrhythmic drug that mediates its effect by interfering with the movement of calcium through the "slow channel."

24   Answer a

Mitral stenosis may be associated with right ventricular failure (resulting from pulmonary hypertension) and hoarseness and dysphagia (resulting from left atrial enlargement). Mitral stenosis is not usually associated with angina.

25   Answer d

The most likely diagnosis of the patient described is acute ventricular septal defect (VSD). The new holosystolic murmur with desaturation and hypotension make VSD the appropriate choice. Most VSDs occur 4 to 7 days after myocardial infarction.

26   Answer d

ACE inhibitors are the antihypertensive agents that would be the best choice for a diabetic patient with hypertension. ACE inhibitors are known to protect the kidneys in patients with diabetes and decrease proteinuria. Several studies have suggested that diuretics and beta blockers may worsen glucose tolerance and insulin resistance.

27   Answer d

Differential diagnoses in a 65-year-old woman who presents with chest pain include pericarditis, cholecystitis, and acute myocardial infarction. Renal calculi would not be a differential diagnosis. Renal calculi would produce flank pain and abdominal pain, not chest pain.

28   Answer b

The most appropriate counseling for the patient described would be to tell the patient that he has a high cholesterol level and he should be further assessed by having fasting LDL and HDL cholesterol levels drawn.

29   Answer d

Common causes of pericarditis include renal failure (without adequate dialysis), metastatic tumors, and viral illnesses. Mediastinitis, which causes infection in the mediastinum, is seldom associated with pericarditis.

30   Answer b

A cause of secondary hypertension is coarctation of the aorta. Patients with coronary artery disease, abdominal aneurysms, and valvular heart disease may have hypertension, but it is not a cause of secondary hypertension.

31   Answer c

The true statement is: Both systolic and diastolic pressures are elevated proximal to the coarctation. Coarctation of the aorta is a congenital deformity of the aorta with a narrowing either proximal or distal to the left subclavian artery. There are abnormal differences in the upper and lower extremity blood pressures with a widened pulse pressure. Congenital defects associated with coarctation may include bicuspid aortic valve. Surgery correction depends on the degree of coarctation.

32   Answer a

The diagnostic test that should be done to confirm the diagnosis of the patient described is MRI. The patient has aortic dissection, and time is of the essence in making the diagnosis. MRI has 95% sensitivity and specificity in detecting aortic dissection. A contrast CT scan does not allow you to see the aortic valve function and involvement of the major branches. A transthoracic echocardiogram is useful in ascertaining valve function, presence of pericardial effusions, and left ventricular function, but cannot visualize the coronary ostia. The chest x-ray may show a widened mediastinum, but is not diagnostic. This chest radiographic finding would heighten your suspicion to further pursue the problem.

33 Answer a

The best pharmacologic agent to control the blood pressure in the patient described is esmolol (Brevibloc). Initial treatment should be aimed at lowering the blood pressure and decreasing the DP/DT, which can be achieved with beta blockers. Sodium nitroprusside (Nipride) can be added if the blood pressure remains elevated after maximal use of beta blockers.

34 Answer b

The most likely diagnosis for the patient described is aortic dissection, given the history of long standing hypertension, and upper back pain with a murmur of aortic insufficiency.

35 Answer c

The initial plan of care for the patient described, who has coronary ischemia, is to administer sublingual nitroglycerin until the patient is pain free. Heparin may also be administered, but not until the nitroglycerin has been administered.

36 Answer b

The patient described, who has left ventricular dysfunction post myocardial infarction, should be placed on warfarin (Coumadin), an ACE inhibitor, and a beta blocker. The ACE inhibitor and beta blocker will help in left ventricular remodeling. Coumadin therapy is recommended in patients with left ventricular ejection fraction less than 30%.

37 Answer a

Ischemic episodes in patients with known coronary disease may be caused by increased myocardial oxygen demands, coronary artery spasm, platelet aggregation, and inadequate (not adequate) vasodilatory reserve.

38 Answer a

The immediate treatment options for the patient described is intra-aortic balloon counterpulsation (IABC). The intra-aortic balloon pump (IABP) may be used initially to stabilize the patient. The IABP adds approximately 800 mL to l L in cardiac output. If the patient does not stabilize, he may need a ventricular assist device. Cardiac transplantation involves a waiting period, and may not be necessary. Use of cardiac muscle stimulation would not be an immediate solution to the patient's myocardial failure. Cardiac muscle stimulation has been done in association with cardiomyoplasty. The training of the cardiac muscle may take up to 6 weeks.

39 Answer d

Causes of complete heart block include myocardial infarction, coronary artery disease, and valvular heart disease (including calcific valvular heart disease).

40 Answer b

The next step in evaluating a patient whose routine chest radiograph reveals cardiomegaly is to obtain a detailed history and perform a complete physical exam. If a chest radiography reveals the patient has cardiomegaly, the patient should be questioned for symptoms of CHF and the physical exam should focus on findings consistent with congestive failure. After further investigation, an echocardiogram should be performed.

41 Answer b

The clinical significance of an S3 heart sound in the 70-year-old patient described is a pathologic finding and may include ventricular failure, ischemic heart disease, and systemic hypertension. It is not a normal variant.

42 Answer c

The initial plan of care for the patient described is to obtain a baseline ECG to see whether the patient is actively ischemic or infarcting. If the ECG is positive, the patient should be referred to the hospital for cardiology evaluation.

43 Answer d

The plan of care for the patient described includes starting folate in an attempt to decrease the homocysteine level, encouraging smoking cessation, and counseling the patient on risk factor modification. The presence of an elevated homocysteine level may be a predictor of development of ischemic heart disease. Given the patient's history of cigarette smoking and family history of coronary disease, the patient should be advised to stop smoking and counseled on risk factor reduction.

44 Answer b

The most likely diagnosis in the patient described and with the ECG changes occurring is an inferior posterior myocardial infarction.

45 Answer a

The next plan of care for the patient described is to admit the patient to the hospital immediately for further evaluation. Based on the presence of Q waves, the most reasonable approach is to have the patient go to a tertiary care center. You could give the patient aspirin and nitrates, but this is not the definitive treatment.

46 Answer a

The most appropriate first intervention for the patient described is to increase the nitroglycerin drip to achieve pain relief and give a dose of a beta blocker. The patient may be experiencing spasm in the vessel recently treated with angioplasty, so increasing the nitroglycerin would be appropriate for pain control. In addition, the patient is not receiving an adequate amount of beta blockers, so giving a dose of a beta blocker would decrease myocardial oxygen demand.

47 Answer d

The appropriate first intervention for the patient described is to obtain an immediate complete blood count (CBC) and order an abdominal CT scan. Your suspicion should be for retroperitoneal bleeding secondary to left femoral manipulation. An immediate CBC should be obtained to see whether the hemoglobin level has dropped; a CT scan will define whether there is bleeding. The cardiologist should also be notified of the patient's condition.

48 Answer b

Reperfusion after thrombolysis is demonstrated by the ST segment elevation resolving quickly, and resolution of Q waves (if the infarct is aborted).

49 Answer c

Current treatments of atrial fibrillation include amiodarone (Cordarone), metoprolol (Lopressor), and diltiazem (Cardizem). Amlodipine (Norvasc) is a calcium channel blocker that may cause reflex tachycardia and is not used to treat atrial fibrillation.

50 Answer b

The hemodynamic profile consistent with cardiogenic shock is a low cardiac index, elevated pulmonary capillary wedge pressure, a low mean arterial pressure as evidenced by hypotension, and signs of left ventricular failure. A hemodynamic profile of a cardiac index of 1.8, wedge pressure of 28, and mean arterial pressure of 60 is consistent with cardiogenic shock.

51 Answer d

Contraindications to thrombolytic therapy in patients with myocardial infarction include abdominal surgery within the past month, heme positive stools, and a history of cerebral bleeding. Thrombolytic therapy is contraindicated in patients with recent surgery and a history of bleeding diathesis. History of pacemaker placement 5 years earlier is not a contraindication.

52 Answer c

Spironolactone (Aldactone) is a potassium-sparing diuretic.

53 Answer c

Symptoms of digoxin (Lanoxin) toxicity include bradycardia and gastrointestinal complications such as diarrhea and nausea. Headaches, severe or not, are not associated with digoxin toxicity.

54 Answer b

The next plan of care for the patient described is to discontinue the enalapril (Vasotec) and start hydralazine (Apresoline). The patient has been on a regime for CHF for the past month. Enalapril, which is an ACE inhibitor, may produce a cough. In addition, CHF may produce a cough, but the patient is compensated. Changing ACE inhibitors will not alleviate the cough if the ACE inhibitor is the cause. The patient should be taken off the enalapril and placed on another vasodilator. If the symptoms persist after changing the ACE inhibitors, check for other possible causes of cough.

55 Answer c

Nonpharmacologic management of CHF includes weight reduction, if applicable, and avoidance of alcoholic beverages and cigarette smoking. It should also include restricting sodium to 2 to 3 g/d (not 5 g/d) to decrease fluid retention.

56 Answer b

The next plan of care for the patient described is to inform the patient of the findings and to plan a carotid duplex for further assessment. The presence of a carotid bruit may imply significant carotid stenosis, so the patient should be referred for a carotid duplex to assess for stenosis. The presence of carotid stenosis could put the patient at risk for stroke during cardiac surgery.

57 Answer c

Routine liver function testing should be done on patients taking lovastatin (Mevacor). Lovastatin may cause hepatic toxicity, so liver function tests should be monitored every 3 to 6 months.

58 Answer d

The most likely diagnosis of the patient described is mediastinitis. The presence of sternal erythema, fever, and pain point to an infectious process. Pericarditis and pleurisy may produce fever and pain but do not involve erythema of the incision. Pneumonia, pericarditis, and pleurisy may all produce fever and pain, but do not involve erythema of the incision.

59 Answer d

Based on the patient's INR findings, you would ascertain that the patient is taking the warfarin (Coumadin) correctly, and there have been no changes in dietary patterns. If so, continue the same warfarin dose, and recheck the INR the next day.

The target INR for patients with atrial fibrillation is 2.0 to 2.5. The patient has been stable, so you would be concerned about correct administration of warfarin and dietary changes. Giving vitamin K is not indicated.

60 Answer d

The first line of treatment for the patient described is corticosteroids. Atrial fibrillation in a patient who has undergone cardiac transplantation usually means rejection and should be initially treated with corticosteroids.

61 Answer c

The primary symptom of diastolic dysfunction is shortness of breath due to pulmonary vascular congestion.

62 Answer b

The most common cause of CHF is myocardial ischemia.

63 Answer b

Treatment of diastolic heart failure includes diuretics, beta blockers, and ACE inhibitors. Diastolic dysfunction is not treated with digoxin (Lanoxin) because of the increase in cardiac contractility.

64 Answer d

The most **likely** diagnosis for the patient described is bacterial endocarditis. The patient has endocarditis and the peripheral manifestation on the torso and palms are from the infection. The palm lesions are Osler nodes.

65 Answer d

Co-trimoxazole (Bactrim) is used as prophylaxis against PCP in the patient who is 3 months post heart transplantation.

66 Answer c

Symptoms of right-sided heart failure include abdominal bloating, nausea, and peripheral edema. Orthopnea is associated with left ventricular failure.

67 Answer c

Your plan of care for the patient described is to obtain a more detailed history about the headaches. Throbbing occipital headaches are common in patients with hypertension, so a more detailed history would be necessary before further interventions are planned.

68 Answer a

Physical exam findings that may be found in patients with essential hypertension include an atrial gallop (S4), hypertensive retinopathy, and a laterally displaced apical impulse (due to left ventricular hypertrophy.)

69 Answer a

Physiologic splitting of the second heart sound is a normal physical finding and is heard during inspiration.

70 Answer d

A patient with a wandering atrial pacemaker will usually have an irregular heart rhythm, a varying PR interval, normal QRS complexes, and heart rates less than 100 beats/min.

71 Answer b

Magnesium is the treatment of choice for torsades de pointes.

72 Answer b

The appropriate next step for the patient described is to start

warfarin (Coumadin), continue the beta blockers and procainamide (Pronestyl), then discharge the patient and arrange
for cardioversion in 4 weeks if not converted. The patient has
new onset of atrial fibrillation but has been in atrial fibrillation for the past 3 days and is at risk for thromboembolic
events if cardioverted. The appropriate treatment plan would
be to continue the same medications and start warfarin, then
plan for cardioversion within the next month.

73 Answer d

Hypertrophic cardiomyopathy is characterized by increased
left ventricular wall thickness (hypertrophy) and may occur
in aortic stenosis and systemic hypertension. It is not characterized by a dilated left ventricle.

74 Answer d

The most appropriate response to the patient who has mitral
valve prolapse with mild mitral regurgitation and is asking
you about her need for antibiotics prior to a dental cleansing
appointment is to tell her: "You should take the antibiotics 1
hour prior to the dental visit." This is the currently recommended endocarditis prophylaxis.

75 Answer b

The pressure gradient between the PAED and the PAWP is
normally 1 to 4 mm Hg.

76 Answer a

The normal PAWP is 6 to 12 mm Hg.

77 Answer c

The "a" wave of the pulmonary artery wedge tracing represents left atrial contraction, the "x" descent represents atrial
relaxation, and the "c" wave (which is usually not visually
appreciated) represents mitral valve closure.

78 Answer b

The instruction that should be given to the patient described
at the time of discharge is to avoid blood pressure measurements in the left arm. There are no indications that the patient
should avoid extreme temperatures, keep the arm elevated at
night, or apply an ace bandage.

79 Answer a

The immediate adverse reactions that may be associated with
muromonab-CD3 (Orthoclone OKT3) are those of anaphylaxis, which include pulmonary edema, fever, and rigors.

80 Answer b

Types of distributive shock, which usually has normal blood
volume, include septic, anaphylactic, and neurogenic shock.
Hypovolemic shock is not a type of distributive shock.

81 Answer b

The initial stage of septic shock is characterized by hypotension. Septic shock is characterized by a hyperdynamic metabolic state, increased cardiac output, and decreased vascular
tone with hypotension.

82 Answer a

The murmur of aortic insufficiency is characterized by a diastolic blowing murmur heard best at the third left intercostal
space.

83 Answer d

Potential complications of prosthetic valve replacements include endocarditis, hemolysis, and paravalvular leak.

84 Answer d

The most likely diagnosis for the patient described is atrial
septal defect. A classic physical exam finding of atrial septal
defect is a fixed split second heart sound.

85 Answer d

The potential complications that may occur as a result of unrepaired atrial septal defect include the development of arrhythmias, cyanosis, and right ventricular failure. Atrial septal defects if unrepaired may cause a dilated right atrium and
ventricle with pulmonary hypertension.

References

Alpert, J: Physiopathology of the Cardiovascular System. Little,
  Brown and Company, Boston, 1984.
Baumgartner, W, et al: The John Hopkins Manual of Cardiac Surgical
  Care. Mosby Year Book, St. Louis, 1994.
Chung, E: ECG Diagnosis: A Self-Assessment Workbook. Blackwell
  Science, Malden, MA, 2000.
Fauci, AS, ed: Harrison's Principles of Internal Medicine, 14th ed.
  McGraw-Hill Book Company, New York, 1998.
Goldman, L, and Braunwald, E: Primary Cardiology. Saunders/
  Harcourt Health Sciences, Philadelphia, 1998.
Goroll, A, et al: Primary Care Medicine Office Evaluation and Man-
  agement of the Adult Patient, 4th ed. Lippincott Williams &
  Wilkins, Philadelphia, 2000.
Harvey, P: Cardiac Pearls. Laennec Publishing, Newton, NJ.
Izzo, J, and Black, H: Hypertension Primer, 2nd ed. American Heart
  Association, Dallas, TX, 1999.
Larosa, J: Cholesterol and atherosclerosis: A controversy resolved.
  Advances for Nurse Practitioners 1998, May:37–41.
Sonnenblick, E: Detecting and treating heart failure: An update on
  strategies. Consultant. January 2000;40(Jan):1.
Wood, S, et. al: Cardiac Nursing, 4th ed. Lippincott Williams &
  Wilkins, Philadelphia, 2000.

4

Pulmonary Problems

1 *A 65-year-old man with alcoholism presents to the emergency department with fever, shortness of breath, and production of purulent sputum. His past medical history is significant for emphysema. Physical exam reveals respiratory rate of 32, and temperature 104°F. Chest x-ray reveals right upper lobe pneumonia. What is the most likely organism responsible for his illness?*

a Influenza A virus
b *Mycoplasma pneumoniae*
c *Klebsiella pneumoniae*
d *Streptococcus pneumoniae*

2 *The treatment of choice for* Mycoplasma *pneumonia is:*

a trimethoprim/sulfamethoxazole (Bactrim).
b amoxicillin (Amoxil).
c penicillin.
d erythromycin (E-mycin).

3 *Which of the following is associated with viral pneumonia?*

a Sudden onset of shaking chills and rigors
b Diffuse, bilateral infiltrates on chest x-ray
c Tachycardia
d Bloody sputum

4 *Spirometry measures all of the following components of lung function* **EXCEPT:**

a forced vital capacity (FVC).
b forced expiratory volume (FEV1).
c arterial saturation.
d mean expiratory flow rate during the middle 50% of the forced expiratory maneuver (FEF 25% to 75%).

5 *If a patient has a low FEV1 to forced vital capacity (FVC) ratio the most likely diagnosis is:*

a normal lung function.
b restrictive lung disease.

c asthma.
d obstructive lung disease.

6 *The major toxic effect of isoniazid (INH) is:*

a ototoxicity.
b hepatitis.
c peripheral neuropathy.
d rash.

7 *The most common adverse reaction to rifampin (Rifadin) is:*

a gastrointestinal upset.
b hepatitis.
c jaundice.
d thrombocytopenia.

8 *A positive skin test for tuberculosis in a patient with human immunodeficiency virus (HIV) infection is one that is greater than:*

a 5 mm.
b 20 mm.
c 10 mm.
d 15 mm.

9 *The organism most responsible for bacterial pneumonia is:*

a *Klebsiella.*
b *Pseudomonas aeruginosa.*
c *Streptococcus.*
d *Haemophilus influenzae.*

10 *Serum cold agglutinins may be used as a diagnostic test for:*

a histoplasmosis.
b Q fever.
c tuberculosis.
d *Mycoplasma.*

11 *Asthma may be characterized by all of the following* **EXCEPT:**

a   air trapping.
b   airway obstruction.
c   airway inflammation.
d   airway hyporesponsiveness.

12 *All of the following are true about exercise-induced asthma* **EXCEPT:**

a   It is caused mainly by smooth muscle constriction.
b   It peaks 20 minutes after the vigorous activity is stopped.
c   Inhaled beta agonists should be used 60 minutes before activity.
d   An exercise challenge test may be used to establish diagnosis.

13 *All of the following are true about Legionnaires' disease* **EXCEPT:**

a   It may be transmitted via contaminated water sources.
b   An increase in outbreaks occur during the winter and spring.
c   It affects middle-aged and elderly persons most.
d   Persons affected may exhibit high fever, cough, and dyspnea.

14 *A 50-year-old man presents to your clinic for further advice concerning an abnormal chest x-ray taken 2 weeks ago. He currently smokes and has a 50 pack per year smoking history. What would be the next step in your evaluation?*

a   Refer the patient to a pulmonary specialist.
b   Order a chest computed tomography (CT) scan.
c   Ask the patient whether he had any other chest x-rays taken and obtain copies of them.
d   Refer the patient for a bronchoscopy.

15 *The medication of choice for treatment of acute exacerbations of asthma and for the prevention of exercise-induced asthma is:*

a   an oral steroid.
b   an inhaled steroid.
c   a beta-2 agonist.
d   cromolyn (Intal).

16 *A 60-year-old school worker comes to the clinic for evaluation of an abnormal chest x-ray. He states he was told he has asbestosis. In your explanation of this disease process all of the following are true* **EXCEPT:**

a   It is a fibrosis of the lung parenchyma or pleura.
b   The severity of asbestos-related pulmonary fibrosis is not related to the total dose of exposure.
c   Extensive pleural thickening has been associated with mesothelioma.

d   Extensive pleural plaques have been associated with lung cancer.

17 *All of the following are associated with chronic cough* **EXCEPT:**

a   cigarette smoking.
b   use of angiotensin-converting enzyme (ACE) inhibitors.
c   postnasal drip.
d   use of aspirin.

18 *In evaluating a person with chronic cough, the differential diagnosis may include:*

a   congestive heart failure.
b   reflux esophagitis.
c   malignancy.
d   all of the above.

19 *A 65-year-old man comes to your office complaining of fever, chest congestion, malaise, and putrid sputum. What is the most likely diagnosis?*

a   Pulmonary edema
b   Lung abscess
c   Tuberculosis
d   Bronchitis

20 *A 70-year-old man is admitted to the hospital with complaints of fatigue and shortness of breath. The chest x-ray reveals a large left pleural effusion. All of the following are criteria for transudative effusion* **EXCEPT:**

a   The ratio of pleural fluid to serum protein is less than 0.5.
b   The ratio of pleural fluid lactate dehydrogenase (LDH) to serum LDH is less than 0.6.
c   The pleural fluid LDH is less than two-thirds of the upper limit of normal for the serum LDH.
d   An elevated white blood cell count is found in pleural fluid.

21 *The most common cause of transudative pleural effusion is:*

a   congestive heart failure.
b   breast cancer.
c   pancreatitis.
d   tuberculosis.

22 *Physical exam findings associated with pleural effusion may include all of the following* **EXCEPT:**

a   neck vein distention.
b   egophony.
c   atrial gallop (S4).
d   tachypnea.

23 *A 35-year-old woman comes to see you for a routine physical exam for a new job. While performing the exam, you note clubbing of both hands. What is the one diagnostic tool that should be obtained for further evaluation?*

a   An echocardiogram
b   A complete blood count
c   A chest x-ray
d   A liver function test

24 *A 55-year-old man has been diagnosed with chronic obstructive pulmonary disease (COPD). All of the following items should be included in his teaching plan* **EXCEPT:**

a   smoking cessation.
b   no exercise.
c   reduction of exposure to known environmental irritants.
d   administration of Pneumovax.

25 *Sarcoidosis is a disease characterized by:*

a   formation of noncaseating granulomas.
b   an association with lung cancer.
c   being more common in whites.
d   an onset that is between age 50 and 65 years.

26 *A 50-year-old woman is diagnosed with Q fever. Q fever is caused by:*

a   *Chlamydia.*
b   *Coxiella burnetii.*
c   cytomegalovirus.
d   *Mycoplasma.*

Questions 27–28 refer to the following scenario:

A 35-year-old woman is admitted with complaints of sharp, pleuritic, right-sided chest pain; and shortness of breath for the past 24 hours. She denies any health problems and is not taking any medications. She currently has her monthly menstrual cycle.

27 *What is the most likely diagnosis?*

a   Pulmonary embolus
b   Pleurisy
c   Pneumonia
d   Spontaneous pneumothorax

28 *The initial diagnostic tool that should be used to diagnose the patient in question 27 is:*

a   a chest CT scan.
b   a magnetic resonance imaging (MRI) of the chest and abdomen.
c   bronchoscopy.
d   a chest x-ray.

29 *A 55-year-old man who smokes two packs of cigarettes per day presents for his annual health physical. He states that he may be interested in quitting smoking because two of his friends died from lung cancer. What is the most important prognostic indicator as to whether or not a person will succeed in smoking cessation efforts?*

a   The commitment of the patient to stop smoking
b   The desire of the family to have the person stop smoking
c   The concurrent use of a nicotine patch
d   The concurrent use of a behavioral modification program

30 *All of the following cancers have been associated with cigarette smoking* **EXCEPT:**

a   lung cancer.
b   esophageal cancer.
c   bladder cancer.
d   colon cancer.

31 *The most common symptom(s) of primary pulmonary hypertension is(are):*

a   dyspnea.
b   easy fatigability.
c   near syncope.
d   all of the above.

32 *A physical examination in the patient with primary pulmonary hypertension may reveal:*

a   a right ventricular heave.
b   lower extremity edema.
c   right-sided third and fourth heart sounds.
d   all of the above.

33 *The initial management of patients with pulmonary hypertension should include:*

a   heart-lung transplantation.
b   oxygen therapy.
c   vasodilators.
d   lung transplantation.

34 *A 55-year-old woman with a history of lung cancer diagnosed 3 months ago and treated with radiation and a left upper lobe lobectomy presents to the emergency department with complaints of shortness of breath and left-sided chest discomfort for the past 2 hours. Vital signs on presentation are: temperature 97.8°F, pulse 120 and regular, respiratory rate 40, blood pressure 100/60, and oxygen saturation of 88% on room air by pulse oximetry. Physical exam reveals a woman in moderate distress, lungs with diminished breath sounds on the left side, heart rate regular with tachycardia, and with no extra sounds. The exam of the abdomen is benign, and the exam of the lower extremities reveals a swollen and painful left calf. What is the most likely diagnosis?*

a Recurrent lung cancer
b Myocardial infarction
c Atrial fibrillation
d Pulmonary embolus

Questions 35–37 refer to the following scenario:

A 65-year-old man is admitted to the hospital with complaints of hemoptysis for the past 2 months. Over the last 2 days, he has been coughing up a cupful of bright red blood, with most of the sputum production in the morning hours. He admits to fatigue and dyspnea on exertion for the past 3 to 4 months. He denies weight loss, night sweats, and fever. Physical exam is unremarkable except for deviation of the trachea to the right, and dullness on percussion of the lung fields. Chest x-ray reveals bilateral lung fibrosis, elevation of the hila, and cavitation in the right upper lung field.

35 *What is the most likely diagnosis?*

a Lung cancer
b Tuberculosis
c Aspergilloma
d Pulmonary fibrosis

36 *Treatment options for aspergilloma with hemoptysis include:*

a pulmonary resection.
b amphotericin B infusion.
c embolization of bronchial arteries.
d all of the above.

37 *The patient is waiting to go to the operating room for treatment of hemoptysis. The staff nurse notifies you that the patient is coughing up large volumes of blood. What measures would you institute until the patient can go to the operative suite?*

a Position patient on his left side.
b Intubate the patient to control the airway.
c Position the patient on his right side.
d Start a dopamine infusion.

38 *Risk factors associated with adult respiratory distress syndrome (ARDS) include all of the following* **EXCEPT:**

a aspiration.
b transfusion of more than 10 U of blood products in a 24-hour period.
c hypertension.
d sepsis.

39 *A 40-year-old man is involved as a passenger in a motor vehicle accident in which the car flipped over several times. In the emergency department, the patient is awake, but groggy. He has a flail chest and multiple bruises without any other fractures or head*

injuries. His vital signs are heart rate of 120, blood pressure 80/50, and respiratory rate of 36. A decision was made to intubate the patient. Chest x-ray reveals left upper lung infiltrate thought to be a pulmonary contusion. Eight hours after admission, arterial blood gas measurement reveals a pH of 7.4, PCO_2 of 39, PO_2 of 50, and an oxygen saturation of 90%. A repeat chest x-ray reveals a "white out" pattern. You decide to add positive end expiratory pressure (PEEP) to the ventilator settings. Potential problems associated with PEEP include all of the following **EXCEPT:**

a hypertension.
b decreased cardiac output.
c pneumothorax.
d barotrauma.

40 *Treatment of idiopathic pulmonary fibrosis (IPF) includes:*

a bronchodilators.
b vasodilators.
c steroids.
d diuretics.

41 *What are the classic pulmonary function test abnormalities seen in the early stages of idiopathic pulmonary fibrosis (IPF)?*

a Reduction in lung volumes
b Normalization of saturation with activity
c Reduction in FEV1/forced vital capacity (FVC) ratio
d Normal diffusing capacity

42 *A 25-year-old man with known human immunodeficiency virus (HIV) disease is seen with complaints of dyspnea, fever, night sweats, and weight loss over the past 2 weeks. Physical exam reveals a man in moderate distress, temperature of 101.5°F, pulse 120, respiratory rate of 28, and blood pressure 90/60. Skin turgor reveals dehydration, and chest exam reveals bibasilar crackles. A chest x-ray reveals diffuse interstitial infiltrates. What is the most likely diagnosis?*

a *Staphylococcus* pneumonia
b Non-Hodgkin's lymphoma
c *Pneumocystis carinii* pneumonia (PCP)
d *H. influenzae*

43 *Which of the following factors may increase the clearance of theophylline?*

a Administration of rifampin (Rifadin)
b Smoking
c Consumption of alcohol (ethanol)
d All of the above

44 *A 30-year-old man complains of nocturnal cough of 2-month duration. He denies any other symptoms. His sister and mother have asthma. You suspect that* the patient may have asthma, but baseline pulmonary function tests and chest x-rays are normal. What is the next step in the evaluation of this patient?

a   Start oral steroids.
b   Start oral theophylline.
c   Obtain an echocardiogram.
d   Perform a methacholine challenge test.

45   *The classic chest x-ray finding of a patient with emphysema is:*

a   flattening of the diaphragms.
b   increased hilar adenopathy.
c   patchy atelectasis.
d   prominence of pulmonary vasculature.

46   *All of the following are true about alpha-1 anti-trypsin deficiency* **EXCEPT:**

a   It is inherited as a dominant trait.
b   It is a rare form of COPD.
c   It is more common in whites.
d   Shortness of breath is common.

47   *Which of the following disorders is associated with alveolar hemorrhage and glomerulonephritis?*

a   Tuberculosis
b   Goodpasture's syndrome
c   Systemic lupus erythematosus
d   Idiopathic pulmonary fibrosis

48   *The diagnosis of Goodpasture's syndrome is made by:*

a   chest x-ray.
b   lung biopsy.
c   chest CT scan.
d   renal biopsy.

49   *Treatment of patients with Goodpasture's syndrome may include all of the following* **EXCEPT:**

a   open lung biopsy.
b   corticosteroids.
c   plasmapheresis.
d   cyclophosphamide (Cytoxan).

50   *A 60-year-old man diagnosed with pulmonary embolus (PE) is receiving heparin therapy. This is his third pulmonary embolus in the past 5 years. You are the nurse practitioner caring for this patient. What would be the indications for referring the patient for inferior vena cava (IVC) filter?*

a   Recurrent PE or deep-vein thrombosis (DVT) despite adequate anticoagulation
b   Allergy to heparin
c   Pulmonary hypertension
d   All of the above

51   *The most common electrocardiogram (ECG) finding in patients diagnosed with pulmonary embolus is:*

a   sinus tachycardia.
b   sinus bradycardia.
c   atrial flutter.
d   right ventricular hypertrophy.

52   *Pulsus paradoxus is commonly associated with:*

a   asthma.
b   emphysema.
c   pulmonary embolus.
d   pneumonia.

53   *Preventative therapy in treatment of tuberculosis should include:*

a   streptomycin therapy for 1 year.
b   INH therapy for 6 months.
c   rifampin therapy for 12 months.
d   bacille Calmette-Guérin (BCG) vaccination.

54   *The most common pulmonary-related acquired immunodeficiency syndrome (AIDS) infection is:*

a   PCP.
b   histoplasmosis.
c   aspergillosis.
d   cytomegalovirus.

55   *The drug of choice for PCP prophylaxis is:*

a   penicillin.
b   trimethoprim-sulfamethoxazole (Bactrim).
c   pentamidine.
d   amphotericin B.

56   *The most common deep fungal infection in patients with HIV infection is:*

a   PCP.
b   histoplasmosis.
c   aspergillosis.
d   cryptococcosis.

57   *A 50-year-old obese man is seen for a routine physical exam. He admits to increased fatigue, sleepiness during the daytime hours, and restlessness during sleeping hours. His wife reports loud snoring which has become worse in the past year. He denies any health problems and is on no medications. He smokes a pack of cigarettes per day. Physical exam reveals normal vital signs, with respiratory rate 18. Lung exam reveals clear lung fields, and trachea midline without adenopathy. What is the most likely diagnosis?*

a   Chronic bronchitis
b   Sleep apnea
c   COPD
d   Asthma

58 *All of the following statements concerning sleep apnea are true* **EXCEPT:**

a Most patients are obese.
b Tracheotomy is the most common treatment.
c There is associated increase in blood pressure.
d Nasal continuous positive airway pressure (CPAP) is the most common treatment.

59 *The treatment of tension pneumothorax is:*

a bronchoscopy.
b insertion of a large bore needle.
c insertion of a chest tube.
d administration of fluids.

60 *A 55-year-old man presents with complaints of shortness of breath with exertion and intermittent wheezing at night. His occupational history is significant for coal mining for the past 25 years. No other health history. He smokes two packs of cigarettes per day. He denies paroxysmal nocturnal dyspnea (PND), orthopnea, fever, chills, and weight loss. Chest x-ray reveals nodular densities with hyperinflation. What is the most likely diagnosis?*

a Asbestosis-related lung disease
b Coal worker's pneumoconiosis
c Asthma
d Tuberculosis

61 *A 60-year-old man is diagnosed with COPD. Which of the following changes would you expect to see on his pulmonary function tests?*

a Decreased forced expiratory volume and increased residual volume
b Decreased residual volume and decreased total lung capacity
c Increased FEV1 and increased total lung capacity
d Increased FVC and decreased total lung capacity.

62 *Complications of cardiopulmonary exercise testing include:*

a hypotension.
b hypoxia.
c cardiac arrhythmia.
d all of the above.

63 *Contraindications to cardiopulmonary exercise testing include:*

a stable angina.
b uncontrolled asthma.
c COPD.
d IPF.

64 *Physical exam findings in the patient with COPD include all of the following* **EXCEPT:**

a distant lung sounds.
b barrel chest deformity.
c decreased diaphragm movement.
d normal tactile fremitus.

65 *Physical exam findings in the patient with pleural effusion include:*

a resonant percussion note.
b increased vesicular breath sounds.
c egophony.
d pleural rub.

66 *A 45-year-old woman is diagnosed with pneumonia with consolidation. What findings would you expect on physical exam?*

a Decreased tactile fremitus
b Dullness on percussion
c Vesicular breath sounds
d Resonance on percussion

67 *Cheyne-Stokes breathing is associated with all of the following conditions* **EXCEPT:**

a congestive heart failure (CHF).
b COPD.
c post stroke.
d drug-induced respiratory depression.

68 *Aspirin-induced asthma may be manifested by all of the following* **EXCEPT:**

a nasal congestion.
b rhinorrhea.
c acute asthma attack.
d epistaxis.

69 *The standard criterion for diagnosing pulmonary embolus is:*

a perfusion lung scan.
b chest x-ray.
c MRI of the thorax.
d pulmonary arteriogram.

70 *Management strategies for the treatment of pulmonary embolus include:*

a thrombolytics.
b heparin.
c insertion of an inferior vena cava (IVC) filter.
d all of the above.

71 *A 68-year-old man was admitted to the unit with a 3-day history of fever to 102°F, malaise, chills, fatigue, and shortness of breath. He was recently discharged from the hospital after being treated for Klebsiella pneumonia for the past 2 weeks. He has a history of hypertension, arthritis, and diabetes mellitus. He smokes 1–1/2 packs of cigarettes daily and* *drinks two 6-packs of beer daily. The chest x-ray reveals right upper lobe area of consolidation with radiolucency. What is the most likely diagnosis?*

a Recurrent pneumonia
b Lung abscess
c Septic pulmonary embolus
d Tuberculosis

72 *Cystic fibrosis (CF) may be manifested by:*

a hyperproteinemia.
b weight gain.
c patchy atelectasis on chest x-ray.
d all of the above.

73 *Which of the following is true concerning cystic fibrosis (CF)?*

a Men affected with CF are sterile.
b Air trapping is seen on chest x-ray.
c Portal hypertension may be present.
d All of the above.

74 *The diagnostic test(s) for cystic fibrosis (CF) is(are):*

a the sweat test.
b a CT scan.
c chest and abdominal CT scans.
d none of the above.

75 *The pulmonary manifestations of cystic fibrosis (CF) should be managed by:*

a postural drainage.
b a cardiopulmonary exercise program.
c bronchodilators.
d all of the above.

76 *The differential diagnosis for anterior mediastinal mass includes:*

a parathyroid tumor.
b retrosternal thyroid.
c bronchogenic cyst.
d thymoma.

77 *A 60-year-old woman presents complaining of shortness of breath and fatigue for the last 2 weeks. She has no other health history. Medications include calcium and multivitamins. A portable anterior chest x-ray was ordered and revealed elevation of the right hemidiaphragm. What is your next step in evaluating this abnormality?*

a Obtain a chest CT scan.
b Obtain a chest x-ray with lateral and decubitus views.
c Obtain an MRI of the chest.
d Obtain a pulmonary arteriogram.

78 *Unilateral diaphragmatic paralysis may:*

a be the result of vagus nerve injury.
b result in patients who are usually very symptomatic and have shortness of breath.
c be the result of phrenic nerve injury.
d all of the above.

79 *Causes of carbon dioxide retention include:*

a brain-stem disease.
b use of morphine derivatives.
c muscular dystrophy.
d all of the above.

80 *The most common symptom of laryngeal disease is:*

a cough.
b hoarseness.
c dysphagia.
d dyspnea.

81 *Cancer of the larynx:*

a is more common in women.
b is highly curable if detected early.
c develops at an average age of 40 years.
d all of the above.

82 *The most common symptom of pulmonary infarction secondary to pulmonary embolus is:*

a hemoptysis.
b cough.
c pleural pain.
d dyspnea.

83 *A 35-year-old woman is 5 days post double lung transplant secondary to cystic fibrosis (CF). The staff nurse notifies you that the patient is acutely short of breath, has tachycardia, and has a temperature of 100.5°F. On physical exam, she is audibly wheezing, with respiratory rate of 32; heart tones are normal. Pulse oximetry revealed room air saturation of 90%. As the acute care nurse practitioner, what is your next step?*

a Check the patient's arterial blood gas results, blood cultures, and chest x-ray, then notify the pulmonologist of the change in condition.
b Arrange for a bronchoscopy.
c Administer high-dose steroids.
d All of the above.

84 *Post lung transplant rejection is diagnosed by:*

a open lung biopsy.
b a decrease in lung spirometry.
c hypoxemia.
d bronchoscopy.

85 *A 50-year-old man is post left lower lobe lobectomy for stage-1 lung cancer. He is 3 days post surgery and you are asked to see him because of milky drainage in his chest tube–chest drainage collection system. What is your next plan of action?*

a Obtain a chest x-ray immediately.
b Obtain a sample of the fluid and send it to the lab for analysis.
c Talk to the surgeon, and plan for the patient to return to surgery.
d Have the patient lie in bed with his left side down.

Answers

1 Answer b

Klebsiella pneumoniae is typically associated with debilitated patients and especially alcoholic patients. It is one of the most frequently occurring pneumonias in ambulatory patients.

2 Answer d

The treatment of choice for *Mycoplasma pneumoniae* is erythromycin (E-mycin).

3 Answer b

Viral pneumonia is more common in immunosuppressed persons and may present with a flulike syndrome including headache, fever, and myalgias. The chest x-ray shows diffuse, patchy infiltrates on chest x-ray.

4 Answer c

Spirometry measures all of the components of lung function except arterial saturation, which may be obtained by arterial blood gas.

5 Answer d

If a patient has a low FEV1 to FVC ratio, the most likely diagnosis is obstructive lung disease.

6 Answer b

The major toxic effect of INH is hepatitis, which seems to increase with older patients. Peripheral neuropathy may occur, but it is uncommon and may be countered by giving pyridoxine (vitamin B6).

7 Answer a

The most common adverse reaction to rifampin (Rifadin) is gastrointestinal upset. Other side effects such as hepatitis, cholestatic jaundice, and thrombocytopenia may occur but are less common.

8 Answer a

A positive skin test for tuberculosis in a patient with HIV infection is one in which the induration is 5 mm or greater; 10 mm or greater for members of high incidence population; and 15 mm or greater for individuals with no identifiable risk factors.

9 Answer c

Streptococcus is the organism most responsible for bacterial pneumonia, accounting for 30% to 50% of all cases.

10 Answer d

Serum cold agglutinins may be used as a diagnostic test for mycoplasma. Cold agglutinins may be present in influenza infections, but high or rising titers are suggestive of *Mycoplasma.*

11 Answer d

Asthma may be characterized by air trapping, airway obstruction, and airway inflammation. It is not characterized by airway hyporesponsiveness. The airway in asthma is hyperresponsive.

12 Answer c

With exercise-induced asthma, inhaled beta agonists should not be used 60 minutes before activity; they should be used 30 minutes before activity. The other statements are true. Exercise-induced asthma is caused mainly by smooth muscle constriction, peaks 20 minutes after stopping the vigorous activity, and an exercise challenge test may be used to establish diagnosis.

13 Answer b

With Legionnaires' disease, it may occur in sporadic cases or epidemics. It does not have a seasonal variation; therefore, there is not an increase in outbreaks during the winter and spring. The other statements are true. It may be transmitted via contaminated water sources, it affects primarily middle-aged and elderly persons, and those may exhibit high fever, cough, and dyspnea.

14 Answer c

A 50-year-old male smoker presents to your clinic with an abnormal chest x-ray, the first step in evaluation is to inquire about subsequent x-rays and obtain them for comparison. If the previous x-ray was normal, the patient should be referred for a chest computed tomography (CT) scan, and to a pulmonary specialist.

15 Answer d

The medication of choice for treatment of acute exacerbations of asthma and for the prevention of exercise-induced asthma is cromolyn (Intal). If patients cannot tolerate cromolyn, then a beta-2–agonist aerosol may be used.

16 Answer b

The severity of asbestos-related pulmonary fibrosis is related to the total dose of exposure; therefore statement b is false. The other statements are true. It is a fibrosis of the lung parenchyma or pleura, extensive pleural thickening has been associated with mesothelioma, and extensive pleural plaques have been associated with lung cancer.

17 Answer d

Chronic cough is associated with cigarette smoking, use of ACE inhibitors, and postnasal drip. It is not associated with the use of aspirin.

18 Answer d

The differential diagnosis in a person with a chronic cough may include CHF, reflux esophagitis, and malignancy.

19 Answer b

The most likely diagnosis in a 65-year-old man with complaints of fever, chest congestion, malaise, and putrid sputum is lung abscess.

20 Answer d

An elevated white blood cell count in the pleural fluid usually means an exudate and may be diagnostic for empyema, not transudative effusion.

21   Answer a

The most common cause of transudative pleural effusion is CHF.

22   Answer c

Pleural effusion may be seen in congestive heart failure and there may be neck vein distention and ventricular gallop (S3), not an atrial gallop (S4). The patient may be tachypneic and have egophony on physical examination.

23   Answer c

A 35-year-old woman with clubbing of both hands should have a chest x-ray performed for further evaluation. The clubbing may represent an asymptomatic pulmonary process. A thorough history should also be obtained concerning other family members with clubbing.

24   Answer b

A 55-year-old man with COPD should have a teaching plan that includes smoking cessation, reduction of exposure to known environmental irritants, administration of Pneumovax, as well as the importance of exercise, including walking and breathing exercises.

25   Answer a

Sarcoidosis is a disease characterized by the formation of noncaseating granulomas. It is 10 times more prevalent in African Americans, and its usual onset is between the ages of 20 and 45 years.

26   Answer b

Q fever is caused by *Coxiella burnetii,* the organisms of which reside mostly in animals such as sheep, goats, and cattle.

27   Answer d

A 35-year-old woman with complaints of sharp, pleuritic chest pain, and shortness of breath for the past 24 hours should be evaluated for a spontaneous pneumothorax. The information from her history that she is menstruating may lead one to think of catamenial pneumothorax, which is a rare disorder associated with right-sided pneumothorax occurring at the time of the menstrual cycle. The exact pathogenesis is not well described, but is thought to be a form of endometriosis.

28   Answer d

The initial tool that should be used to diagnose the patient with a spontaneous pneumothorax is a chest x-ray. A chest CT scan is used later in defining the lung and pleural pathology.

29   Answer a

The most important prognostic indicator as to whether or not a person will succeed in smoking cessation efforts is the commitment of the patient. The desire of the family, concurrent behavioral modification, and nicotine patch use may be helpful, but the patient's desire to stop is the singular most important predictor.

30   Answer d

Cigarette smoking has not been linked to colon cancer. It has been linked to lung, esophageal, and bladder cancers.

31   Answer d

The most common symptoms of primary pulmonary hypertension are dyspnea, easy fatigability, and near syncope. The symptoms are usually effort related and may also be related to an inability to increase cardiac output with activity. There may also be a long period when the patient may be asymptomatic.

32   Answer d

Physical examination findings in patients with primary pulmonary hypertension may reveal signs of right heart failure, which may include a right ventricular heave, lower extremity edema, and right-sided third and fourth heart sounds.

33   Answer b

The initial management of patients with pulmonary hypertension should include oxygen therapy, especially patients who have a room air blood gas arterial oxygen tension measurement less than 55 mm Hg.

34   Answer d

A 55-year-old woman with a previous diagnosis of lung cancer presenting to the emergency room with tachycardia, tachypnea, pleuritic chest pain, hypoxemia, and painful calf most likely has pulmonary embolus. Tachycardia is found in 50% of these patients and tachypnea in 90% of the patients.

35   Answer c

A patient with complaints of hemoptysis, dyspnea, and fatigue with lung cavitation is suggestive of aspergilloma. Tuberculosis is possible, but the patient does not have fever, night sweats, and weight loss.

36   Answer d

Treatment options of aspergilloma with hemoptysis include pulmonary resection, amphotericin B infusion, and embolization of bronchial arteries.

37   Answer c

Stabilization of the patient with hemoptysis before operative intervention includes positioning the patient on the side of the suspected source of the bleeding to minimize pooling of blood to the unaffected side. This patient has cavitation in the right upper lung field; therefore positioning the patient on his right side would be a measure to take.

38   Answer c

Risk factors associated with adult respiratory distress syndrome (ARDS) include aspiration, transfusion of blood products, and sepsis. Hypotension, rather than hypertension, is another potential risk factor.

39   Answer a

Potential problems associated with PEEP include hypotension, not hypertension, as well as decreased cardiac output, pneumothorax, and barotrauma.

40   Answer c

Treatment of IPF includes the use of steroids to try to suppress active, ongoing alveolar and interstitial inflammation.

41   Answer a

The classic pulmonary function test abnormalities seen in the early stages of IPF are reduced lung volumes.

42   Answer c

The most likely diagnosis in a 25-year-old man with known HIV disease, and complaints of dyspnea, fever, night sweats, and weight loss, along with a chest x-ray showing diffuse infiltrates is PCP.

43   Answer d

Factors that may increase the clearance of theophylline include the administration of rifampin, consumption of alcohol (ethanol), and smoking. All of these factors cause enzyme induction of P450.

44 Answer d

The next step in evaluation of a 30-year-old man with nocturnal cough and suspected asthma would be to perform a bronchial challenge test using methacoline (methacholine challenge test). If this test is normal, asthma is excluded.

45 Answer a

The classic chest x-ray finding in a patient with emphysema is flattening of the diaphragms.

46 Answer a

Alpha-1 antitrypsin deficiency is inherited as a recessive trait, not a dominant trait. It is a rare form of COPD and presents with shortness of breath. It is more prevalent in whites.

47 Answer b

Goodpasture's syndrome is associated with alveolar hemorrhage and glomerulonephritis. The syndrome is antibody-mediated, attacking the basement membranes.

48 Answer d

The diagnosis of Goodpasture's syndrome is made by renal biopsy.

49 Answer a

Treatment of Goodpasture's syndrome may include corticosteroids, plasmapheresis, and cyclophosphamide (Cytoxan). An open lung biopsy is generally not indicated.

50 Answer d

A patient with recurrent PE or DVT, despite adequate anticoagulation, allergy to heparin, and pulmonary hypertension would all be indications for referral of a patient for consideration of IVC filter for treatment of pulmonary embolus.

51 Answer a

The most common ECG finding in patients diagnosed with pulmonary embolus is sinus tachycardia.

52 Answer a

Pulsus paradoxus is commonly associated with asthma.

53 Answer b

Preventive therapy in treatment of tuberculosis is INH for 6 months. It has been proven to be effective in decreasing the risk of developing active disease in 70% of patients.

54 Answer a

The most common pulmonary-related AIDS infection is PCP. It occurs in approximately 75% of HIV-infected individuals.

55 Answer b

The drug of choice for PCP prophylaxis is trimethoprim/sulfamethoxazole (Bactrim).

56 Answer d

The most common deep fungal infection in patients with HIV infection is cryptococcosis, which occurs in approximately 10% of these patients.

57 Answer b

The most likely diagnosis in an obese patient with increased fatigue, sleepiness during the daytime hours, and snoring is sleep apnea. The most common symptoms of patients with sleep apnea are daytime sleepiness due to inability to sleep at night. Patients with COPD and desaturation at night may also have similar symptoms.

58 Answer b

The most common treatment for sleep apnea is CPAP, not tracheotomy. Patients with sleep apnea are often obese and have hypertension.

59 Answer b

The treatment of tension pneumothorax is the insertion of a large bore needle in the second intercostal space on the affected side.

60 Answer b

The most likely diagnosis for this patient is coal worker's pneumoconiosis based on the occupational history in the coal mining business and the chest x-ray findings of nodular density.

61 Answer a

In patients with COPD, decreased FEV1 and increased residual volume may be seen on spirometry.

62 Answer d

Complications of cardiopulmonary testing may include hypotension, hypoxia, and cardiac arrhythmia.

63 Answer b

Contraindications to cardiopulmonary testing include uncontrolled asthma.

64 Answer d

Physical exam findings in the patient with COPD include distant lung sounds, barrel chest deformity, decreased diaphragm movement, and decreased (not normal) tactile fremitus.

65 Answer c

Physical exam findings in the patient with pleural effusion include egophony. The percussion note is usually dull to flat, and vesicular breath sounds are decreased rather than increased.

66 Answer b

Physical exam findings in the patient with pneumonia and consolidation include dullness on percussion, as well as increased tactile fremitus and bronchial breath sounds.

67 Answer b

Cheyne-Stokes breathing is a central form of apnea associated with congestive heart failure, post stroke, and drug-induced respiratory depression. It is not associated with COPD.

68 Answer d

Aspirin-induced asthma may be manifested by nasal congestion, rhinorrhea, and acute asthmatic attack. It is not associated with epistaxis.

69 Answer d

The standard criterion for diagnosing pulmonary embolus is pulmonary arteriogram. A perfusion lung scan may be suggestive but is not diagnostic.

70 Answer d

Management strategies for the treatment of pulmonary embolus include administration of thrombolytics and heparin, and insertion of an IVC filter.

71 Answer b

The most likely diagnosis in the patient described with a recent gram-negative pneumonia is lung abscess.

72 Answer c

CF may be manifested by patchy atelectasis on chest x-ray. Additional findings include failure to thrive with weight loss, decreased protein stores, cough, and frequent bowel movements.

73 Answer d

CF is an autosomal recessive disease characterized by pancreatic and pulmonary dysfunction. Patients with CF will be sterile. Air trapping is seen on chest x-ray and there is portal hypertension.

74 Answer a

The most accurate diagnostic test for CF is the sweat test.

75 Answer d

The pulmonary manifestations of CF should be managed by postural drainage, a cardiopulmonary exercise program, and bronchodilators if there is bronchospasm.

76 Answer c

The differential diagnosis for anterior mediastinal mass includes bronchogenic cyst. Retrosternal thyroid, parathyroid tumor, and thymoma are differential diagnoses for a superior mediastinal mass.

77 Answer b

An anterior chest x-ray finding of elevated right hemidiaphragm should be further evaluated with a chest x-ray with lateral and decubitus views. Elevation of the right hemidiaphragm may be secondary to upward displacement of intra-abdominal processes.

78 Answer c

Unilateral diaphragmatic paralysis is usually the result of phrenic nerve injury. Patients are usually asymptomatic.

79 Answer d

Causes of carbon dioxide retention include brain-stem disease, use of morphine derivatives, and muscular dystrophy. Other causes include Pickwickian syndrome, chest wall abnormalities, Guillain-Barré syndrome, and diseases of the myoneural junction.

80 Answer b

Hoarseness is the most common symptom of laryngeal disease. Other symptoms such as cough, dysphagia, and dyspnea may also be present.

81 Answer b

Cancer of the larynx is highly curable if detected early. It is more common in men and usually develops around age 60 years.

82 Answer a

The most common symptom of pulmonary infarction secondary to pulmonary embolus is hemoptysis.

83 Answer a

A patient post lung transplant is in acute respiratory distress, the exact mechanism is not clear. You must exclude infectious processes and rejection. The appropriate step would be to assess the patient's arterial blood gas results to rule out hypoxemia, check blood cultures, and check the chest x-ray, then notify the attending physician of the change in the patient's status.

84 Answer d

Post lung transplantation rejection is diagnosed by bronchoscopy.

85 Answer b

The appropriate action for evaluation of milky drainage from the chest tube–chest drainage collection system is to obtain a sample of the fluid and send it to the lab for analysis.

Bibliography

Cote, C, and Celli, B: Answers to nine key questions of COPD. Contemporary Internal Medicine 10(March):3, 1998.

Criner, G, and D'Alonzo, G: Pulmonary Pathophysiology. Fence Creek Publishing, Madison, CT, 1999.

Goroll, A, et al: Primary Care Medicine Office Evaluation and Management of the Adult Patient, ed 4. Lippincott Williams & Wilkins, Philadelphia, 2000.

Hunninghake, GW: Approaches to the treatment of pulmonary fibrosis. Am J Respir Crit Care Med 151:915, 1995.

Traveline, J: Pulmonary Function Testing using a spirometer. Hosp Med, 1994.

Weinberger, S: Principles of Pulmonary Medicine, ed. 3. Harcourt, Philadelphia, 1998.

5

Endocrine Problems

1 *Type 1 diabetes mellitus:*

a generally manifests in late adulthood.
b is more common than type 2 diabetes.
c is associated with pregnancy.
d generally manifests in childhood.

2 *The most common complication of diabetes is:*

a neuropathy.
b retinopathy.
c myocardial infarction.
d renal failure.

3 *The most prevalent risk factor for type 2 diabetes is:*

a obesity.
b hypertension.
c steroid use.
d renal failure.

4 *The major risk factor for the development of thyroid cancer is:*

a external irradiation of the head and neck.
b hyperthyroidism.
c hypothyroidism.
d diabetes mellitus.

5 *Symptoms of hypothyroidism include:*

a lethargy.
b menorrhagia.
c weight gain.
d all of the above.

6 *Graves' disease is associated with all of the following* **EXCEPT:**

a hypothyroidism.
b diffuse goiter.
c exophthalmos.
d pretibial myxedema.

7 *The two most common causes of hypercalcemia are:*

a Paget's disease and hyperthyroidism.
b renal failure and adrenal insufficiency.
c sarcoidosis and malignancy.
d malignancy and hyperparathyroidism.

8 *Hypercalcemia emergency is best treated with:*

a prednisone.
b intravenous phosphate.
c calcitonin.
d an intravenous fluid of normal saline solution alternating with dextrose solution.

9 *Medically significant hypoglycemia is diagnosed on the basis of:*

a a blood glucose level less than 50 mg/dL, symptoms consistent with hypoglycemia, and resolution of symptoms after ingestion of carbohydrates.
b lack of coordination, headache, and blurred vision.
c anxiety, flushing, and coma.
d pallor, confusion, and weakness.

10 *Neuroendocrine tumors that may be associated with hypoglycemia include all of the following* **EXCEPT:**

a myeloma.
b carcinoid tumor.
c pheochromocytoma.
d neurofibroma.

11 *A 50-year-old man presents with a 6-month history of muscle aches, headaches, sweating, decreased libido, and low back pain. He is taking no medications and states he had no health concerns before the past 6 months. Physical exam reveals a well-nourished man with wide spacing between his teeth, coarse skin, and enlarged hands, which are sweaty. Vital signs are normal. What is the most likely diagnosis?*

a Diabetes insipidus (DI)
b Graves' disease.
c parathyroid hyperplasia.
d acromegaly.

12 *The best screening test for the diagnosis of acromegaly is measurement of the:*

a prolactin level.
b testosterone level.
c luteinizing hormone (LH) level.
d somatomedin C level.

13 *The preferred diagnostic imaging tool for assessing the pituitary is:*

a a skull x-ray.
b a MRI scan.
c a CT scan with contrast.
d none of the above.

14 *Multinodular goiter is associated with:*

a a thyroid bruit.
b young persons.
c older persons.
d pregnancy.

15 *A 35-year-old woman is 4 months postpartum and presents with complaints of fatigue, weight loss, decreased exercise tolerance, and nervousness. Family history is positive for hyperthyroidism in her mother and sister. Physical exam reveals a thin anxious female. Vital signs revealed normal temperature, pulse 110, blood pressure 100/65, and respiratory rate 20. Her skin is moist and warm. Hair is thin. Thyroid exam reveals a symmetrically enlarged thyroid gland with a bruit. No exophthalmos. Cardiac, pulmonary, and abdominal exam results are normal. She is hyperreflexic and has proximal muscle weakness in her thighs. What is the most likely diagnosis?*

a Postpartum depression
b Multinodular goiter
c Graves' disease
d Subacute thyroiditis.

16 *Silent thyroiditis is:*

a condition that can occur post pregnancy.
b an autoimmune process.
c manifested by an enlarged thyroid gland.
d all of the above.

17 *In hyperthyroidism, the:*

a total thyroxine (T_4) and triiodothyronine (T_3) are decreased.
b total T_4 is decreased.
c total T_4 and T_3 are increased.
d thyroid-stimulating hormone (TSH) is increased.

18 *What diagnostic tool should be used to distinguish silent thyroiditis from Graves' disease?*

a TSH levels
b Radioactive iodine uptake test
c Thyroid-binding globulins
d None of the above

19 *Causes of an elevated prolactin level may include:*

a a pituitary tumor.
b breast stimulation.
c hypothyroidism.
d all of the above.

20 *A female with an elevated prolactin level may exhibit:*

a amenorrhea.
b hair loss.
c weight loss.
d all of the above.

21 *The most common manifestation of Cushing's syndrome is:*

a muscle weakness.
b obesity.
c hypertension.
d hyperpigmentation.

22 *Metabolic abnormalities seen in adrenal insufficiency include:*

a hypokalemia.
b hyponatremia.
c hyperglycemia.
d alkalosis.

23 *A 40-year-old man with diabetes insipidus (DI) presents to the emergency department. DI is characterized by:*

a small volumes of dilute urine.
b urinary osmolarity less than 250 mOsm/kg.
c a low serum osmolarity.
d hyperkalemia.

24 *A female patient with type 2 diabetes is scheduled for a cardiac catheterization within the next 7 days. Her medication regime includes metformin (Glucophage) 500 mg TID. What instructions would you give her regarding her medication?*

a Continue the medication; do not stop it.
b Stop the medication 7 days before the catheterization.
c Do not take the medication on the morning of the catheterization only.
d Stop the medication 3 days before catheterization.

25 *A 50-year-old female with type 2 diabetes is currently on insulin therapy. She is taking 35 U of neu-*

tral protamine Hagedorn (NPH) insulin with 4 U of regular insulin in the morning. She brings you a listing of her self–blood glucose monitoring readings to the office (shown in the following table). She is following an 1800-calorie diabetic diet, and she has no somatic complaints. What would you do?

Table for Question 25

Day	Fasting	Before Lunch	Before Dinner	Bedtime
1	180	240	250	180
2	165	190	230	170
3	200	220	260	180

a Leave insulin the same.
b Increase the morning regular insulin.
c Increase the morning regular and NPH insulin.
d Consider adding an oral agent.

26 *The cornerstone of therapy for all patients with type 2 diabetes who are obese is:*

a administration of insulin therapy.
b weight reduction.
c a combination of oral agents and insulin.
d administration of an oral agent.

27 *A patient with diabetes who is also hypertensive should be on which classification of medications?*

a Beta blockers
b Angiotensin-converting enzyme (ACE) inhibitors
c Calcium channel blockers
d Thiazide diuretics

28 *Hemoglobin A_{1C} (HbA_{1C}):*

a allows assessment of glucose control for the past week.
b should be used in lieu of glucose monitoring in patients with type 1 diabetes.
c allows assessment of glucose control over a 2- to 3-month period.
d levels less than 8% suggest a glucose level in the excess of 300 mg/dL.

29 *All of the following may lead to worsening hyperglycemia during insulin therapy* **EXCEPT:**

a occult infection.
b insulin resistance.
c Somogyi's phenomenon.
d decreased caloric intake.

30 *The Somogyi phenomenon observed in patients with diabetes is:*

a characterized by nocturnal hypoglycemia.
b characterized by nocturnal hyperglycemia.
c treated by gradually increasing the insulin.
d treated by adding an oral agent.

31 *The most common cause of hypothyroidism in the adult is:*

a trauma.
b an alteration in prolactin.
c thyroid surgery.
d primary hypothyroidism.

32 *The most important laboratory test to assess the hypothalamic-pituitary-thyroid (HPT) axis is the:*

a serum T_4 level.
b TSH level.
c T_3 resin uptake(T_3RU).
d thyroid hormone index.

33 *The treatment of choice for hypothyroidism is:*

a a beta blocker.
b levothyroxine.
c radioactive iodine.
d surgery.

34 *A 45-year-old woman is diagnosed with Graves' disease. What is the most common treatment?*

a Radioactive iodine (I131)
b Propylthiouracil (PTU)
c Surgery
d None of the above

35 *Risk factors for the development of osteoporosis include:*

a a poor dietary calcium intake.
b smoking.
c immobilization.
d all of the above.

36 *A 25-year-old woman has anorexia nervosa. You explain to her that she is at risk of death because of:*

a ventricular arrhythmias.
b renal failure.
c respiratory failure.
d hypercalcemia.

37 *The most common cardiac manifestation of Graves' disease is:*

a bradycardia.
b tachycardia.
c atrial flutter.
d a diastolic murmur.

38 *A young married couple comes to see you about their inability to conceive. What is the initial plan of care?*

a Order a pelvic ultrasound for the woman.
b Obtain a semen specimen from the man.
c Instruct the woman to check daily body temperatures.
d Obtain a detailed health history from both.

39 *A 28-year-old woman has had four miscarriages, and you suspect luteal phase defects. What is the standard test for diagnosing luteal phase defects?*

a Thyroid function test
b Laparoscopy
c Prolactin levels
d Endometrial biopsy

40 *Causes of menstrual abnormalities include:*

a thyroid disease.
b ovarian failure.
c pregnancy.
d all of the above.

41 *Which test may be used to screen for pituitary adenoma?*

a TSH
b Prolactin
c CT scan
d Follicle-stimulating hormone (FSH)

42 *A 40-year-old woman complains of abdominal bloating, and amenorrhea for the past 2 months. What diagnostic test would you order to rule out pregnancy?*

a Prolactin level
b Beta chorionic gonadotropin
c Abdominal ultrasound
d Thyroid function test

43 *A 50-year-old woman with history of type 1 diabetes mellitus is brought to the emergency department. Her family members tell you that she has had fever, chills, cough with production of yellow sputum, and nausea and vomiting for the past 4 days. She has not been able to eat for the past 2 days and therefore has not taken her insulin for the past 2 days. The patient is lethargic, but arousable, pulse 120, respiratory rate 32, and blood pressure of 100/60. Her past medical history is significant for hypertension, hyperlipidemia, and diabetes since age 30. Laboratory data are sodium 150, potassium 5.0, chloride 110, and bicarbonate 15. What is the patient's acid-base status?*

a Normal
b Metabolic acidosis
c Respiratory acidosis
d Metabolic alkalosis

44 *Signs and symptoms of vitamin A intoxication include:*

a anemia.
b hepatomegaly.
c coarse hair.
d all of the above.

45 *A 30-year-old man is found to have bilateral gynecomastia, small testes, infertility, and deficient secondary sex features. What is the most likely diagnosis?*

a Klinefelter's syndrome
b Breast carcinoma
c Hepatic cirrhosis
d Testicular tumor

46 *Which laboratory test(s) should be done if you suspect Klinefelter's syndrome?*

a LH and FSH
b TSH
c Prolactin level
d All of the above

47 *A 50-year-old woman presents with complaints of polydipsia and polyuria. The differential diagnosis for this patient may include:*

a diabetes mellitus.
b diabetes insipidus.
c diuretic use.
d all of the above.

48 *In diabetes insipidus (DI), urine osmolarity is:*

a normal.
b decreased.
c slightly increased.
d markedly increased.

49 *Treatment of a patient with central DI includes:*

a dopamine.
b epinephrine.
c desmovasopressin (DDAVP).
d Nonsteroidal anti-inflammatory drugs (NSAIDs).

50 *Conditions that may cause nephrogenic DI include:*

a Hypercalcemia
b Hyperkalemia
c Pituitary surgery
d All of the above

51 *The most common cause of erectile dysfunction is:*

a peripheral vascular disease.
b diabetes mellitus.
c hypothyroidism.
d bladder dysfunction.

52 *A 45-year-old woman is scheduled for a hysterectomy and has been taking steroids for the past 5 years* *for Cushing's disease. What should be done preoperatively?*

a   Give hydrocortisone 100 mg intravenously while waiting to go to the operating room.
b   Hold steroids until after surgery.
c   Hold steroids for 2 days before surgery.
d   Hold the steroids for 1 week before surgery.

53   *Criteria for diagnosing primary aldosteronism include:*

a   diastolic hypertension.
b   low renin levels.
c   hypersecretion of aldosterone which is not suppressed during volume loading.
d   all of the above.

54   *Primary aldosteronism due to an adenoma is best treated by:*

a   surgical excision.
b   salt restriction.
c   administration of spironolactone (Aldactone).
d   all of the above.

55   *Adrenocorticotrophic hormone (ACTH) stimulation testing is used to diagnose:*

a   thyroid disease.
b   Addison's disease.
c   pituitary tumor.
d   all of the above.

56   *The diagnosis of pheochromocytoma is confirmed by:*

a   the presence of hypertension.
b   a 24-hour urine collection for catecholamine metabolites.
c   an elevation in creatinine levels.
d   the presence of hypocalcemia.

57   *Stein-Leventhal syndrome is characterized by:*

a   polycystic ovary disease.
b   insulin resistance.
c   obesity.
d   all of the above.

58   *A 65-year-old man presents with hypocalcemia. You tap on the front of the patient's ear at the angle of the jaw and the patient's lateral facial muscles contract. What is this sign?*

a   Chvostek's sign.
b   Trousseau's sign.
c   Mueller's sign.
d   None of the above.

59   *A 50-year-old woman presents with an acute attack of gout. What is the most commonly used treatment?*

a   Prednisone
b   NSAIDs
c   Probenecid
d   Colchicine

60   *Which of the following medications may lead to hyperuricemia?*

a   Furosemide (Lasix)
b   Aspirin
c   Ethanol
d   All of the above

61   *A common symptom associated with enlargement of the sella turcica is:*

a   nausea.
b   headache.
c   blindness.
d   weight loss.

62   *The most common cause of pituitary infarction is:*

a   radiation.
b   pituitary adenoma.
c   postpartum necrosis.
d   meningioma.

63   *Clinical features of diabetes insipidus (DI) include polyuria, excessive thirst, and:*

a   nausea.
b   weight loss.
c   polydipsia.
d   muscle atrophy.

64   *The treatment of choice in patients with diabetes insipidus (DI) is:*

a   dopamine.
b   DDAVP
c   Insulin
d   Prednisone

65   *The cause(s) of the syndrome of inappropriate antidiuretic hormone secretion (SIADH) include:*

a   pneumonia.
b   lung carcinoma.
c   skull fractures.
d   all of the above.

66   *A 35-year-old woman presents with complaints of easy fatigability, weight gain around the abdomen, no menstrual period for the past 3 months, and easy bruisability. A serum pregnancy test result is negative. Vital signs reveal pulse 84 and blood pressure 160/100. What disease should be considered in your differential diagnosis?*

a   Pregnancy (because the serum test result may be a false-negative).
b   Cushing's syndrome.

c Hypothyroidism.
d Pheochromocytoma.

67 *The treatment of choice for patients with familial combined hyperlipidemia is:*

a gemfibrozil (Lopid).
b lovastatin (Mevacor).
c fish oils.
d nicotinic acid.

68 *In the patient taking spironolactone (Aldactone), which of the following electrolytes should be closely monitored?*

a Sodium
b Potassium
c Chloride
d Calcium

69 *The cardinal symptom of Addison's disease is:*

a asthenia.
b anorexia.
c weight loss.
d diarrhea.

70 *Initial treatment of adrenal crisis includes:*

a An infusion of 5% dextrose in water (D5W) followed by 100 mg of cortisol.
b 1 g solumedrol.
c an epinephrine infusion.
d an infusion of dobutamine.

71 *The principal electrolyte abnormality in primary aldosteronism is:*

a hypomagnesemia.
b hyperkalemia.
c hyponatremia.
d hypokalemia.

72 *What is one of the primary interventions for the patient with diabetic ketoacidosis?*

a Insulin administration
b Potassium administration
c Sodium bicarbonate administration
d Normal saline infusions

73 *Which of the following medications may lead to development of glucose intolerance and diabetes?*

a Prednisone
b Ibuprofen (Motrin)
c Metoprolol (Lopressor)
d Digoxin (Lanoxin)

74 *You suspect a 50-year-old woman with type 1 diabetes may be experiencing the dawn phenomenon. What do you do to confirm your suspicion?*

a Check her glucose level before bedtime.
b Check her glucose level before breakfast.
c Check her glucose level at dinner time.
d Check her glucose level at 3:00 AM.

75 *Treatment of the dawn phenomenon would include:*

a decreasing the evening dose of insulin.
b increasing the evening dose of insulin.
c increasing the morning dose of insulin.
d decreasing the morning dose of insulin.

76 *Long-term complications of diabetes mellitus include:*

a retinopathy.
b neuropathy.
c diabetic nephropathy.
d all of the above.

77 *Obesity is defined as:*

a a body mass index more than 20% above ideal body weight.
b a body mass index more than 40% above ideal body weight.
c a body mass index more than 50% above ideal body weight.
d none of the above.

78 *A 65-year-old woman presents with complaints of a swollen, painful right great toe, which awakened her from sleep. She denies any previous episodes. Her past medical history includes hypertension and she is taking verapamil, bumetanide (Bumex), and atenolol. On examination, she has a temperature of 100°F, pulse 60, blood pressure 140/90. Erythema and swelling of the right great toe are found with tenderness extending to the ankle. What is the most likely diagnosis?*

a Osteomyelitis
b Acute gout
c Cellulitis
d Osteoarthritis

79 *Patients with asymptomatic hyperuricemia are best treated with:*

a colchicines.
b allopurinol (Zyloprim).
c indomethacin (Indocin).
d none of the above.

80 *Diagnosis of acute gout may be made by:*

a a serum uric acid level.

b synovial fluid analysis.
c a 24-hour urine analysis.
d all of the above.

81 *Risk factors for development of osteoporosis include:*

a cigarette smoking.
b a low skeletal mass.
c postmenopausal state.
d all of the above.

82 *The most common cause of abnormal uterine bleeding in patients greater than 40 years of age is:*

a diabetes mellitus.
b hypothyroidism.
c uterine cancer.
d anovulation.

83 *Medications that may cause osteoporosis include:*

a thyroid hormone.
b steroids.
c heparin.
d all of the above.

84 *The most frequent cause of chronic hypocalcemia is:*

a hypoalbuminemia.
b diarrhea.
c acidosis.
d anorexia.

85 *Which of the following is most important in the development of atherosclerosis?*

a High-density lipoprotein (HDL)
b Very low density lipoprotein (VLDL)
c Triglycerides
d Low-density lipoprotein (LDL)

Answers

1   Answer d
Type 1 diabetes mellitus generally manifests in childhood and early adulthood. It is not more common than type 2 diabetes and is not associated with gestational diabetes.

2   Answer b
The most common complication of diabetes is retinopathy. The presence of retinopathy increases with the duration of diabetes.

3   Answer a
The most prevalent risk factor for type 2 diabetes is obesity. It has been estimated that 80% of adults with diabetes are obese. Obesity decreases the concentration of insulin receptors in the tissue. Steroids and renal failure may cause impairment of glucose tolerance.

4   Answer a
The major risk factor that has been linked to the development of thyroid cancer is previous irradiation of the head and neck.

5   Answer d
Symptoms of hypothyroidism include lethargy, menorrhagia, and weight gain.

6   Answer a
Graves' disease is not associated with hypothyroidism. Patients with Graves' disease are hyperthyroid and have diffuse toxic goiter, exophthalmos, and pretibial myxedema.

7   Answer d
The two most common causes of hypercalcemia are malignancy and hyperparathyroidism.

8   Answer d
Hypercalcemic emergency is best treated with an intravenous fluid of normal saline solution alternating with D5W. The correction of hypercalcemia may require consumption of 10 to 15 L of fluid. After the calcium level decreases, long-term therapy may consist of oral phosphates and the use of glucocorticoids. Calcitonin may be used singularly or in combination with glucocorticoids for emergent treatment of hypercalcemia.

9   Answer a
Medically significant hypoglycemia is diagnosed on the basis of a blood glucose level less than 50 mg/dL, symptoms consistent with hypoglycemia, and resolution of symptoms after ingestion of carbohydrates. Symptoms of incoordination, headache, blurred vision, anxiety, flushing, coma, pallor, confusion, and weakness may all indicate hypoglycemia but are not diagnostic.

10   Answer a
Neuroendocrine tumors that may be associated with hypoglycemia include carcinoid tumor, pheochromocytoma, and neurofibroma. Myeloma is not a neuroendocrine tumor; it is a hematologic tumor.

11   Answer d
The most likely diagnosis for the patient described is acromegaly. Acromegaly is a clinical prodrome that results from excessive growth hormone production and may be secondary to a pituitary tumor. The symptoms may consist of headache, visual disturbances, muscle aches, decreased libido, excessive sweating, coarse skin, and widely spaced teeth with an underbite.

12   Answer d
The best screening test for the diagnosis of acromegaly is the measurement of the somatomedin C level. This is a liver protein and assesses the action of the growth hormone. Prolactin level is used to measure pituitary function; LH and testosterone levels are used to assess the reproductive axis of the pituitary.

13   Answer b
The preferred diagnostic imaging tool for assessing the pituitary is the MRI scan, because it can define the landmarks and tumor involvement. This information is useful for surgical resection. The CT scan may detect larger masses but is less sensitive for smaller masses. The skull radiograph is of no use.

14   Answer c
Multinodular goiter is associated with older persons and is usually not associated with thyroid bruit or pregnancy.

15   Answer c

The most likely diagnosis for the patient described is Graves' disease. The patient's clinical history and physical exam are most consistent with hyperthyroidism secondary to Graves' disease. The family history of thyroid disease suggests an autoimmune pattern. In multinodular goiter and subacute thyroiditis, a bruit over the thyroid is not heard. Multinodular goiter does not have a symmetrically enlarged gland, but rather a nodular pattern. Subacute thyroiditis usually produces a painful thyroid gland and usually associated with a recent viral illness. The patient could be suffering from postpartum depression, but it would not produce the physical exam findings of hyperreflexia, enlarged thyroid gland, and proximal muscle weakness.

16   Answer d

Silent thyroiditis is an autoimmune process that can occur after pregnancy in approximately 5% of the population and it is manifested by an enlarged thyroid gland.

17   Answer c

In hyperthyroidism, total T_4 and T_3 levels are increased and the TSH level is suppressed.

18   Answer b

The diagnostic tool that should be used to distinguish silent thyroiditis from Graves' disease is the radioactive iodine uptake test. In Graves' disease, there is an overproduction of thyroid hormone and resultant excessive uptake of iodine into the gland. In silent thyroiditis, there is excessive release of thyroid hormone into systemic circulation suppressing thyroid stimulating hormone, caused by damage to thyroid follicular cells. The radioactive uptake in silent thyroiditis is very low.

19   Answer d

Causes of an elevated prolactin level may include a pituitary tumor, frequent breast stimulation, hypothyroidism, chronic renal failure, liver failure, and many medications including amphetamines, tricyclics, opiates, and methyldopa.

20   Answer a

A female with an elevated prolactin level may exhibit amenorrhea. The patient may experience hirsutism rather than hair loss and may have no change in weight.

21   Answer b

The most common manifestation of Cushing's syndrome is obesity. Other features may include proximal weakness, hyperpigmentation with easy bruisability, and diastolic hypertension.

22   Answer b

Metabolic abnormalities seen in adrenal insufficiency include hyponatremia secondary to renal tubular loss of sodium ions. In adrenal insufficiency, there is decrease in cortisol, which helps to regulate intracellular and extracellular potassium and sodium. Patients with adrenal insufficiency will be hyperkalemic, hypoglycemic, and may have acidosis.

23   Answer b

DI is characterized by urinary osmolarity less than 250 mOsm/kg. The patient urinates large quantities of dilute urine and will have an elevated serum osmolarity. With the increased urination, it is possible that hypokalemia, rather than hyperkalemia, will ensue.

24   Answer d

For the patient described, you should instruct the patient to stop the medication at least 3 days before the catheterization. The use of metformin (Glucophage) and the contrast dye from the catheterization may put the patient at risk for acute renal failure.

25   Answer c

The treatment for the elevated blood glucose levels for the patient described would be to increase the morning regular insulin dosage in hopes of decreasing the before-lunch blood glucose level, and to increase the morning NPH insulin dosage in hopes of decreasing the before-dinner blood glucose level. Some consideration may be given to adding a before-dinner insulin regime.

26   Answer b

The cornerstone of therapy for all patients with type 2 diabetes who are obese is weight reduction; the intention is to reduce the patient's requirements for insulin.

27   Answer b

A patient with diabetes who is also hypertensive should be on an ACE inhibitor to reduce proteinuria and the resultant diabetic nephropathy. Beta blockers may mask the signs and symptoms of hypoglycemia. Thiazide diuretics may worsen glucose tolerance. Calcium channel blockers may lead to a decrease in cardiac output, which may worsen renal function in the patient.

28   Answer c

Hemoglobin A_{1C} (HbA$_{1C}$) allows for assessment of glucose control over a 2- to 3-month period. This test can be used in lieu of glucose monitoring in the patient with type 2 diabetes. A value less than 8% suggests a glucose level less than 200 mg/dL.

29   Answer d

Occult infection, insulin resistance, and the Somogyi phenomenon may all lead to worsening hyperglycemia during insulin therapy; a decreased caloric intake will not. An increased caloric intake may lead to worsening diabetic control.

30   Answer a

The Somogyi phenomenon observed in patients with diabetes is characterized by nocturnal hypoglycemia and often goes undetected. Some of the symptoms associated with the phenomenon are night sweats; poor sleep patterns, and morning headache. It is treated by gradually decreasing the insulin dosage.

31   Answer d

The most common cause of hypothyroidism in the adult patient is primary hypothyroidism. It occurs most often between the ages of 40 to 65 years and is most common in women.

32   Answer b

The most important test to assess the HPT axis is the TSH level. Most diseases of the thyroid gland are caused by the gland itself rather than the pituitary or hypothalamus. In the development of thyroid disease, TSH is the first value to become abnormal.

33   Answer b

The treatment of choice for hypothyroidism is levothyroxine. Radioactive iodine, a beta blocker, and surgery may be used to treat hyperthyroidism.

34   Answer a

The most common treatment for Graves' disease is radioactive iodine. It is a highly effective form of treatment and usually is only given in a single dose, but may take up to 2 months to work.

35 Answer d

Risk factors for the development of osteoporosis are poor dietary calcium intake, especially early in life; smoking; and immobilization. Other factors associated with osteoporosis are a positive family history, malnutrition, caffeine intake, use of steroids, high phosphate intake, and alcohol intake.

36 Answer a

Patients with anorexia nervosa are at risk for death due to ventricular arrhythmias. The arrhythmias are usually secondary to electrolyte abnormalities such as hypomagnesemia, hypokalemia, and hypocalcemia. Patients may also suffer congestive heart failure, which may lead to arrhythmias.

37 Answer b

The most common cardiac manifestation of Graves' disease is tachycardia.

38 Answer d

The initial plan of care for a couple unable to conceive is to obtain a thorough medical history of both persons, including a sexual history. After a thorough history, obtaining a semen specimen from the male would be the next step in the evaluation.

39 Answer d

The standard test for diagnosing luteal phase defects is endometrial biopsy.

40 Answer d

Causes of menstrual abnormalities include thyroid disease, ovarian failure, pituitary tumors, and pregnancy.

41 Answer b

The test that may be used to screen for pituitary adenoma is prolactin.

42 Answer b

The diagnostic test to rule out pregnancy in this patient is beta chorionic gonadotropin.

43 Answer b

The patient described has metabolic acidosis. The patient also has diabetes with poorly controlled glucose secondary to illness and is dehydrated.

44 Answer d

Signs and symptoms of vitamin A intoxication include anemia, hepatomegaly, coarse hair, splenomegaly, leukopenia, sparse hair, and hyperlipidemia.

45 Answer a

The most likely diagnosis for this patient is Klinefelter's syndrome. Klinefelter's syndrome usually presents with gynecomastia, which occurs in puberty, small and firm testes, infertility and deficient secondary sex characteristics. Breast carcinoma usually presents with unilateral gynecomastia. Hepatic cirrhosis may present with loss of sexual libido, bilateral gynecomastia, and testicular atrophy. Testicular tumor would not produce the lack of secondary sex features but might cause atrophy of the testes.

46 Answer a

The laboratory tests that should be done if you suspect Klinefelter's syndrome are monitoring levels of LH and FSH. These levels would be elevated in Klinefelter's syndrome.

47 Answer d

The differential diagnosis in a patient with polydipsia and polyuria includes diabetes mellitus, DI, and side effects of diuretic use.

48 Answer b

In DI, urine osmolarity is decreased. The patient usually urinates in excess of 3 L/d diluted urine.

49 Answer c

Treatment of patients with central DI includes the use of DDAVP. NSAIDs may be helpful in patients with nephrogenic DI because they inhibit renal prostaglandins and reduce water delivery to the distal tubules.

50 Answer a

Conditions that may cause nephrogenic DI include hypercalcemia. Hypercalcemia may cause damage to the renal tubule and hence cause difficulty with concentration of urine. The antidiuretic hormone is usually normal, but there is impaired renal tubular concentration. Hypokalemia may cause nephrogenic DI. Pituitary surgery may cause central DI.

51 Answer b

The most common cause of erectile dysfunction is diabetes mellitus.

52 Answer a

The steroids should be given intravenously on call to the operating room for a patient on chronic steroid therapy. The stress of surgery may cause addisonian crisis:

53 Answer d

Criteria for diagnosing primary aldosteronism include diastolic hypertension, circulating low renal levels, and hyposecretion of aldosterone, which is not suppressed during volume loading.

54 Answer a

Primary aldosteronism secondary to an adenoma is best treated by surgical excision. Dietary restriction of salt and administration of spironolactone (Aldactone), which is an aldosterone antagonist, may also be used.

55 Answer b

ACTH stimulation testing is used to diagnose Addison's disease.

56 Answer b

Diagnosis of pheochromocytoma is confirmed by a 24-hour urine for catecholamine metabolites (vanillylmandelic acid, the metanephrines, and the unconjugated catecholamines).

57 Answer d

Stein-Leventhal syndrome is characterized by polycystic ovary disease, amenorrhea, and obesity with insulin resistance. It is thought to be transmitted as an X-linked trait.

58 Answer a

Indicating hypocalcemia, Chvostek's sign occurs when you tap on the front of the patient's ear at the angle of the jaw and the patient's lateral facial muscles contract. Trousseau's sign, another sign of hypocalcemia, is demonstrated by inflating a blood pressure cuff to occlude blood supply to the arm, then deflating the cuff. If the patient is hypocalcemic, the patient's hand and fingers start to contract.

59 Answer b

The most commonly used treatment for gout is the administration of NSAIDs. The goal is to terminate the acute attack by decreasing the inflammatory response. NSAIDs have replaced colchicine as the most common treatment. Colchicine is also effective as first line treatment for acute gout. Agents such as probenecid have no anti-inflammatory properties, but may be helpful in decreasing urate levels.

60   Answer d

Medications that may lead to hyperuricemia include furosemide (Lasix), aspirin, and ethanol. Furosemide induces volume depletion and may lead to enhanced tubular reabsorption of uric acid and decreased uric acid filtration. The mechanisms through which aspirin and ethanol lead to hyperuricemia are not clearly understood.

61   Answer b

A common symptom associated with enlargement of the sella turcica of the pituitary gland is headache. Other symptoms that may be present include weight gain, visual field defects, and elevated blood pressure.

62   Answer c

The most common cause of pituitary infarction is postpartum pituitary necrosis, which may be due to hemorrhagic shock. During pregnancy, the anterior pituitary gland is enlarged and is vulnerable to infarction during excessive bleeding. Radiation, pituitary adenoma, and meningioma may lead to pituitary dysfunction but not infarction.

63   Answer c

Clinical features of DI include polyuria, excessive thirst, and polydipsia.

64   Answer b

The treatment of choice in patients with diabetes insipidus is DDAVP.

65   Answer d

Causes of SIADH may include pneumonia, lung carcinoma (particularly oat-cell carcinoma), and skull fractures.

66   Answer b

The disease that should be considered in your differential diagnosis is Cushing's syndrome. The symptoms of truncal obesity, fatigue, bruising, amenorrhea, and hypertension suggest Cushing's syndrome. The serum pregnancy test result is negative, so pregnancy is unlikely. The fatigue and weight gain may be associated with hypothyroidism. Pheochromocytoma is unlikely, but the patient is hypertensive, however has no vasomotor symptoms.

67   Answer d

The treatment of choice for patients with familial combined hyperlipidemia is nicotinic acid. Nicotinic acid lowers VLDL apo-B synthesis.

68   Answer b

Potassium should be closely monitored in the patient taking spironolactone (Aldactone). Spironolactone is a potassium-sparing diuretic.

69   Answer a

The cardinal symptom of Addison's disease is asthenia. The weakness associated with Addison's disease is slowly progressive and debilitating. Other symptoms that may occur include anorexia, weight loss, nausea and vomiting, abdominal pain, salt craving, and syncope.

70   Answer a

The initial treatment of adrenal crisis is directed at repletion of sodium and water deficits and increasing circulating glucocorticoids, so the initial treatment would be an infusion of D5W and the administration of cortisol.

71   Answer d

The principal electrolyte abnormality in primary aldosteronism is hypokalemia.

72   Answer a

The patient with diabetic ketoacidosis (DKA) is hyperglycemic and needs glucose control. Decreasing the glucose level will correct the acidosis. In a patient with DKA, repletion of potassium and volume is important in the management of the condition, but it will not correct the acidosis. Administration of sodium bicarbonate is controversial.

73   Answer a

Prednisone may lead to the development of glucose intolerance and diabetes.

74   Answer d

To confirm your suspicion of the dawn phenomenon, you should check the 3:00 AM glucose level.

75   Answer b

The dawn phenomenon is thought to result from the waning of insulin action in the early morning hours and mediated by nocturnal output of growth hormone. It is best treated by increasing the evening dose of insulin to prevent early morning hypoglycemia.

76   Answer d

Long-term complications of diabetes mellitus include retinopathy, neuropathy, diabetic nephropathy, and atherosclerosis.

77   Answer a

Obesity is defined as body mass index greater than 20% above ideal body weight.

78   Answer b

The most likely diagnosis is acute gout. The patient has acute inflammation and pain in one joint. The most commonly affected joint in gout is the first metatarsophalangeal joint.

79   Answer d

Patients with asymptomatic hyperuricemia are best not treated unless the patient has a history of uric acid stones or gouty attacks.

80   Answer b

Diagnosis of acute gout may be made by microscopically identifying crystals from synovial joint fluid. The serum uric acid level may be elevated, but is not specific for an acute gout attack. A 24-hour analysis of the urine may be helpful in evaluating hyperuricemia.

81   Answer d

Risk factors for the development of osteoporosis includes cigarette smoking, alcohol intake, sedentary lifestyle, a low skeletal mass, white race, and postmenopausal state.

82   Answer d

The most common cause of abnormal uterine bleeding in patients older than 40 years of age is anovulation. Dysfunctional uterine bleeding may be associated with endocrine disorders such as diabetes and thyroid disorders. Uterine cancer is a cause of uterine bleeding but not the most common.

83 Answer d

Medications that may cause osteoporosis include thyroid hormone, steroid use, heparin (prolonged use), phenobarbital, and phenytoin (Dilantin).

84 Answer a

The most common cause of chronic hypocalcemia is hypoalbuminemia.

85 Answer d

LDL is most important in the development of atherosclerosis.

Bibliography

American Diabetes Association: Management of dyslipidemia in adults with diabetes. Diabetes Care 22:S56–S59, 1999.

American Diabetes Association: Standards of medical care for patients with diabetes mellitus. Diabetes Care 21:S23–S31, 1998.

Elliott B: Diagnosing and treating hypothyroidism. Nurse Practitioner. 25:92–105, 2000.

Gomberg-Maitland M: Thyroid hormone and cardiovascular disease. Am Heart J 1998;135:187–196.

Goroll, A, et al: Primary Care Medicine Office Evaluation and Management of the Adult Patient, 4th ed. Lippincott Williams & Wilkins, Philadelphia, 2000.

Gutowski C: Understanding new pharmacologic therapy for type 2 diabetes. Nurse Practitioner, 1999.

Warren-Boulton E. An update on primary care management of type 2 diabetes. Nurse Practitioner 34:12, 14–33, 1999.

6

Neurologic Problems

1 *A 50-year-old woman presents to the emergency department with complaints of acute onset of left sided facial pain, inability to close her left eye, increasing tearing of the left eye, and left ear pain that developed over the past 12 hours. She denies any other health problems and is currently taking no medications. What is the most likely diagnosis?*

a   Meningitis
b   Bell's palsy
c   Temporal arteritis
d   Multiple sclerosis

2 *Bell's palsy is a result of damage to cranial nerve:*

a   V.
b   III.
c   II.
d   VII.

3 *Common symptoms of temporal arteritis include:*

a   headache.
b   scalp tenderness.
c   jaw claudication.
d   all of the above.

4 *The most feared complication of temporal arteritis is:*

a   facial paralysis.
b   blindness.
c   diplopia.
d   chronic headache.

5 *The first symptom of cervical radiculopathy is:*

a   headache.
b   visual disturbances.
c   arm pain.
d   syncope.

Questions 6–7 refer to the following scenario:

A 25-year-old woman presents with complaints of severe headache, nausea and vomiting, and neck pain for the past 2 days. She has no other health history and denies alcohol and drug use. Physical exam reveals a woman who appears ill: temperature 101°F, pulse 120, blood pressure 100/60.

6 *What is your next step in the care of this patient?*

a   Obtain a further history.
b   Obtain a neurology consult.
c   Order a head computed tomography (CT) scan.
d   Plan for a lumbar puncture.

7 *What is the most likely diagnosis of the patient?*

a   Cluster headache
b   Meningitis
c   Brain abscess
d   Brain tumor

8 *Carpal tunnel syndrome is characterized by all of the following symptoms* **EXCEPT:**

a   arm pain.
b   arm paresthesias.
c   arm numbness.
d   back pain.

9 *A patient with carpal tunnel syndrome has a positive Tinel's sign. What is Tinel's sign?*

a   Pain in the elbow with extension
b   Pain produced by tapping on the wrist, or anywhere along the median nerve
c   Pain in the shoulder with hand grasp
d   Absent ulnar pulse on the affected side

10 *The most common site of ulnar entrapment is:*

a   the shoulder.

b the wrist.
c the elbow.
d none of the above.

11 *A 55-year-old man presents with complaints of fever to 101°F for the past week, with rhinorrhea, chest congestion, cough, and fatigue. He also complains of decreased appetite with nausea and vomiting for the past 3 days. Today, he noted progressive symmetrical weakness in his lower extremities. Physical exam revealed ill-appearing male with temperature 100°F, pulse 120, respiratory rate 16, and blood pressure 100/60. Heart and lung exam results were normal. Neck exam revealed shotty anterior cervical adenopathy. Neurologically, the patient had decreased upper arm reflexes. What is the most likely diagnosis?*

a Multiple sclerosis
b Guillain-Barré syndrome
c Cerebrovascular accident (CVA)
d Peripheral neuropathy

12 *The most common demyelinating disease of the central nervous system is:*

a multiple sclerosis.
b myasthenia gravis.
c dementia.
d Parkinson's disease.

13 *A 60-year-old man presents with tremor. What historical question may help to classify the tremor?*

a Does it awaken you at night?
b Does it happen on only one side of the body or both sides?
c Does it cause your body to shake?
d None of the above.

14 *Medications that may be associated with tremors include all of the following* **EXCEPT:**

a lithium.
b theophylline.
c beta-adrenergic agents.
d digoxin (Lanoxin).

15 *Tremors associated with a specific task is best treated with:*

a lorazepam (Ativan).
b propranolol (Inderal).
c alprazolam (Xanax).
d botulinum toxin.

16 *A 40-year-old woman presents to the emergency department with complaints of diplopia, inability to raise her eyelid, blurred vision, dysphagia, and dysarthria over the past 12 hours. She has no previous health history. Physical exam reveals temperature 98°F, pulse 60, respiratory rate 18, and blood pressure*

120/70. Neurologic exam reveals bilateral lid lag, decreased visual fields, dilated pupils reactive to light, and bilateral lower extremity weakness. What is the most likely diagnosis?

a Botulism
b Guillain-Barré syndrome
c Myasthenia gravis
d CVA

17 *One of your patients is a 55-year-old woman who had a colon resection for colon carcinoma. On postoperative day #3, you are notified that the patient has left facial droop and is unable to move her left arm and leg. Vital signs reveal pulse 88, respiratory rate 20, and blood pressure 160/100. Her past medical history is significant for hypertension, obesity, and hypothyroidism. Current medications include levothyroxine sodium (Synthroid), metoprolol tartrate (Lopressor), enaprilat (Vasotec), and heparin 5000 U every 12 hours subcutaneously. Head CT scan revealed an acute stroke, and the neuroradiologist wants to administer thrombolytic therapy. What in this patient's history would be a contraindication to thrombolytics?*

a Obesity
b Recent colon resection
c Hypertension
d Heparin administration

18 *Treatment of migraine headaches may include:*

a nonsteroidal anti-inflammatory drugs (NSAIDs).
b beta blockers.
c tricyclic antidepressants.
d all of the above.

19 *All of the following statements are true about common migraine headache* **EXCEPT:**

a it is more common in young women.
b it may be associated with nausea and vomiting.
c the headache may last for hours and be relieved by sleep.
d it has unilateral orbital pain lasting from 30 to 90 minutes.

20 *A 75-year-old man is suspected of having dementia. Which laboratory test(s) should be ordered as part of his evaluation?*

a Head CT scan
b Thyroid function test
c Vitamin B12 levels
d All of the above

21 *The primary cause of nontraumatic dementia is:*

a Parkinson's disease.
b alcoholic dementia.
c Alzheimer's disease.
d seizure disorder.

22 *All of the following statements are true about tension headache* **EXCEPT:**

a   it is more common in women.
b   it is usually triggered by fatigue.
c   it has steady aching in the occipital and upper neck region.
d   it is associated with photophobia.

23 *A medication that may be used to treat migraine headaches which may be given subcutaneously as well as nasally is:*

a   sumatriptan (Imitrex).
b   naproxen (Naprosyn).
c   dihydroergotamine (D.H.E. 45).
d   prednisone.

24 *A 50-year-old woman presents with severe headache with abrupt onset over the past 2 hours. She describes it as the worst headache ever. Her past medical history is significant for hypertension for the past 2 years, treated with enalaprilat (Vasotec). No other health history was significant. Physical exam inclusive of neurologic, cardiac, and lung exam is normal. Vital signs were pulse 76, respiratory rate 16, and blood pressure 150/90. What is the most likely diagnosis?*

a   Meningitis
b   Trigeminal neuralgia
c   Migraine headache
d   Subarachnoid hemorrhage

25 *Which segmental level of the spine is tested with the biceps reflex?*

a   Cervical 7, 8
b   Lumbar 3, 4
c   Cervical 5, 6
d   Lumbar 2, 3, 4

26 *Which cranial nerve controls hearing and balance?*

a   VII
b   VIII
c   IX
d   None of the above

27 *A patient with unilateral loss of smell without history of nasal disease suggests:*

a   papilledema.
b   drug use.
c   tonsillar abscess.
d   frontal lobe lesion.

28 *Causes of ataxia include:*

a   cerebellar disease.
b   loss of position sense.

c   intoxication.
d   all of the above.

29 *A 50-year-old man who had kidney transplantation is taking prednisone; neural physical examination reveals symmetrical weakness of proximal leg muscles. What do these findings suggest?*

a   Polyneuropathy
b   Myopathy
c   Bursitis
d   Cranial nerve XI damage

30 *A disease process that may cause loss of vibratory sense is:*

a   diabetes.
b   hypertension.
c   gout.
d   hypothyroidism.

31 *Classic symptoms of Parkinson's disease include tremor at rest, bradydyskinesia, and:*

a   lower extremity weakness.
b   shuffling gait.
c   visual loss.
d   personality change.

32 *The treatment of choice for patients diagnosed with trigeminal neuralgia is:*

a   carbamazepine (Tegretol).
b   phenytoin (Dilantin).
c   carbidopa (Sinemet).
d   levodopa.

33 *A 40-year-old woman is suspected of having myasthenia gravis. What diagnostic test should be performed to support your diagnosis?*

a   CT scan.
b   Magnetic resonance imaging (MRI) of the head.
c   Electroencephalogram (EEG).
d   Tensilon test.

34 *Treatment options for patients with myasthenia gravis include:*

a   pyridostigmine (Mestinon).
b   azathioprine (Imuran).
c   prednisone.
d   all of the above.

35 *A 25-year-old woman is admitted to the intensive care unit with complaints of diarrhea, abdominal pain, temperature to 102°F, periorbital edema, myalgias, and general malaise. She has no previous health history, is taking no medications, and has no history of alcohol or drug use. She attended a picnic 24 hours before and had* *eaten a roast ham sandwich and ribs, which she stated were medium rare. What is the most likely diagnosis?*

a Meningitis.
b Myotonic dystrophy.
c Polymyositis.
d Trichinosis.

36 *A disease associated with thiamine deficiency, malnutrition, and alcoholism is:*

a amnesia.
b Korsakoff's disease.
c Parkinson's disease.
d simple partial seizure.

37 *Broca's aphasia is characterized by:*

a impaired spontaneous speech.
b fluent speech.
c damage to the cerebral cortex.
d all of the above.

38 *A 30-year-old woman involved in a motor vehicle accident is brought to the emergency department. She has suspected head and neck injuries, but she is awake and oriented. She has a cervical collar in place. Cervical spine films have been ordered. What precautions should be taken?*

a Remove the cervical collar and perform the radiographs.
b Obtain radiographs of the cervical spine and have the patient flex and extend her head.
c Take the radiographs with the collar on and off.
d None of the above.

39 *A 40-year-old man is admitted with a closed head injury after a motorcycle accident. While monitoring the patient in the intensive care unit, you note that he has only voided 20 mL/hr for the past 2 hours. Laboratory data reveal a serum sodium level of 125. The clinical situation is most consistent with:*

a diabetes insipidus.
b syndrome of inappropriate antidiuretic hormone (SIADH).
c Cushing's syndrome.
d hyperparathyroidism.

40 *Absence of blinking signifies a problem with cranial nerve:*

a II.
b III.
c VII.
d V.

41 *Differential diagnosis for syncope may include:*

a anxiety.
b aortic valve disease.

c hypoglycemia.
d all of the above.

42 *A 60-year-old woman presents to the emergency department with acute onset of right-sided paralysis over the past hour. Her past medical history is significant for hypertension, and type 2 diabetes mellitus. Current medications include diltiazem (Cardizem) and glipizide (Glucotrol). Vital signs were pulse 64, respiratory rate 20, blood pressure 190/100, and afebrile. Physical exam revealed right-sided hemiplegia with a right hemianopsia with deviation of eyes to the left side. Lung exam results were normal. Cardiac exam revealed regular rate and rhythm with normal first and second heart sounds with the presence of atrial gallop. Electrolytes and complete blood count were normal. The most likely diagnosis is:*

a posterior cerebral artery stroke.
b watershed infarct.
c left middle cerebral artery stroke.
d none of the above.

43 *The most common site of intracranial vascular thrombosis is the:*

a middle cerebral artery.
b anterior cerebral artery.
c carotid artery.
d vertebral artery.

44 *The diagnostic tool of choice for a patient with an acute stroke is a(n):*

a MRI scan.
b head CT scan.
c lumbar puncture.
d EEG.

45 *The most common risk factor associated with stroke is:*

a cigarette smoking.
b migraine headaches.
c advancing age.
d hypertension.

46 *A 70-year-old woman is hospitalized for treatment of a diabetes-related foot ulcer. The staff nurse notifies you that the patient is unable to move her left arm and leg. She also has slurred speech. These symptoms lasted 5 days and then completely resolved. The most likely diagnosis is:*

a completed stroke.
b transient ischemic attack (TIA).
c reversible ischemic neurologic disability (RIND).
d all of the above.

47 *The pharmacologic treatment of choice for the prevention of TIAs is:*

a a beta blocker.
b a calcium channel blocker.
c dipyridamole (Persantine).
d aspirin.

48 *What laboratory test should be obtained to support the diagnosis of a patient with suspected temporal arteritis?*

a Complete blood count
b Erythrocyte sedimentation rate (ESR)
c Thyroid-stimulating hormone (TSH)
d Calcium level

49 *The treatment of choice for temporal arteritis is:*

a prednisone.
b indomethacin (Indocin).
c phenytoin (Dilantin).
d aspirin.

50 *A 75-year-old woman has been diagnosed with Parkinson's disease. What is the preferred treatment for patients with severe symptoms?*

a L-dopa (Levodopa)
b Metoprolol (Lopressor)
c Haloperidol (Haldol)
d Amantadine (Symmetrel)

51 *Acoustic neuroma may progress to:*

a palsy of cranial nerve VI.
b palsy of cranial nerve VIII.
c palsy of cranial nerve V.
d none of the above.

52 *Neurosyphilis is characterized by all of the following* **EXCEPT:**

a chancre.
b ataxic gait.
c memory loss.
d apathy.

53 *A 50-year-old woman is in the neurosurgical unit 1 day after undergoing a craniotomy. She develops Cushing's response. What is Cushing's response?*

a An early sign of increasing intracranial pressure (ICP)
b A sign of decreasing ICP
c A late sign of increasing ICP
d A sign associated with a good neurologic recovery

54 *A 25-year-old man is admitted after a motor vehicle accident. He has periorbital ecchymosis ("raccoon eyes"), otorrhea, and rhinorrhea. These physical findings suggest:*

a basilar skull fracture.
b acute stroke.

c subdural hematoma.
d all of the above.

55 *Dorsiflexion of the great toe with fanning of the other toes is:*

a Romberg's sign.
b Kernig's sign.
c Brudzinski's sign.
d Babinski's response.

56 *Scissors gait is associated with:*

a Parkinson's disease.
b spastic paresis of the legs.
c loss of position sense.
d hyperextension of the legs.

57 *Decerebrate rigidity is manifested by a(n):*

a abducted arms.
b extended neck.
c flexed upper arms.
d internally rotated legs.

58 *Thoracic outlet syndrome is associated with:*

a shortness of breath.
b sensory loss and weakness in the hand.
c ischemia to the shoulder and arm.
d pleural effusions.

59 *All of the following statements about simple partial seizures are true* **EXCEPT:**

a There is loss of consciousness.
b It may be treated with phenytoin (Dilantin).
c Over 50% of patients will have an abnormal EEG.
d There are focal neurologic events.

60 *A 50-year-old man found on the street is brought into the emergency department in a depressed neurologic state. He has an elevated blood alcohol level. When would you expect him to have alcohol withdrawal seizures?*

a 5 to 6 days after admission.
b 2 to 3 hours.
c 6 to 48 hours.
d 4 to 6 hours.

61 *Side effects associated with phenytoin (Dilantin) include:*

a peripheral neuropathy.
b gingival hyperplasia.
c ataxia.
d all of the above.

62 *A 60-year-old man with a 40-year history of heavy alcohol consumption is diagnosed with alcoholic* *dementia. All of the following are characteristics of alcoholic dementia* **EXCEPT:**

a ataxia.
b confusion.
c seizures.
d cognitive dysfunction.

63 *Symptoms associated with multi-infarct dementia include:*

a hand clumsiness.
b dysarthria.
c confusion.
d all of the above.

64 *Treatment options for patients with multi-infarct dementia include:*

a antiplatelet therapy.
b anticoagulation.
c reduction of risk factors.
d all of the above.

65 *A distal pattern of muscle weakness may be associated with:*

a subdural hematoma.
b muscular dystrophy.
c amyotrophic lateral sclerosis.
d polymyositis.

66 *A 50-year-old man has been diagnosed with amyotrophic lateral sclerosis (ALS). Which of the following statements concerning ALS is true?*

a It is more common in women.
b Bulbar symptoms such as hoarseness and respiratory failure may occur.
c Sphincter muscles may be affected.
d The prognosis is good.

67 *Duchenne's muscular dystrophy is:*

a more common in women.
b associated with mortality in the fifth decade of life.
c associated with absence of dystrophin in the muscle membrane.
d characterized by ataxia.

68 *Argyll-Robertson pupils are associated with:*

a neurosyphilis.
b TIAs.
c brain tumors.
d lung cancer.

69 *Ménière's disease is characterized by:*

a vertigo.
b tinnitus.

c unilateral sensation in the ears.
d all of the above.

70 *A 40-year-old man presents for annual physical exam. You perform Romberg's maneuver. What is Romberg's maneuver?*

a Having the patient discern two separate tactile stimulations.
b Having the patient hop on one leg.
c Using a tuning fork, tapping it, and placing it over a joint, then asking the patient to identify conclusion of vibration.
d Observing steadiness while the patient stands with feet together and eyes open, then closed.

71 *A 25-year-old woman is diagnosed with bacterial meningitis. She has a positive Kernig's sign. What is a positive Kernig's sign?*

a Passive flexion of the head while supine, which elicits flexion of the thighs and legs
b Straight leg raising, which produces pain in the back
c Flexion of the thigh to 90 degrees, which produces pain with leg extension
d Pain with tapping of the median nerve

72 *A 50-year-old patient on your service is suspected of having meningitis. The neurologist has planned a lumbar puncture (LP). All of the following statements are true concerning lumbar puncture* **EXCEPT:**

a it may be used to administer intrathecal antibiotics.
b it should not be performed in patients with papilledema.
c patients may develop headaches after the procedure.
d a head CT scan should be performed before all LPs.

73 *A 65-year-old man presents with 2-month history of left shoulder and upper back pain that has been unremitting. He is unable to find a comfortable position. He has received some relief with narcotics but has not been pain free for the past 2 months. He also complains of loss of appetite and a 10-pound weight loss. Past medical history include hypertension and 50-pack-per-year smoking history. Physical exam is unremarkable except for pain with range of motion of left shoulder. Sensory exam is intact. What is the most likely diagnosis?*

a Spondylosis
b Metastatic disease to the spine
c Cervical disk herniation
d Arthritis

74 *The most common symptom of vertebrobasilar insufficiency is:*

a   tinnitus.
b   ataxia.
c   headache.
d   vertigo.

75   *A 68-year-old woman presents to the emergency department with a head injury after falling off a ladder while painting her kitchen. She has generalized tonic-clonic seizures. What is the treatment of choice to treat the seizures?*

a   Phenytoin (Dilantin)
b   Carbamazepine (Tegretol)
c   Phenobarbital
d   Depakote (Valproate)

76   *A 75-year-old woman presents for a routine physical examination. Her past medical history is significant for hypertension, and hyperlipidemia, and her current medications include enalapril maleate (Vasotec) and atorvastatin calcium (Lipitor). Physical exam reveals a right carotid bruit. She denies any symptoms of stroke or transient ischemic attack. What is your next step in evaluation of the bruit?*

a   Order a head CT scan.
b   Order a carotid doppler study.
c   Have the patient return in 3 months to evaluate the bruit.
d   Order a cardiac echocardiogram.

77   *A 75-year-old woman is diagnosed with a subarachnoid hemorrhage after falling down steps. She has developed obstructive hydrocephalus. What would be the first sign of increased ICP?*

a   Dilated pupils
b   Altered level of consciousness
c   Development of seizures
d   Fixed pupils

78   *The most common acid-base disorder that is seen in patients with status epilepticus is:*

a   metabolic acidosis.
b   metabolic alkalosis.
c   respiratory alkalosis.
d   none of the above.

79   *You are monitoring cerebral perfusion pressure (CPP) in a 40-year-old male patient after craniotomy. What is the normal range for CCP?*

a   10 to 20 mm Hg
b   20 to 30 mm Hg
c   50 to 130 mm Hg
d   180 to 200 mm Hg

80   *A 30-year-old man with human immunodeficiency virus (HIV) infection develops a rapidly pro-* *gressive dementia. What are the common symptoms of HIV dementia?*

a   Peripheral neuropathy
b   Paralysis of the upper extremities
c   Confusion and psychosis
d   Muscle twitching

81   *Which diagnostic modality is used to document hydrocephalus?*

a   EEG
b   LP
c   CT scan
d   Cerebral arteriogram

82   *A 25-year-old woman is diagnosed with meningococcal meningitis. What finding would you expect on physical exam?*

a   Dilated pupils
b   Petechiae
c   Janewa's lesions
d   Osler's nodes

83   *Symptoms associated with a medulloblastoma include:*

a   vomiting.
b   frequent falls.
c   unilateral hearing loss.
d   all of the above.

84   *Which of the following tumors may occur in the pineal area of the brain?*

a   Astrocytoma
b   Pituitary adenoma
c   Acoustic neurofibroma
d   Medulloblastoma

85   *Clinical signs that may be associated with pinealoma are:*

a   unreactive pupils.
b   blindness.
c   hearing loss.
d   seizures.

Answers

1   Answer b

The most likely diagnosis is Bell's palsy. The history of unilateral facial pain with inability to close eye with increased tearing and left ear pain suggests this diagnosis. Bell's palsy occurs as a result of inflammation to cranial nerve VII and frequently is preceded by a respiratory viral infection. Temporal arteritis may cause severe headaches and may lead to blindness if left untreated. Multiple sclerosis may produce the visual symptoms, but it is usually bilateral rather than unilateral. Meningitis usually produces headache with photophobia.

2 Answer d

Bell's palsy is a result of inflammation and edema to cranial nerve VII.

3 Answer d

Common symptoms of temporal arteritis include a throbbing dull headache, scalp tenderness, and jaw claudication.

4 Answer b

The most feared complication of temporal arteritis is blindness. Blindness results from occlusion of the ophthalmic artery.

5 Answer a

The first symptom of cervical radiculopathy is headache, which is thought to be secondary to irritation of the upper cervical root.

6 Answer a

The next step in the care of this patient is to obtain a further history. The patient presents with a febrile illness with meningeal signs. Further information is required, and the patient will probably need a neurologic consultation.

7 Answer b

The most likely diagnosis of the patient with a 2-day history of fever, headache, nausea, vomiting, and neck pain is meningitis.

8 Answer d

Carpal tunnel syndrome is characterized by all of the symptoms except back pain. Symptoms commonly associated with carpal tunnel are arm pain, paresthesias, and numbness.

9 Answer b

A positive Tinel's sign is present when tapping on the wrist or anywhere along the median nerve reproduces pain in the wrist.

10 Answer c

The most common site of ulnar entrapment is the elbow.

11 Answer b

The most likely diagnosis is Guillain-Barré syndrome. Guillain-Barré syndrome is a progressive ascending paralysis that results from decreased myelin at the nerve root and the peripheral nerves. It often is preceded by a viral illness. Multiple sclerosis is associated with motor deficits that are initially unilateral and ocular symptoms. CVA may present with weakness, but it is usually unilateral. Peripheral neuropathy usually has sensory impairment before motor deficits.

12 Answer a

The most common demyelinating disease of the central nervous system is multiple sclerosis. Demyelination may occur in the optic nerves, spinal cord, brain stem, cerebellum, and periventricular areas.

13 Answer b

The question in the history that may help to classify tremors is one that will determine whether the tremor is symmetrical or unilateral.

14 Answer d

Medications that may be associated with tremors include beta-adrenergic agents, stimulants, theophylline, and lithium. Digoxin (Lanoxin) is not associated with tremors.

15 Answer d

Tremors associated with a specific task are best treated with botulinum toxin. Botulism is caused by a neuromuscular junction toxin produced by *Clostridium botulinum.* The toxin can be purified and injected into muscle to reduce excessive contractions.

16 Answer a

The most likely diagnosis is botulism. Botulism is characterized by involvement of the cranial nerve including diplopia, ptosis, blurred vision, dysphagia, and dysarthria. The patient may have dilated fixed pupils. The Centers for Disease Control and Prevention (CDC) lists the features of botulism as the absence of fever, normal mental status, normal pulse, no sensory dysfunction, and symmetrical neurologic dysfunction. Myasthenia usually presents with fatigue but will have all the ocular symptoms. Guillain-Barré syndrome may present with bilateral weakness but will not be associated with the ocular symptoms. A CVA is usually unilateral.

17 Answer b

A contraindication to the use of thrombolytics in this patient is the recent colon resection, which was performed 3 days before the event. Other contraindications to thrombolytics include possible hemorrhage on CT scan, pretreatment systolic blood pressure above 185 mm Hg, or diastolic blood pressure above 110 mm Hg, therapeutic IV heparin administration within the past 48 hours, seizures at the onset of the stroke, thrombocytopenia, and hyperglycemia.

18 Answer d

Treatment of migraine headaches may include the use of NSAIDs, beta blockers, and tricyclic antidepressants.

19 Answer d

Common migraine headache is more frequently found in young women, may be associated with nausea and vomiting, may last for hours, and may be relieved by sleep. Cluster headaches usually produce unilateral orbital pain lasting from 30 to 90 minutes.

20 Answer d

Laboratory tests that should be ordered as part of the evaluation of dementia include imaging of the brain either by MRI or CT scan, assessment of thyroid function, and vitamin B12 levels. Other initial laboratory tests may include the Rapid Plasma Reagin, complete blood count, chemistry profile, and ESR.

21 Answer c

The primary cause of nontraumatic dementia is Alzheimer's disease.

22 Answer d

Tension headache is a generalized, steady aching headache that is most intense in the occipital area and upper neck. It is more common in women and usually triggered by fatigue, stress, or noise. Tension headaches are usually not associated with photophobia, which is most common with migraine headaches.

23 Answer a

A medication that may be used to treat migraine headaches that may be given subcutaneously as well as nasally is sumatriptan (Imitrex). The usual dosage subcutaneously is 6 mg with a maximum of 12 mg in 24 hours. Orally, the maximum dosage for 24 hours is 200 mg. Nasally, the dosage is usually 5 to 20 mg, with a total of 40 mg maximum for 24 hours.

24 Answer d

The most likely diagnosis is subarachnoid hemorrhage. Subarachnoid hemorrhage is associated with abrupt onset, and with what is usually described as the "worst headache ever" and may quickly progress to confusion, collapse, and coma. Meningitis is usually associated with febrile illness and stiffness of the neck. Trigeminal neuralgia is associated with facial pain. Migraine headache is associated with visual disturbances and with nausea.

25 Answer c

The level of the spine that is tested with the biceps reflex is around cervical vertebrae 5 and 6.

26 Answer b

Cranial nerve VIII controls hearing (the cochlear division) and balance (vestibular division).

27 Answer d

Unilateral loss of smell without history of nasal disease suggests a frontal lobe lesion of the brain.

28 Answer d

Causes of ataxia include cerebellar disease, loss of position sense, and intoxication.

29 Answer b

The findings of symmetrical weakness of proximal leg muscles suggest myopathy. That the patient has undergone organ transplantation and is taking steroids further suggests myopathy, because steroids may produce myopathy. Symmetrical weakness of distal muscles may suggest polyneuropathy. Cranial nerve XI is the spinal accessory nerve and it relates to the sternomastoid muscle and upper portion of the trapezius.

30 Answer a

One disease process that may cause loss of vibratory sense is diabetes, which produces a peripheral neuropathy with attendant loss of vibratory sense. Other diseases that may cause loss of vibratory sense include alcoholism and posterior column disease. Aging may also be associated with loss of vibratory sense.

31 Answer b

Classic symptoms of Parkinson's disease include tremor at rest, bradydyskinesia, shuffling gait, masked facies, and stooped posture. Other symptoms that may occur include depression, dysarthria, dysphagia, and dizziness with position changes.

32 Answer a

The treatment of choice for patients diagnosed with trigeminal neuralgia is carbamazepine (Tegretol). Although an anticonvulsant, carbamazepine is thought to decrease the pain associated with this disorder. Phenytoin sodium may be used as adjunctive therapy in combination with carbamazepine. Carbidopa and levodopa are used in management of Parkinson's disease.

33 Answer d

The diagnosis of myasthenia gravis should be supported with a Tensilon test. The Tensilon test consists of administering edrophonium intravenously not to exceed 10 mg to see whether neurologic function improves. A chest CT scan may be performed to assess for hyperplasia of the thymus or thymoma.

34 Answer d

Treatment options for patients with myasthenia gravis include pyridostigmine (Mestinon), azathioprine (Imuran) and pred-nisone (steroids). Other therapies may include thymectomy, irradiation, and the use of plasmapheresis.

35 Answer d

The most likely diagnosis is trichinosis. *Trichinella spiralis,* a gastrointestinal parasite, is responsible for trichinosis, which is usually related to eating undercooked pork. The infection may manifest itself with gastrointestinal disturbances, fever, periorbital edema, myalgias, and general malaise. Muscle biopsy and demonstration of eosinophilia establish the diagnosis.

36 Answer b

Korsakoff's disease is associated with thiamine deficiency, malnutrition, and alcoholism.

37 Answer a

Broca's aphasia is characterized by impaired spontaneous speech that is not fluent, dysprosodic, and telegraphic. The cognitive skills of repetition, naming, reading, and writing are impaired. The most common cause of Broca's aphasia is an infarct involving the left middle cerebral artery.

38 Answer d

If you suspect neck or head trauma, extreme caution should be taken. The neck should not be moved until full views of the cervical spine are taken and evaluated to rule out spinal instability. If there has been a cervical spine injury and the neck is manipulated, cervical cord injury may occur.

39 Answer b

SIADH is one of the complications of closed head injury and results in abnormal secretion of antidiuretic hormone. This response causes reabsorption of water from the renal tubules and dilution of sodium concentration leading to hyponatremia.

40 Answer d

Absence of blinking or the corneal reflex signifies a problem with cranial nerve V.

41 Answer d

Differential diagnosis for syncope may include anxiety, panic disorders, aortic stenosis, or hypoglycemia.

42 Answer c

The most likely diagnosis is left middle cerebral artery stroke. Symptoms of acute thrombotic event involving the middle cerebral artery include hemiplegia, hemianopsia, paresthesia, and deviation of the eyes toward the side of the lesion.

43 Answer a

The most common site of intracranial vascular thrombosis is the middle cerebral artery.

44 Answer b

The diagnostic tool of choice for a patient with an acute stroke is a head CT scan. CT scan helps to differentiate an infarct from a cerebral bleed. MRI is a valuable tool, especially in detecting smaller strokes and cerebellar and brain-stem lesions; it has not, however, replaced the CT scan for this purpose.

45 Answer d

The most common risk factor associated with stroke is hypertension. Other risk factors that have been associated with stroke include advancing age, diabetes mellitus, ischemic heart disease, oral contraceptive use, cigarette smoking, and migraine headaches.

46 Answer c

The most likely diagnosis is RIND, which is a neurologic deficit that lasts longer than 24 hours but less than 3 weeks. TIA is a neurologic deficit that resolves within 24 hours. Completed stroke results in permanent deficits.

47 Answer d

The pharmacologic treatment of choice for the prevention of TIAs is the use of aspirin therapy. Beta blockers and calcium channel blockers have no role in the prevention of TIAs. Dipyridamole has not been proven to be effective in treating TIAs.

48 Answer b

The laboratory test that should be obtained to support the diagnosis of temporal arteritis measures ESR. The ESR is a sensitive test in a patient suspected of having temporal arteritis. Hypothyroidism may be associated with temporal arteritis, so the TSH should be checked; however, it is not diagnostic for temporal arteritis.

49 Answer a

The treatment of choice for temporal arteritis is prednisone. The course of treatment with prednisone may vary from 4 weeks to 2 years, dependent on the severity of the condition.

50 Answer a

The preferred treatment for patients with severe symptoms associated with Parkinson's disease is L-dopa (Levodopa). L-dopa is a precursor to dopamine in the basal ganglia. The effectiveness of L-dopa may decrease after several years of use.

51 Answer b

Acoustic neuroma may progress to cranial nerve VIII palsy. Acoustic neuromas are slow-growing tumors and may be large before symptoms develop. Symptoms may include deafness, headache, facial paresthesia, ataxia, and tinnitus.

52 Answer a

Neurosyphilis is characterized by ataxic gait, memory loss, and apathy. Chancre is a manifestation of the first stage of syphilis.

53 Answer c

Cushing's response is a late sign of ICP, which indicates brain compression, and is associated with a poor outcome.

54 Answer a

The findings of periorbital ecchymosis ("raccoon eyes"), otorrhea, and rhinorrhea in a patient after trauma suggest basilar skull fracture. The presence of rhinorrhea and otorrhea that is bloody further indicates a laceration of the dura, putting the patient at risk for infection.

55 Answer d

Dorsiflexion of the great toe with fanning of the other toes is Babinskis response, which indicates upper motor neuron disease. Brudzinski's and Kernig's signs are meningeal signs. Romberg's sign is used to assess balance.

56 Answer b

Scissors gait is associated with spastic paresis of the legs with short steps. This gait is typically stiff.

57 Answer b

Decerebrate rigidity is manifested by neck extension, rigidity of the jaws, extension of the elbows with pronation of the forearms, and plantar flexion. It is usually caused by a lesion in the midbrain or pons, but may be associated with metabolic derangements.

58 Answer b

Thoracic outlet syndrome is an abnormality of the first rib, which may lead to pressure on the subclavian artery or brachial plexus. The presenting symptoms may include sensory loss and weakness in the hand, with color changes.

59 Answer a

Simple partial seizures are focal neurologic events that are not associated with loss of consciousness. Patients with simple partial seizures will have abnormal EEG results in over 50% of patients and may be treated with phenytoin (Dilantin).

60 Answer c

The patient with alcohol withdrawal seizures is most likely to exhibit seizures 6 to 48 hours after admission, with a peak at 12 to 24 hours. Alcohol withdrawal seizures are more likely to occur in patients with known seizure disorder.

61 Answer d

Side effects associated with phenytoin (Dilantin) include peripheral neuropathy, gingival hyperplasia, and ataxia. Other side effects may include dysarthria, nystagmus, osteomalacia, anemia, and hypertrichosis.

62 Answer c

Characteristics of alcoholic dementia include ataxia, confusional state, and cognitive dysfunction. The cognitive deficits may be secondary to thiamine deficiency and damage to brain structures. Seizures are not characteristic of alcoholic dementia.

63 Answer d

Symptoms associated with multi-infarct dementia include hand clumsiness, dysarthria, and confusion. Also, on physical exam, the patient may demonstrate a positive Babinski reflex.

64 Answer d

Treatment options for patients with multi-infarct dementia include antiplatelet therapy, anticoagulation, and reduction of risk factors.

65 Answer c

A distal pattern of muscle weakness may be associated with ALS. Muscular dystrophy and polymyositis may produce proximal muscle weakness. Subdural hematoma will produce a weakness of the extensor muscles in the upper extremities and the flexor muscles in the lower extremities.

66 Answer b

ALS is a motor neuron disease that is more common in men and begins with gradual onset of weakness beginning in the distal limbs and migrating proximally to the trunk and cranial musculature. Patients may note limb twitching; the sphincter muscles are not involved. Other symptoms may include dysphagia, hoarseness, respiratory failure, hyperreflexia, and spasticity. The prognosis is poor, with mean life span less than 4 years.

67 Answer c

Duchenne's muscular dystrophy is characterized by absence of dystrophin in the muscle membrane; is associated with atrophy and weakness of the muscles; occurs only in men, and is usually fatal in the second to third decade of life from infectious, cardiac, or pulmonary complications.

68 Answer a

Argyll-Robertson pupils are associated with neurosyphilis.

69   Answer d

Ménière's disease is characterized by abrupt attacks of vertigo and may be associated with tinnitus, unilateral pressure sensation in the ears, and hearing deficit.

70   Answer d

Romberg's maneuver is observation of steadiness while the patient stands with feet together and eyes open, then closed. If marked unsteadiness is noted and falling with eyes closed occurs, this implies that there may be a posterior lesion, and if the eyes are open with unsteadiness, it implies a cerebellar lesion.

71   Answer c

Kernig's sign is a meningeal sign. With the patient lying supine to 90 degrees and the thigh flexed, if, when you attempt extension of the leg, pain and spasm ensues, the sign is considered positive. Passive flexion of the head while supine and flexion of the thighs and legs is Brudzinski's sign. Straight leg raising suggest sciatic nerve irritation. Pain with tapping of the median nerve is Tinel's sign and is present with carpal tunnel syndrome.

72   Answer d

LP is a tool commonly used to diagnose meningitis but may also be diagnostic in encephalitis and intracerebral bleeding. LP may be used in certain situations to administer intrathecal antibiotics, and patients may develop postprocedure headaches. Patients with papilledema and focal neurologic signs should have a head CT scan done before an LP is performed.

73   Answer b

The most likely diagnosis for this patient is metastatic disease to the spine. The clinical presentation of anorexia and weight loss in a 50-pack-per-year smoker suggests malignancy. Metastatic disease of the spine may arise from the breast, bone, lung, and prostate and may produce excruciating pain.

74   Answer d

The most common symptom of vertebrobasilar insufficiency is vertigo. Other symptoms that may be identified include tinnitus, diplopia, perioral numbness, dysphagia, visual field defects, and motor deficits.

75   Answer d

The treatment of choice for tonic-clonic seizures is depakote (Valproate). Other agents such as phenytoin (Dilantin), carbamazepine (Tegretol), and phenobarbital may be used, but depakote is the agent of choice.

76   Answer b

The next step in the evaluation of a patient with an asymptomatic bruit is carotid Doppler study to assess whether there is blockage in the carotid arteries.

77   Answer b

The first sign of increasing ICP in a patient with obstructive hydrocephalus is alteration in the level of consciousness. Other symptoms may include dilated pupils and seizure activity, but these will occur after there is a change in mental status.

78   Answer a

The patient with status epilepticus has metabolic acidosis. The patient with seizure activity has repetitive spasms of the muscle, which may cause anaerobic metabolism, which may lead to metabolic acidosis.

79   Answer c

The normal range for CCP is 50 to 130 mm Hg.

80   Answer c

The most common symptoms associated with HIV-related dementia are confusion and psychosis. Peripheral neuropathy and upper extremity paralysis are uncommon.

81   Answer c

The diagnostic modality utilized to document hydrocephalus is the CT scan, which allows you to visualize the ventricles.

82   Answer b

A patient with meningococcal meningitis will have petechiae on examination secondary to septicemia. Janeway's lesions and Osler's nodes are associated with endocarditis.

83   Answer d

Medulloblastoma is a rapidly growing tumor, which may arise in the cerebellum and may present with malaise, vomiting, headaches, stumbling, frequent falling, and unilateral hearing loss.

84   Answer a

Astrocytoma may occur in the pineal area of the brain. Other tumors that may arise from this region include teratoma, germinoma, pineocytoma, and pineoblastoma.

85   Answer a

Clinical signs that may be associated with pinealoma are slightly dilated and unreactive pupils. Other signs may include paralysis of the upward gaze, headache, and gait instability. If the tumor progressively enlarges, it may cause visual loss and diabetes insipidus.

Bibliography

Devinsky, O, et al: Neurologic Pearls. FA Davis, Philadelphia, 2000.

Dunphy, L: Management Guidelines for Adult Nurse Practitioners. F. A. Davis, Philadelphia, 1999.

Goroll, A, et al: Primary Care Medicine Office Evaluation and Management of the Adult Patient, 4th ed. Lippincott Williams & Wilkins, Philadelphia, 2000.

Haley, K, and Blair, D: Trigeminal neuralgia. Am J Nurse Practitioners, January 2000, pp. 9–11.

Schretzma, D. Acute ischemic stroke. Nurse Practitioner 24:71–88, 1999.

7

Renal, Genitourinary, and Gynecologic Problems

1 *All of the statements concerning prostate cancer are true* **EXCEPT:**

a   it is more common in Caucasian men.
b   it increases with age.
c   it is rare in people under age 50 years.
d   it may be asymptomatic for many years.

2 *The most common cause of gross hematuria in men over age 60 years is:*

a   bladder cancer.
b   urinary tract infection (UTI).
c   benign prostatic hyperplasia.
d   renal calculi.

3 *A 30-year-old woman with a 6-month history of three UTIs associated with hematuria is seen at the clinic. What should be your plan of care?*

a   Refer to a urologist for evaluation.
b   Continue to follow the patient; if the patient has two more episodes, refer to a urologist.
c   Refer for abdominal ultrasound.
d   No further intervention is needed.

4 *Which of the following symptoms are associated with benign prostatic hypertrophy (BPH)?*

a   Urinary frequency
b   Nocturia
c   Slowing of the urinary stream
d   All of the above

5 *A 75-year-old man has been started on finasteride (Proscar) for BPH. How does this drug work in treating this disorder?*

a   It increases androgen stimulation of the prostate gland.
b   It inhibits luteinizing hormone (LH) secretion.
c   It inhibits dehydrotestosterone (DHT).
d   It inhibits 5-alpha reductase.

6 *Selective alpha-1 antagonists are utilized in the treatment of BPH to reduce vesicle outlet resistance. Which of the following medications are alpha-1 antagonists?*

a   Doxazosin (Cardura) and terazosin (Hytrin)
b   Prazosin (Minipress) and doxazosin
c   Enalapril (Vasotec) and doxazosin
d   Spironolactone (Aldactone) and doxazosin

7 *Which of the following conditions may increase prostate-specific antigen (PSA)?*

a   Prostatitis
b   Testicular torsion
c   Testicular cancer
d   Bladder cancer

8 *The clinical presentation associated with acute bacterial prostatitis includes:*

a   dysuria.
b   tender prostate gland.
c   urinary frequency.
d   all of the above.

9 *A 60-year-old man is scheduled to have a transurethral prostatectomy (TURP) for prostate cancer. What is one of the more common potential complications associated with this procedure?*

a   Gynecomastia
b   Impotence

c Cystitis
d Bladder neck contractures

10 *Initial management of acute bacterial prostatitis may include:*

a prostate biopsy.
b TURP.
c warm sitz baths.
d intravenous antibiotics.

11 *What is the most common systemic disease associated with erectile dysfunction?*

a Hypertension
b Diabetes
c Gout
d Chronic renal failure

12 *The most common acid-base disturbance associated with chronic renal failure is:*

a metabolic acidosis.
b metabolic alkalosis.
c respiratory acidosis.
d respiratory alkalosis.

13 *Which of the following is a urologic emergency?*

a Variocele
b Testicular torsion
c Prostatitis
d Hydrocele

14 *The most common treatable form of secondary hypertension is:*

a pheochromocytoma.
b coarctation of the aorta.
c hyperaldosteronism.
d renal artery stenosis.

15 *Which of the following may cause prerenal azotemia?*

a BPH
b Nephrolithiasis
c Gastrointestinal loss secondary to nasogastric suction
d Renal artery stenosis

16 *Urine findings in acute renal failure may include:*

a urinary osmolarity greater than 500 mOsm/kg.
b urinary sodium levels less than 20 mEq/L.
c normal urinary sediment.
d urinary osmolarity less than 400 mOsm/kg.

17 *The treatment of choice for uncomplicated cystitis in a young woman is:*

a trimethoprim sulfamethoxazole (Bactrim).
b amoxicillin/clavulanate (Augmentin).

c ampicillin (Omnipen).
d gentamicin.

18 *The electrocardiogram (ECG) findings associated with hyperkalemia include:*

a the presence of U waves.
b tachycardia.
c shortened PR intervals.
d elevated T waves.

19 *Symptoms that may be associated with hypercalcemia include:*

a anxiety.
b myopathy.
c constipation.
d urinary retention.

20 *Stress incontinence is defined as incontinence associated with a(n):*

a increased abdominal pressure on the bladder that may occur with coughing, sneezing, exercising, or lifting objects.
b strong desire to void without access to a bathroom.
c over-distended bladder.
d UTI.

21 *Neurologic disorders, such as multiple sclerosis, may cause which type of urinary incontinence?*

a Stress urinary incontinence
b Urge urinary incontinence
c Transient urinary incontinence
d Overflow urinary incontinence

22 *All of the statements concerning total body water are true EXCEPT:*

a 50% of total body weight is water.
b it is divided into intracellular, interstitial, and intravascular compartments.
c it increases with age.
d the intracellular fluid compartment accounts for 40% of body weight.

23 *The most common cause of metabolic acidosis in patients after surgery is:*

a nasogastric suction.
b renal tubular dysfunction.
c circulatory dysfunction with lactic acidosis.
d hypothermia.

24 *Which of the following screening tools for prostate cancer is recommended for men over age 50 years?*

a Prostate biopsy
b Prostate ultrasound

c Digital rectal examination (DRE) and serum PSA
d Serum PSA

25 *A 40-year-old man is diagnosed with epididymitis secondary to sexually transmitted disease. The organism(s) most likely responsible for epididymitis is(are):*

a Pseudomonas.
b *Chlamydia trachomatis* and *Neisseria gonorrhea*.
c human papilloma virus (HPV).
d *Haemophilus* ducreyi.

26 *All of the following statements concerning HPV are true* **EXCEPT:**

a incubation periods can be 3 to 8 months.
b cryotherapy has been shown to completely irradicate HPV infection.
c poor hygiene may be a contributing factor.
d unprotected sexual contact may be a contributing factor.

27 *A 60-year-old woman with type 1 diabetes mellitus and end-stage renal disease on hemodialysis requests antacids for treatment of dyspepsia. Which of the following may be safely prescribed?*

a Aluminum hydroxide (Amphojel)
b Magnesium hydroxide (Maalox)
c Milk of magnesia
d Psyllium (Metamucil)

28 *Normal urinary protein excretion per 24 hours is:*

a less than 150 mg.
b between 150 mg and 200 mg.
c between 200 mg and 250 mg.
d between 250 mg and 300 mg.

29 *Differential diagnosis for significant proteinuria may include:*

a nephrotic syndrome.
b diabetes mellitus.
c CHF.
d all of the above.

30 *Which of the following may be useful in monitoring testicular cancer?*

a PSA
b CD4 count
c Urine cytology
d Human chorionic gonadotropin (HCG) and alpha-fetoprotein

31 *The most common type of renal calculi in the United States is:*

a struvite.
b cystine.

c uric acid.
d calcium oxalate.

32 *A 50-year-old man is diagnosed with uric acid renal calculi. Treatment of uric acid renal calculi includes:*

a limitation of dietary purines.
b allopurinol (Zyloprim) therapy.
c thiazide diuretics.
d calcium restriction.

33 *The antihypertensive treatment of choice for patients with marked proteinuria is the use of:*

a diuretics.
b calcium channel blockers.
c beta blockers.
d ACE inhibitors.

34 *Treatment for hyperphosphatemia in patients with chronic renal failure includes use of:*

a vitamin D.
b calcium citrate.
c sodium bicarbonate.
d erythropoietin.

35 *Which of the following statements is* **NOT** *true concerning bladder carcinoma?*

a It is more prevalent in patients over age 60 years.
b Most carcinomas are squamous cell tumors.
c Gross hematuria may be the initial symptom.
d Use of cyclophosphamide (Cytoxan) is a risk factor.

36 *The most common symptom associated with renal cell carcinoma is:*

a painless hematuria.
b flank pain.
c weight gain.
d fever.

37 *The most common complication of renal transplantation is:*

a postischemic acute tubular necrosis.
b urinary tract obstruction.
c allograft dysfunction.
d renal artery thrombosis.

38 *Which of the following electrolyte imbalances may potentiate digoxin (Lanoxin) toxicity?*

a Hypokalemia
b Hyperkalemia
c Hypocalcemia
d Hypermagnesemia

39 *A 40-year-old man is on continuous ambulatory peritoneal dialysis (CAPD) and presents to the emergency department with complaints of abdominal pain and fever to 102°F. Peritonitis is suspected. What is the most common pathogen responsible for bacterial peritonitis?*

a Pseudomonas
b *Staphylococcus epidermidis*
c Group B streptococcus
d Klebsiella

40 *Which of the following health problems is commonly associated with urinary tract infections?*

a Hypertension
b Tuberculosis
c Polycythemia
d Diabetes mellitus

41 *A 20-year-old female college student complains of yellowish vaginal discharge and vaginal itching for the past week. Examination of the genitalia reveals an inflamed cervix and red papules on the labia and vagina. What is the most likely diagnosis?*

a Uterine cancer
b Cervical cancer
c Candida vaginitis
d Trichomonal vaginitis

42 *Which of the following renal diseases is associated with deafness?*

a Goodpasture's syndrome
b Alport syndrome
c Amyloidosis
d Lupus nephritis

43 *Which of the following renal diseases is associated with arthritis?*

a Amyloidosis
b Sarcoidosis
c Lupus nephritis
d Pyelonephritis

44 *All of the following statements concerning glomerular filtration rate (GFR) are false* **EXCEPT:**

a it is the amount of urine filtered through the nephrons per unit of time.
b it is the best index of functioning renal mass.
c the normal GFR for women is 70 to 90 mL/min.
d GFR and renal function are inversely proportional.

45 *A 65-year-old woman presents with hematuria and is suspected of having a bladder tumor. What is a useful diagnostic study in evaluating this suspected tumor?*

a Abdominal ultrasound
b Abdominal computed tomography (CT) scan

c Intravenous pyelogram
d Cystoscopy

46 *A 45-year-old man who has had abdominal surgery has now developed acute renal failure with a creatinine of 4.5 mg/dL and blood urea nitrogen (BUN) of 100. Indications for dialysis include:*

a hyperkalemia.
b metabolic acidosis.
c encephalopathy.
d all of the above.

47 *What is the most common cause of death in patients with acute renal failure?*

a Hyperkalemia
b Cerebrovascular accident (CVA)
c Infection
d Perforated gastric ulcer

48 *An adverse effect that may be associated with renal-dose dopamine (Intropin) is:*

a bradycardia.
b myocardial contusion.
c bowel ischemia.
d urinary retention.

49 *The most common cause of glomerulonephritis is:*

a idiopathic nephritis.
b IgA nephropathy.
c polyarteritis nodosa.
d subacute bacterial endocarditis.

50 *Clinical manifestations of rapidly progressive glomerulonephritis (RPGN) include:*

a fever, chills, and flank pain.
b hematuria, proteinuria, and red cell casts.
c urinary retention and hematuria.
d flank pain and hematuria.

51 *Treatment options for patients with RPGN include:*

a renal transplantation.
b total lymphoid irradiation.
c plasmapheresis and glucocorticoids.
d cyclosporine.

52 *The pathologic hallmark of RPGN is:*

a urinary sediment.
b white blood cells in the urine.
c hyaline casts.
d crescent formation on the renal biopsy.

53 *A 65-year-old woman with a long history of hypertension presents with complaints of fatigue, nausea, and vomiting for the past day, and decreased uri-*

nary output. During the hospitalization, she develops hemoptysis, expectorating approximately 50 mL of blood. Laboratory tests are positive for circulating anti–glomerular-basement membrane (anti-GBM) antibodies and glomerulonephritis. What is the most likely diagnosis?

a Systemic lupus erythematosus
b Polyarteritis nodosa
c Goodpasture's syndrome
d Wegener's granulomatosis

54 *A 50-year-old woman has been diagnosed with nephrotic syndrome. Management of nephrotic syndrome may include:*

a a high-protein diet and beta blockers.
b ACE inhibitors, dietary protein restriction, and nonsteroidal anti-inflammatory drugs (NSAIDs).
c a low-fat diet and diuretics.
d a high-protein diet and calcium channel blockers.

55 *The most common type of urinary incontinence in the older patient is:*

a stress incontinence.
b functional incontinence.
c urge incontinence.
d complex incontinence.

56 *Which of the following medications is most commonly associated with urinary incontinence in the older patient?*

a Calcium channel blockers
b Alpha blockers
c Antihistamines
d Diuretics

57 *Contributing factors to incontinence in the older patient include:*

a an increased bladder capacity.
b the loss of the kidneys' ability to concentrate urine.
c bladder exercises.
d an increased activity level.

58 *Which of the following statements concerning estrogen replacement in the postmenopausal period is **TRUE**?*

a There is an increased risk of breast cancer.
b There is an increased incidence of endometrial cancer.
c Estrogen should not be used in the post-menopausal period
d Breast cancer is not a contraindication to estrogen replacement.

59 *Which of the following is **NOT** a risk factor for pelvic inflammatory disease (PID)?*

a Multiple sexual encounters
b Unprotected sexual contact
c Use of barrier contraceptives
d Previous history of PID

60 *A 45-year-old woman with dysfunctional uterine bleeding (DUB) is seen at the clinic. Differential diagnosis for DUB in this age group includes:*

a anovulation.
b uterine fibroids.
c endometrial cancer.
d all of the above.

61 *The anemia(s) associated with chronic renal failure is(are):*

a microcytic anemia.
b macrocytic anemia.
c normochromic and normocytic anemias.
d hyperchromic and macrocytic anemias.

62 *The anemia associated with chronic renal failure is caused by:*

a decreased synthesis of erythropoietin by the kidney.
b lack of vitamin D.
c iron deficiency.
d malnutrition.

63 *Which laboratory test(s) is(are) used to assess for iron-deficiency anemia in a patient with chronic renal failure?*

a Reticulocyte count
b Erythropoietin level
c Transferrin saturation and serum ferritin
d Red blood cell (RBC) count

64 *What is the most common complication that may occur during hemodialysis?*

a Hypokalemia
b Hypotension
c Nausea and vomiting
d Sepsis

65 *Possible causes of pruritus in patients undergoing dialysis include:*

a hyperparathyroidism.
b dry skin.
c elevated plasma histamine levels.
d all of the above.

66 *Which of the following is an absolute contraindication to peritoneal dialysis?*

a CHF
b Polycystic kidney disease

c   Pericardial effusion
d   Colostomy

67   Which of the following symptoms are associated with peritonitis?

a   Rectal pain
b   Visibly cloudy effluent and abdominal pain
c   Constipation
d   Right-upper-quadrant abdominal pain

68   A 50-year-old woman is receiving peritoneal dialysis. The nurse notifies you that her inflow fluid balance is greater than her outflow balance. What is the potential etiology of this problem?

a   Short dwell times
b   Hypotonic dialysate
c   Kinked tubing
d   All of the above

69   A 55-year-old man with a history of hypertension, gout, hypothyroidism, and type 1 diabetes mellitus has end-stage renal failure and is receiving hemodialysis. The patient is asking about receiving a renal transplantation. What in the patient's history is an absolute contraindication to renal transplantation?

a   Hypertension
b   Type 1 diabetes mellitus
c   Age
d   Gout

70   What is the minimal level of creatinine clearance for a person who is a living relative kidney donor?

a   25 mL/min
b   70 mL/min
c   50 mL/min
d   None of the above

71   What is the most common viral infection that occurs in the first 6 months in the patient after renal transplantation?

a   Cytomegalovirus (CMV)
b   Epstein-Barr virus (EBV)
c   Herpes simplex virus (HSV)
d   Human papilloma virus (HPV)

72   The normal anion gap is:

a   10 to 15.
b   less than 5.
c   20 to 30.
d   50 to 75.

73   The most common cause of narrow-gap acidosis in the adult is:

a   a pancreatic fistula.
b   renal tubular acidosis.

c   constipation.
d   chronic hyperalimentation.

74   The most effective method to treat hyperkalemia is to give:

a   2 g of magnesium.
b   2 ampules of D_{50} and 10 units of insulin.
c   1 ampule of sodium bicarbonate.
d   1 ampule of calcium gluconate.

75   The most common cause of severe hyponatremia (serum sodium level less than 125 mEq/dL) is:

a   diuretic use.
b   renal failure.
c   metabolic acidosis
d   syndrome of inappropriate secretion of antidiuretic hormone (SIADH).

76   Which of the following neurologic signs may occur when the serum sodium is less than 120 mEq/dL?

a   Tremors
b   Seizures
c   Tinnitus
d   Nystagmus

77   The treatment of choice for uncomplicated cystitis in women is to give:

a   an oral fluoroquinolone.
b   oral trimethoprim sulfamethoxazole (Bactrim).
c   ampicillin (Omnipen).
d   a cephalosporin.

78   The most common cause of recurrent UTI in male patients is:

a   a renal calculus.
b   BHP.
c   chronic bacterial prostatitis.
d   epididymitis.

79   A 40-year-old man presents with complaints of a unilateral, painless scrotal mass. What is the most likely diagnosis?

a   Nephrotic syndrome
b   Testicular torsion
c   Epididymitis
d   Spermatocele

80   The most common site of hernias in men is the:

a   femoral area.
b   inguinal area.
c   abdominal area.
d   none of the above.

81 *A 70-year-old woman with a suspected allergic medication reaction is seen at the clinic. What is the most likely urinary finding?*

a Proteinuria
b Hematuria
c Urine eosinophils
d Leukoesterase

82 *A 40-year-old male driver who is wearing an approved seat safety belt is involved in an automobile accident and suspected to have an extraperitoneal bladder rupture. What is the proposed mechanism of this injury?*

a Seat belt injury to the abdomen
b Compression of the bladder by the diaphragm
c Bladder perforation secondary to a pelvic fracture
d Lower back injury

83 *Loop diuretics work by:*

a promoting potassium wasting.
b blocking sodium reabsorption in the ascending loop of Henle.
c decreasing phosphate and glucose levels.
d promoting sodium secretion into the distal tubule.

84 *Which diagnostic test is recommended in patients with possible bladder rupture?*

a Retrograde cystogram
b Magnetic resonance imaging (MRI) of the pelvis
c Bone scan
d Abdominal ultrasound

85 *A 55-year-old woman with chronic renal failure has a suspected vascular access infection. What is the appropriate management?*

a Obtain blood cultures and give vancomycin (Vancocin) 1 g intravenously.
b Order an ultrasound of the vascular access site.
c Plan for surgical removal of the vascular access.
d Monitor the patient's temperature and obtain blood cultures.

Answers

1 Answer a
Prostate cancer is one of the most common cancers in men and is more prevalent in African-American than Caucasian men. It occurs more often as people age, is rare in people under age 50 years, and may be asymptomatic for many years.

2 Answer c
The most common cause of gross hematuria in men over age 60 years is BPH. Differential diagnosis for gross hematuria may include bladder and renal cancer, as well as renal calculi in this age group. Patients with UTIs may have hematuria, but it is usually not gross.

3 Answer a
A patient with recurrent UTIs associated with hematuria should be referred to a urologist for further evaluation.

4 Answer d
Urinary frequency, nocturia, and slowing of urinary stream are all symptoms associated with BPH.

5 Answer d
Finasteride (Proscar) inhibits 5-alpha reductase, which decreases androgen stimulation of the prostate gland and decreases the prostate size, thus improving symptoms in a vast majority of patients. Androgen suppressors may inhibit luteinizing hormone (LH) and dehydrotestosterone (DHT) secretion with improvement in symptoms of BPH.

6 Answer a
Alpha-1 antagonists that are utilized to treat BPH include doxazosin (Cardura) and terazosin (Hytrin). Other agents are prazosin (Minipress) and flomax.

7 Answer a
PSA may be elevated in several conditions other than prostate cancer, including prostatitis, BPH, trauma, prostate biopsy, and prostatic infarction.

8 Answer d
The clinical presentation of acute bacterial prostatitis includes dysuria, febrile state, tender and often enlarged prostate gland, and urinary frequency.

9 Answer b
One of the more common potential complications associated with TURP is impotence. Other complications include incontinence, need for prolonged Foley catheter insertion, and anastomotic stricture. Cystitis and bladder neck contractures may be associated with radiation therapy used to treat prostate cancer. Gynecomastia may be associated with estrogen therapy or alpha antagonists.

10 Answer d
Initial management of acute bacterial prostatitis includes intravenous antibiotics, which may require hospitalization. There is no role for prostate biopsy nor transurethral prostatectomy in the management of acute bacterial prostatitis. Warm sitz baths may provide symptomatic relief in patients with nonbacterial prostatitis.

11 Answer b
The most common systemic disease associated with erectile dysfunction is diabetes. Erectile dysfunction is present in approximately 50% of patients with diabetes.

12 Answer a
The most common acid-base disturbance associated with renal failure is metabolic acidosis.

13 Answer b
A urologic emergency, testicular torsion is the twisting of the testis and spermatic cord that may result in venous obstruction, arterial compromise, and eventual loss of testicular function, which leads to infertility.

14 Answer d
The most common treatable form of secondary hypertension is renal artery stenosis, accounting for approximately 5% of the population with hypertension. Pheochromocytoma is a

neuroendocrine tumor and a rare form of secondary hypertension. Hyperaldosteronism is a rare form of secondary hypertension and may be secondary to bilateral adrenal hyperplasia or adrenocortical adenoma. Coarctation of the aorta is a congenital abnormality of the aorta with differences of blood pressure in the upper and lower extremities.

15   Answer c

Prerenal azotemia may result from gastrointestinal loss secondary to nasogastric suction, which may lead to dehydration. BPH and nephrolithiasis may lead to postrenal azotemia. Renal artery stenosis may cause intrarenal azotemia.

16   Answer d

Urinary findings in acute renal failure may include urinary osmolarity less than 400 mOsm/kg. Urinary sodium is usually more than 40 mEq/L, and the urinary sediment usually consists of granular cast or debris.

17   Answer a

Treatment of choice for uncomplicated cystitis in a young woman is trimethoprim sulfamethoxazole (Bactrim DS). The responsible organism for cystitis is usually *Escherichia coli* (*E. coli*) and is highly susceptible to this drug.

18   Answer d

The ECG findings associated with hyperkalemia include elevated T waves. U waves, bradycardia, and prolonged PR intervals are associated with hypokalemia.

19   Answer b

Symptoms that may be associated with hypercalcemia include myopathy, confusion, lethargy, urinary frequency, coma, nausea, and vomiting.

20   Answer a

Stress incontinence is defined as incontinence associated with an increased abdominal pressure on the bladder that may occur with coughing, sneezing, exercising, or lifting objects. Urge incontinence is associated with a strong desire to void without access to a bathroom. Incontinence associated with an over-distended bladder is overflow incontinence. Transient incontinence is associated with treatable factors such as UTI.

21   Answer b

Neurologic disorders such as multiple sclerosis, may cause sensory loss to the bladder, thus resulting in urge urinary incontinence. Urge urinary incontinence is characterized by leakage of urine caused by strong and sudden sensations of bladder urgency.

22   Answer c

Total body water decreases with age and is related to decreasing lean muscle mass.

23   Answer c

The most common cause of metabolic acidosis in patients who have had surgery is circulatory dysfunction, which may occur from tissue hypoxia and anaerobic metabolism with resultant lactic acidosis. Nasogastric suction may lead to metabolic alkalosis. Renal tubular dysfunction may cause metabolic acidosis. Hypothermia may occur as a result of metabolic alkalosis.

24   Answer c

Screening tools for prostate cancer recommended for men over age 50 years are a digital rectal examination (DRE) and serum prostate-specific antigen (PSA) test.

25   Answer b

The organisms most likely responsible for epididymitis in the patient described are *Chlamydia trachomatis* and *Neisseria gonorrhea*. *Pseudomonas* may be associated with epididymitis related to prostatitis. Human papilloma virus is associated with genital warts. *Haemophilus ducreyi* is the organism associated with chancroid.

26   Answer b

HPV is not curable at this point; external genital and perianal warts may be treated with cryotherapy.

27   Answer a

Aluminum hydroxide (Amphojel) may be safely prescribed for treatment of dyspepsia in a patient with end-stage renal disease on hemodialysis. Aluminum hydroxide also works as a phosphate binder and will decrease phosphorus level, which are elevated in chronic renal failure. Products containing magnesium should be avoided in end-stage renal disease because of the potential for further increasing magnesium levels. Psyllium (Metamucil) has no role in treating dyspepsia.

28   Answer a

Normal urinary protein excretion per day is less than 150 mg, with the mean being 40 to 50 mg/d.

29   Answer d

Significant proteinuria may occur secondary to several disease processes such as nephrotic syndrome, diabetes mellitus, and CHF.

30   Answer d

HCG and alpha-fetoprotein levels may be useful in monitoring testicular cancer but are not diagnostic of cancer. PSA may be useful for screening for prostate cancer. CD4 count may be useful in monitoring HIV infection. Urine cytology has no role in monitoring testicular cancer.

31   Answer d

The most common type of renal calculi in the United States is calcium oxalate calculi.

32   Answer b

Treatment of uric acid renal calculi includes allopurinol (Zyloprim) therapy, alkalization of urine, and hydration. Thiazide diuretics and calcium restriction are treatments for calcium-containing stones. Limitation of dietary purines is helpful in treating xanthine stones.

33   Answer d

The antihypertensive treatment of choice for patients with marked proteinuria is the use of ACE inhibitors.

34   Answer b

Treatment for hyperphosphatemia in patients with chronic renal failure includes the use of calcium citrate, which is given three times a day. Vitamin D may be used to treat hypocalcemia. Sodium bicarbonate is used to treat acidosis. Erythropoietin injections are utilized to treat the anemia associated with chronic renal failure.

35   Answer b

Most bladder carcinomas are transitional cell carcinoma, accounting for approximately 90% of bladder tumors. All of the other statements are true. Bladder carcinoma is more prevalent in patients over the age of 60 years; gross hematuria may be the patient's initial symptom; and the patient's use of cyclophosphamide (Cytoxan) is a risk factor.

36 Answer a

The most common symptom associated with renal cell carcinoma is painless hematuria.

37 Answer c

The most common complication of renal transplantation is allograft dysfunction, which may lead to graft loss.

38 Answer a

Hypokalemia may potentiate digoxin (Lanoxin) toxicity.

39 Answer b

The most common pathogen responsible for bacterial peritonitis is *Staphylococcus epidermidis*, thought to be secondary to contamination of the catheter.

40 Answer d

Diabetes mellitus is commonly associated with UTIs.

41 Answer d

The most likely diagnosis for the patient described is *Trichomonal vaginitis*, which is characterized by yellowish copious vaginal discharge, pruritus, and a cherry-red–appearing cervix.

42 Answer b

Alport syndrome is associated with deafness.

43 Answer c

Lupus nephritis is associated with arthritis.

44 Answer b

The statement that GFR is the best index of functioning renal mass is true. GFR is the amount of plasma, not urine, filtered through glomeruli per unit of time. The normal range for women is 90 to 100 mL/min, not 70 to 90 mL/min, and GFR and renal function are closely correlated, not inversely proportional.

45 Answer d

The most useful diagnostic study in evaluating a suspected bladder tumor is cystoscopy. If the cystoscopy is nondiagnostic, then you can proceed with abdominal and pelvic CT scans.

46 Answer d

Indications for dialysis for the patient described include hyperkalemia, metabolic acidosis, and encephalopathy. Other indications may include anorexia, nausea and vomiting, hyponatremia, volume overload, and uremic pericarditis with pericardial effusions.

47 Answer c

The most common cause of death in patients with acute renal failure is infection.

48 Answer c

An adverse effect that may be associated with renal dose dopamine (Intropin) is bowel ischemia, but it is an uncommon occurrence. Other adverse effects may include peripheral ischemia, myocardial ischemia, tachycardia, and cardiac arrhythmia.

49 Answer b

The most common cause of glomerulonephritis is IgA nephropathy.

50 Answer b

Clinical manifestations of RPGN include hematuria, proteinuria, and red cell casts. The disease may rapidly progress to renal failure.

51 Answer c

Treatment options for patients with RPGN include the use of plasmapheresis, glucocorticoids, and cyclophosphamide.

52 Answer d

The pathologic hallmark of RPGN is crescent formation on the renal biopsy. Crescent formation is a nonspecific response to injury of the glomerular wall, which may lead to impaired filtration.

53 Answer c

The most likely diagnosis for the patient described is Goodpasture's syndrome based on the findings of hemoptysis, glomerulonephritis, and anti-GBM antibodies.

54 Answer b

Management of nephrotic syndrome may include ACE inhibitors, dietary protein restriction, and careful use of nonsteroidal anti-inflammatory drugs. These therapies are aimed at reducing proteinuria.

55 Answer c

The most common type of urinary incontinence in the elderly patient is urge incontinence. Urge incontinence, which is termed detrusor hyperreflexia, is usually manifested by leakage of urine with strong and sudden sensations in the bladder.

56 Answer d

Diuretics are commonly associated with urinary incontinence in the elderly. Other medications that have been implicated include sedatives, muscle relaxants, ethanol, and hypnotics.

57 Answer b

Loss of the kidneys' ability to concentrate urine is a contributing factor to incontinence in the elderly. A decreased bladder capacity and decreased activity level may also contribute to incontinence. Bladder exercises are one of the treatments of incontinence.

58 Answer b

Estrogen replacement therapy in the postmenopausal period has been associated with an increased incidence of endometrial cancer, but the incidence may be blunted with use of progesterone in conjunction with estrogen. Breast cancer is an absolute contraindication to estrogen replacement, but estrogen replacement is not a risk factor for breast cancer.

59 Answer c

Use of barrier contraceptives, such as condoms, is not a risk factor for PID; rather it is a protective factor. Risk factors associated with PID include multiple sexual partners, unprotected sex, and previous history of PID.

60 Answer d

Differential diagnosis for DUB in women over the age of 40 years includes anovulation, uterine fibroids, endometrial cancer, and uterine polyps.

61 Answer c

The anemias associated with chronic renal failure are normochromic and normocytic anemias.

62   Answer a

The anemia associated with chronic renal failure is caused by a decreased synthesis of erythropoietin by the kidney.

63   Answer c

The laboratory tests used to assess for iron-deficiency anemia in a patient with chronic renal failure are transferrin saturation and serum ferritin. The transferrin saturation correlates with the amount of iron available to the bone marrow for the red blood cells. The serum ferritin level correlates with iron stores in the reticuloendothelial system.

64   Answer b

The most common complication that may occur during hemodialysis is hypotension. The cause of hypotension may be secondary to too rapid fluid removal, myocardial infarction, bleeding, sepsis, pericardial tamponade, CHF, or administration of antihypertensives.

65   Answer d

Possible causes of pruritus in patients undergoing dialysis include hyperparathyroidism, dry skin, and elevated plasma histamine levels.

66   Answer d

Colostomy is an absolute contraindication to peritoneal dialysis.

67   Answer b

Peritonitis is manifest by visible cloudy effluent and abdominal pain. Other symptoms may include fever, diarrhea, nausea, and abdominal guarding.

68   Answer d

A greater fluid inflow balance than outflow balance in a patient receiving peritoneal dialysis may be attributed to short dwell times, hypotonic dialysate, or kinked tubing.

69   Answer b

An absolute contraindication to renal transplantation is type 1 diabetes mellitus.

70   Answer b

The minimal level of creatinine clearance for a person who is a living related renal donor is 70 mL/min.

71   Answer a

The most common viral infection in a patient during the first 6 months after renal transplantation is CMV.

72   Answer a

The normal anion gap is 10 to 15.

73   Answer b

The most common cause of narrow-gap acidosis in the adult is renal tubular acidosis. Other causes of narrow-gap acidosis include pancreatitis, diarrhea, chronic hyperalimentation, Addison's disease, large quantities of normal saline, and ureterosigmoidostomy.

74   Answer b

The most effective method of treating hyperkalemia is to give 2 ampules of D_{50} and 10 units of insulin. Glucose and insulin work by moving glucose into the cell, thus carrying potassium along with it. Magnesium may lower potassium level, but must be used cautiously in the hyperkalemic patient in whom

renal function may not be normal. Sodium bicarbonate may be effective if the patient is acidotic. Calcium chloride may be given to reverse the potassium effects on the heart.

75   Answer d

The most common cause of severe hyponatremia is SIADH.

76   Answer b

When a patient is severely hyponatremic (serum sodium is less than 120 mEq/dL), seizures, confusion, and coma may ensue.

77   Answer a

The treatment of choice for uncomplicated cystitis in young women is an oral fluoroquinolone.

78   Answer c

The most common cause of recurrent UTI in men is chronic bacterial prostatitis.

79   Answer d

The most likely diagnosis for the patient described is a spermatocele. A spermatocele is a spermatozoa-filled cyst of the epididymis. The patient with nephrotic syndrome will have bilateral scrotal swelling. Testicular torsion and epididymitis will present as painful and tender scrotal tenderness.

80   Answer b

The most common site of hernias in men is the inguinal area. The hernias may be direct or indirect. Direct hernias originate above the inguinal ligament, whereas indirect hernias occur laterally.

81   Answer c

Urine eosinophils may indicate an allergic reaction. Proteinuria may be seen with hematuria, glomerulonephritis, and nephrotic syndrome. Leukoesterase is usually seen with UTI.

82   Answer c

The most likely cause of extraperitoneal bladder rupture is bladder perforation secondary to a pelvic fracture.

83   Answer b

Loop diuretics work by blocking sodium reabsorption in the ascending loop of Henle, and may lead to a brisk diuresis. Loop diuretics may lead to glucose intolerance. Thiazide diuretics promote sodium excretion into the distal tubules.

84   Answer a

A patient with suspected bladder rupture should have a retrograde cytogram in which an indwelling (Foley) catheter is inserted and the bladder is filled with contrast material. Films are obtained before and after contrast removal.

85   Answer a

Appropriate management for a patient with suspected vascular access infection includes obtaining blood cultures and giving 1 g of vancomycin (Vancocin) intravenously. The effect of vancomycin will last approximately 5 to 7 days in a patient on dialysis. The patient may ultimately require removal of the vascular access device.

Bibliography

Androgue, HJ, Madias, NE: Management of life-threatening acid-base disorders. N Engl J Med 338:107–111, 1998.

Bernie, J, Kambo, A, and Monga, M: Urinary lithiasis: Current treatment options. 40:14, 2340–2346, December 2000.

Dunphy, L: Management Guidelines for Adult Nurse Practitioners. FA Davis, Philadelphia, 1999.

Goroll, A, et al: Primary Care Medicine Office Evaluation and Management of the Adult Patient, 4th ed. Lippincott Williams & Wilkins, Philadelphia, 2000.

Greenberg, A: Primer on Kidney Diseases, 2nd ed. Academic Press, San Diego, 1998.

Brenner, BM: Brenner and Rector's the Kidney, 6th ed. Harcourt, Philadelphia, 2000.

Wilson, RA: Extrahepatic manifestations of chronic viral hepatitis. Am J Gastroenterol 92:4–17, 1997.

8

Gastrointestinal Problems

Questions 1–3 refer to the following scenario:

A 21-year-old woman presents to the emergency department with complaints of severe abdominal pain along with nausea and vomiting for the past 3 hours. She states she ate food with a tomato sauce for lunch and thinks she has food poisoning. She has no previous history of these symptoms. Her last menstrual period was 2 weeks ago, and her health history consists of exercise-induced asthma. Physical examination reveals a young woman in moderate distress: temperature 100, pulse 100, blood pressure 110/60. Abdominal exam reveals abdominal guarding and a positive psoas sign.

1 *What should be your initial plan of care for the patient described?*

a   Obtain and check a complete blood count.
b   Obtain an abdominal ultrasound.
c   Have a barium enema performed.
d   Obtain an abdominal computed tomography (CT) scan.

2 *What is the most likely diagnosis of the patient described in question #1?*

a   Acute cholecystitis
b   Ectopic pregnancy
c   Perforated gastric ulcer
d   Acute appendicitis

3 *Management of the patient described in question #1 should include:*

a   an immediate surgical consultation.
b   administration of morphine to decrease the pain.
c   a follow-up exam in 7 days.
d   an abdominal CT scan.

4 *Appendicitis is more common in:*

a   women.
b   persons between the ages of 10 and 30 years.
c   during the winter months.
d   all of the above.

5 *A positive psoas sign is:*

a   pain or tenderness in the right lower quadrant (RLQ) when palpated.
b   rebound tenderness.
c   increased pain when the patient attempts to flex the thigh when counterpressure (resistance) is applied above the knee.
d   when a rectal exam causes pain in the left lower abdomen.

6 *All of the following signs and symptoms are associated with acute appendicitis* **EXCEPT:**

a   abdominal rigidity.
b   a positive Murphy's sign.
c   abdominal guarding.
d   a positive psoas sign.

7 *An 80-year-old woman presents with severe colicky abdominal pain and fecal vomiting for the past 12 hours. What is the most likely diagnosis?*

a   Acute pancreatitis
b   Gastric ulcer
c   Diverticulitis
d   Small-bowel obstruction

8 *A 65-year-old man presents with complaints of left lower quadrant (LLQ) abdominal pain, poor appetite, and constipation. Physical exam reveals hypoactive bowel sounds and tenderness in the LLQ. Rectal exam* reveals brown stool, hematest negative, and left-sided tenderness on rectal exam. The patient has a temperature of 100.5°F. What is the most likely diagnosis?

a Small-bowel obstruction
b Diverticulitis
c Large-bowel obstruction
d Ischemic bowel

9 A 70-year-old man presents for a routine physical examination. His past medical history is significant for hypertension and gout. He complains of a 6-week history of indigestion after meals relieved with 2 tablespoons of calcium carbonate (Maalox). He denies weight loss or a change in appetite. His current medications include aspirin 325 mg daily, enalapril maleate (Vasotec) 10 mg twice daily, and one multivitamin daily. Physical exam reveals a pulse of 80 and blood pressure 130/70. Cardiac, abdominal, and lung exams are normal. Rectal exam reveals brown stool, which was positive for blood. What is the next step in evaluation of this patient?

a Instruct the patient to look at bowel movements for blood and report back if further blood is noted.
b Instruct the patient to stop taking aspirin.
c Have the patient return in 1 week for a repeat rectal exam.
d Refer the patient to a gastroenterologist for further evaluation.

10 A 28-year-old woman with known human immunodeficiency virus (HIV) disease presents with complaints of fever, weight loss, anorexia, and dysphagia. She also complains of burning in the chest. All of the symptoms have been present for the past week. Physical exam reveals a cachectic woman in no acute distress: temperature 100°F, respiratory rate 20, and blood pressure 110/60. HEENT evaluation reveals anterior cervical adenopathy and oral thrush. Heart, abdominal, and lung exams are normal. What is the most likely diagnosis?

a Esophageal mass
b Gastroesophageal reflux disease (GERD)
c Peptic ulcer disease
d Candida esophagitis

11 A 35-year-old woman presents with complaints of colicky right upper quadrant (RUQ) pain occurring 1 to 2 hours after meals. She has no health problems. She weighs 160 lbs and is 60 inches tall. What is the most likely diagnosis?

a Ovarian cyst
b Cholelithiasis
c GERD
d Peptic ulcer disease

12 What is the initial diagnostic tool for evaluating cholelithiasis?

a Abdominal CT scan
b Abdominal x-ray
c Magnetic resonance imaging (MRI) of the abdomen
d Abdominal ultrasound

13 Causes of constipation include all of the following **EXCEPT:**

a hypercalcemia.
b hyperkalemia.
c opiates.
d irritable bowel syndrome (IBS)

14 The most common cause of acute diarrhea is:

a laxative abuse.
b pancreatic insufficiency.
c ulcerative colitis.
d viral gastroenteritis.

15 A 50-year-old woman presents with complaints of watery diarrhea stools for the past 3 days. She states that she is having 5 to 6 stools per day and feels exhausted. She denies any health problems or previous history of diarrhea. She states she was taking a 10-day prescription of clindamycin (Cleocin) for an abscessed tooth. She finished the course of antibiotics 7 days ago. What is the most likely diagnosis?

a Pseudomembranous colitis
b Crohn's disease
c IBS
d Ischemic colitis

16 Crohn's disease is characterized by all of the following **EXCEPT:**

a diarrhea.
b LLQ abdominal pain.
c weight loss.
d rectal bleeding.

17 Systemic involvement of Crohn's disease may include:

a diabetes mellitus.
b hypothyroidism.
c ankylosing spondylitis.
d peripheral neuropathy.

18 A 60-year-old man has been diagnosed with diverticulosis and you are developing a teaching plan. When discussing the teaching plan, you would advise the patient to:

a avoid foods with seeds.
b eat a high carbohydrate diet.
c decrease dietary fiber.
d take twice weekly enemas.

19 *The major complications of diverticular disease include all of the following* **EXCEPT:**

a obstruction.
b hematemesis.
c perforation.
d bleeding.

20 *Peptic ulcer disease is:*

a more common in women.
b associated with aspirin use.
c more common during the winter months.
d all of the above.

21 *A 45-year-old man is diagnosed with ascites. On physical exam for ascites:*

a dullness shifts to the more dependent side.
b rebound tenderness occurs.
c there is RLQ tenderness.
d abdominal rigidity may be palpated.

22 *A hepatic bruit suggests:*

a ascites.
b carcinoma of the liver.
c peritonitis.
d mesenteric ischemia.

23 *IBS is characterized by all of the following* **EXCEPT:**

a an increased incidence in male patients.
b chronic constipation.
c pencil-like pasty stools.
d chronic abdominal pain.

24 *Megacolon is characterized by:*

a colonic distention.
b diarrhea.
c nausea and vomiting.
d RUQ tenderness.

25 *An 80-year-old woman is diagnosed with adynamic ileus. All of the following are true about adynamic ileus* **EXCEPT:**

a it usually requires surgical intervention.
b the prognosis is good.
c it can be treated with decompression.
d none of the above.

26 *A 60-year-old woman is diagnosed with* Clostridium difficile *pseudomembranous colitis. What is the drug of choice for treatment of this condition?*

a Cefuroxime (Zinacef)
b Intravenous vancomycin (Vancocin)
c Metronidazole (Flagyl)
d Diphenoxylate (Lomotil)

27 *A patient treated with oral metronidazole for* C. difficile *colitis for 7 days continues to have 6 to 7 diarrhea stools per day and crampy abdominal pain. What is your next intervention?*

a Continue the oral metronidazole for another 7 days.
b Start the patient on oral vancomycin.
c Refer the patient for a colonoscopy.
d Start intravenous metronidazole.

28 *Which of the following medications are contraindicated in* C. difficile *colitis because toxic megacolon may occur?*

a Bismuth subsalicylate (Pepto-Bismol)
b Magnesium hydroxide (Maalox)
c Loperamide (Imodium)
d All of the above

29 *A 35-year-old obese woman who has had a cholecystectomy 5 days ago complains of abdominal bloating and pain. You suspect a bile duct leak. Which of the following diagnostic tests may be used to assist in management of this complication?*

a Abdominal ultrasound
b Abdominal CT scan
c Hepatobiliary scans
d All of the above

30 *The gold standard for assessment of patients with chronic hepatitis is(are):*

a liver function tests.
b an abdominal CT scan.
c an enzyme immunoassay.
d a liver biopsy.

31 *All of the following are true about hepatitis C* **EXCEPT:**

a it may be transmitted by contaminated supplies used in body piercing.
b it may be transmitted by sexual contact.
c the acute phase may be accompanied by anorexia and fatigue.
d liver function tests are normal.

32 *The hallmark symptom of acute pancreatitis is:*

a projectile vomiting.
b left upper quadrant (LUQ) abdominal pain.
c diarrhea.
d fever.

33 *The most important laboratory value in the diagnosis of pancreatitis is:*

a serum amylase.
b serum bilirubin.

c an elevated white blood cell count.
d an elevated calcium level.

34 *A 60-year-old alcoholic man is admitted with acute pancreatitis. His initial management should include:*

a a surgical consultation for pancreatic resection.
b having the patient take nothing by mouth (NPO) and initiating total parental nutrition.
c peritoneal lavage.
d pain control with morphine.

35 *Small-bowel obstruction may lead to:*

a reverse peristalsis.
b malnutrition.
c atelectasis.
d all of the above.

36 *Clinical findings of large-bowel obstruction include all of the following* **EXCEPT:**

a abdominal distention.
b bowel perforation.
c pneumonia.
d sepsis.

37 *The most common mode of transmission of* Giardia lamblia *is:*

a water.
b food.
c sexual contact.
d from personal contacts, for example, day-care workers.

38 *The medication used to treat giardiasis is:*

a erythromycin (Erythrocin).
b metronidazole.
c ciprofloxacin (Cipro).
d penicillin.

39 *Volvulus of the intestines most frequently involves the:*

a stomach.
b sigmoid flexure.
c jejunum.
d cecum.

40 *A 45-year-old woman presents with complaints of diarrhea, cramping feeling in the abdomen with defecation, facial flushing after eating, and palpitations. What is the most likely diagnosis?*

a Pheochromocytoma
b Peptic ulcer disease
c Ulcerative colitis
d Carcinoid syndrome

41 *The classic triad of symptoms associated with abdominal aortic aneurysm (AAA) include all of the following* **EXCEPT:**

a hypotension.
b pulsatile abdominal mass.
c low back pain.
d hypertension.

42 *A 68-year-old man is admitted to the hospital for elective AAA repair. His past medical history includes hypertension, type 2 diabetes, hypothyroidism, and arthritis. Three days postoperative, you are called to see the patient because he has a temperature of 102 °F. On examination, you find a small amount of serosanguineous drainage from the abdominal incision, tenderness of the abdominal incision, and decreased breath sounds at both lung bases. As the acute care nurse practitioner, what is your initial step in the management of this patient?*

a Notify the vascular surgeon.
b Obtain blood and wound cultures and start a broad spectrum antibiotic.
c Obtain an ultrasound of the abdomen.
d Obtain a chest x-ray.

43 *Which of the following statements concerning aortic graft infections is* **TRUE?**

a Antibiotics will usually eradicate the infection.
b Surgery is required to definitively treat the infection.
c Graft infections occur only late in the course.
d Most graft infections are caused by klebsiella.

44 *Ultrasound screening for AAA should be done for which of the following patients?*

a A 45-year-old woman
b A 60-year-old man with hypertension
c A 45-year-old male smoker
d A 60-year-old woman with diabetes

45 *The most common cause(s) of pancreatic disease is(are):*

a alcoholism.
b gallbladder disease.
c prescription medication use.
d all of the above.

46 *The initial presentation of IBS commonly occurs in which age group?*

a Children
b The elderly
c Adolescents
d Young adults

47 *IBS is commonly associated with which type of anemia?*

a Macrocytic anemia
b Aplastic anemia
c Microcytic anemia
d Sickle cell anemia

48 *A 25-year-old woman with a history of Crohn's disease presents with abdominal pain, fever, and nausea. An abdominal x-ray reveals air under the diaphragm. What is your next plan of care?*

a Obtain a stat surgical consultation, and start antibiotics.
b Order a Fleet's enema.
c Plan for admission to the intensive care unit.
d All of the above.

49 *A 40-year-old morbidly obese woman states she wants to have a jejuno-ileal bypass. You counsel her about the complications of this procedure, which include:*

a diarrhea.
b malabsorption.
c bile salt deficiency.
d all of the above.

50 *Which of the following statements about appendicitis in the elderly is* **TRUE**?

a The mortality is less than 5%.
b They usually present with perforation.
c RLQ pain is always present.
d The incidence is less than 1%.

51 *Risk factors for peptic ulcer disease include:*

a cigarette smoking.
b use of aspirin.
c intake of alcohol.
d all of the above.

52 *Duodenal ulcer is characterized by which of the following?*

a It is more common in women.
b It is associated with a high incidence of malignancy.
c Weight loss is common.
d Eating food will relieve the pain and discomfort.

53 Helicobacter pylori *(H. pylori) infection is:*

a more common in children.
b associated with squamous cell carcinoma.
c diagnosed by gastric biopsy.
d diagnosed with blood serologies.

54 *Treatment of* H. pylori *infection includes all of the following* **EXCEPT:**

a antacids.
b antibiotics.
c proton pump inhibitors.
d histamine-2 (H2) antagonists.

55 *A 60-year-old man with diabetes presents with complaints of midsternal chest burning, dysphagia, and a bitter taste in his mouth. He states these symptoms usually occur at night when he lies down to sleep. What is the most likely diagnosis?*

a Cholecystitis
b Pancreatitis
c Abdominal aneurysm
d GERD

56 *A 75-year-old woman presents with complaints of gnawing abdominal pain with radiation to the back, and weight loss (an unintentional 20 lb over the past 2 months). On physical exam there is abdominal wasting, poor skin turgor, icteric scleras, an LUQ bruit, and hepatomegaly. What is the most likely diagnosis?*

a Cirrhosis
b Pancreatic cancer
c Gastritis
d IBS

57 *The most common presenting complaint in peptic ulcer disease is:*

a vomiting.
b dyspepsia.
c anorexia.
d fatigue.

58 *Which of the following abnormalities would be seen in severe diarrhea?*

a Hyperkalemia
b Hyponatremia
c Hypercalcemia
d Metabolic acidosis

59 *The most common viral organism that causes diarrhea in the United States is:*

a *Giardia lamblia.*
b adenovirus.
c rotavirus.
d cytomegalovirus.

60 *All of the following are true about hepatitis A* **EXCEPT:**

a the average incubation period is 3 months.
b it can be diagnosed with IgM anti-hepatitis A virus (anti-HAV).
c it causes an elevation of the serum aminotransferase (AST).
d mortality is rare.

61 *A 35-year-old female health-care worker has suffered a needle stick from a patient known to have hepatitis B. What should be the plan of care for this health-care worker?*

a Give the hepatitis B vaccine immediately.
b Obtain baseline liver function tests.
c Give the hepatitis B vaccine within 1 week.
d Give hepatitis B immune globulin (HBIG) and hepatitis B vaccine immediately.

62 *A 22-year-old homeless man presents to the clinic with complaints of colicky abdominal pain, fever, nausea, and aching in the arm and leg muscles. Physical exam reveals a rigid abdomen without tenderness, normal bowel sounds, and no abdominal bruits. Vital signs are temperature 99°F, pulse 80, respiratory rate 18, and blood pressure 110/70. Musculoskeletal exam reveals equal motor strength with intact sensation. History reveals that the patient's dietary habits are poor, with him eating only once a day. He has been homeless for 6 months and sometimes sleeps in abandoned buildings. What is the most likely diagnosis?*

a Hepatitis
b Lead poisoning
c Gastritis
d Ileus

63 *Which of the following markers is indicative of acute hepatitis A infection?*

a Hepatitis A IgM positive
b Hepatitis A IgM negative
c Hepatitis A IgG negative
d Hepatitis A IgG positive

64 *A 30-year-old woman is seen in the office and states she is traveling to a place where hepatitis A is common, and she wants to receive a vaccination for her trip. She states she is leaving in 3 days. What is your plan of care?*

a Give her a hepatitis A vaccination and tell her she is protected.
b Give her a hepatitis A vaccination and tell her she is not protected.
c Start interferon (Roferon).
d Start interferon and ribavirin (Rebetron).

65 *Hepatitis B is characterized by all of the following* **EXCEPT:**

a it is common in health-care workers.
b the incubation period is 10 days.
c it may be associated with arthralgia and fatigue.
d there may be a chronic carrier state.

66 *Hepatitis C:*

a is the most common chronic blood-borne infection in the United States.

b is not associated with injection drug use.
c can be transmitted via breastfeeding.
d has not been transmitted via organ transplantation.

Questions 67–68 refer to the following scenario:

A 55-year-old woman presents to the emergency department with complaints of bright red bleeding from the rectum over the past 24 hours along with dizziness and a feeling that she is going to pass out. She states that she has hemorrhoids and thought the bleeding was caused by her hemorrhoids because she was constipated and was straining prior to the onset of bleeding. The patient denies any health problems and takes no medicine, except Motrin for the past 4 days for a sprained ankle. Physical exam reveals a pale woman, afebrile, pulse 100 lying and 120 standing, respiratory rate 20, and blood pressure 120/70 lying and 100/60 standing. Heart, lung, and abdominal exams are benign. Rectal exam reveals external hemorrhoids with bright red blood in the rectal vault but no palpable masses.

67 *What differential diagnosis should be considered?*

a Diverticulosis
b Colonic arterial venous malformations (AVMs)
c Upper gastrointestinal (GI) bleeding
d All of the above

68 *What would be your immediate plan of care?*

a Perform a colonoscopy.
b Draw blood for a hemoglobin and hematocrit and start IV fluids.
c Obtain an abdominal CT scan.
d Order a barium enema.

69 *The most common cause of acute lower GI bleeding is:*

a angiodysplasia in the colon.
b colonic carcinoma.
c hemorrhoids.
d diverticulosis.

70 *Mallory-Weiss tears are:*

a caused by forceful retching.
b a cause of upper GI bleeding.
c mucosal lacerations near the gastroesophageal (GE) junction.
d all of the above.

71 *Causes of acute liver injury include:*

a infections.
b exposure to toxins.
c ischemia.
d all of the above.

72 *Which hepatic enzyme suggests alcoholic liver disease?*

a AST
b ALT
c Bilirubin
d Albumin

73 A 25-year-old woman is seen at the clinic with complaints of severe midgastric abdominal pain for the past 4 days. She states she went to the emergency department 2 days ago and was told she had reflux symptoms and was started on a trial of ranitidine hydrochloride (Zantac) with some relief. She states that she has bouts of diarrhea and constipation with abdominal pain for the past 3 months, and that defecation relieves the pain. She reports no weight loss. Her physical exam is benign. What is the most likely diagnosis?

a Diverticulitis
b Ulcerative colitis
c GERD
d IBS

74 Treatment of IBS may include all of the following EXCEPT:

a tricyclic antidepressants.
b antispasmodics.
c increased fiber in the diet.
d narcotics.

75 Rome criteria for diagnosing IBS includes:

a weight loss.
b anemia.
c alternating diarrhea and constipation.
d nocturnal abdominal pain.

76 All of the following are causes of malabsorption EXCEPT:

a pancreatic insufficiency.
b celiac sprue.
c bacteria overgrowth.
d Salmonella.

77 Acute diarrhea is characterized by diarrhea that:

a lasts 6 months.
b lasts less than 6 weeks.
c is bloody.
d is caused by a parasite.

78 Which medications may cause constipation?

a Analgesics
b Calcium channel blockers
c Diuretics
d All of the above

79 A 55-year-old man presents to you with complaints of constipation for the past 8 weeks, and a 10-lb unintentional weight loss. He has no complaints of abdominal pain or melena. What is your initial plan of care?

a Obtain a more detailed history.
b Order stool for occult blood.
c Refer to a gastroenterologist.
d Order a colonoscopy.

80 Treatment for constipation includes all of the following EXCEPT:

a a low-fiber diet.
b psyllium (Metamucil).
c docusate (Colace).
d an increased fluid intake.

81 Causes of secretory diarrhea include:

a ulcerative colitis.
b IBS.
c esophageal cancer.
d pancreatitis.

82 Abdominal pain with coughing suggests:

a GERD.
b peptic ulcer disease.
c cholecystitis.
d peritoneal inflammation.

83 The most common cause of a protuberant abdomen is:

a an umbilical hernia.
b abdominal fat.
c an abdominal tumor.
d hepatomegaly.

84 Hypoactive bowel sounds may be associated with:

a an ileus.
b an abdominal tumor.
c diarrhea.
d an early intestinal obstruction.

85 An enlarged, irregular liver suggests:

a hepatitis A.
b congestive heart failure.
c hepatitis C.
d hepatic malignancy.

Answers

1 Answer a

A 21-year-old woman who presents with fever, abdominal pain, nausea, and vomiting with physical findings consistent with appendicitis should have a complete blood count done.

If the patient has leukocytosis, this is highly suggestive of appendicitis. Abdominal ultrasound and CT scan may be used in diagnosing appendicitis, but are a waste of time in this situation. Barium studies are contraindicated because if the appendix has ruptured, the barium may leak into the peritoneum.

2   Answer d

The most likely diagnosis of the patient described in question #1 is acute appendicitis. The presentation of this patient with abrupt abdominal pain associated with nausea and vomiting is highly suggestive of appendicitis. Also the patient has guarding, a low-grade temperature, and a positive psoas sign. Acute cholecystitis may have all the symptoms but does not usually have abdominal guarding and a positive psoas sign. The patient had a menstrual cycle 2 weeks ago, so ectopic pregnancy is unlikely.

3   Answer a

Management of the patient presented in question #1 should include an immediate surgical consultation for a possible emergency appendectomy.

4   Answer b

Appendicitis is more common in persons between the ages of 10 and 30 years.

5   Answer c

A positive psoas sign is increased pain caused by irritation of the psoas muscle by an inflamed appendix. It occurs when the patient attempts to flex the thigh when counterpressure (resistance) is applied above the knee.

6   Answer b

A positive Murphy's sign is not associated with acute appendicitis; rather it is associated with acute cholecystitis.

7   Answer d

An 80-year-old patient with severe colicky abdominal pain and fecal vomiting most likely has small-bowel obstruction. With small-bowel obstruction the presenting symptom is usually colicky pain, and the intestine contracts to overcome the obstruction, which leads to vomiting of fecal materials.

8   Answer b

The most likely diagnosis for the patient described is diverticulitis. The clinical presentation of the patient with diverticulitis includes LLQ abdominal tenderness, left-sided tenderness on rectal exam, fever, anorexia, and constipation.

9   Answer d

The next step in the evaluation of the patient described would be to refer the patient to a gastroenterologist for further evaluation. It would also be appropriate for the patient to stop the aspirin, but the cause of the blood in the stool needs to be determined.

10   Answer d

The most likely diagnosis for the patient described is candida esophagitis. The clinical history and the presence of oral thrush suggest candida esophagitis.

11   Answer b

The most likely diagnosis for the patient described is cholelithiasis. The presentation of abdominal pain after meals and the fact that she is obese makes cholelithiasis the most likely diagnosis.

12   Answer d

The initial diagnostic tool for evaluating cholelithiasis is an abdominal ultrasound.

13   Answer b

Causes of constipation include hypercalcemia, opiates, and IBS. Hyperkalemia is not a cause of constipation. Hypokalemia may cause constipation by producing a generalized ileus.

14   Answer d

The most common cause of acute diarrhea is viral gastroenteritis. Pancreatic insufficiency, ulcerative colitis, and laxative abuse may cause chronic diarrhea.

15   Answer a

The most likely diagnosis for the patient described is pseudomembranous colitis. *C. difficile* develops when the normal flora is suppressed with antibiotics. The antibiotics usually associated with *C. difficile* are ampicillin and clindamycin.

16   Answer b

Crohn's disease is not characterized by LLQ abdominal pain. It is associated with diarrhea, RLQ abdominal pain, weight loss, and rectal bleeding.

17   Answer c

Systemic involvement of Crohn's disease may include ankylosing spondylitis. Other systemic diseases may include arthritis, uveitis, and erythema nodosum.

18   Answer a

The teaching plan of a patient diagnosed with diverticulosis should include advising the patient to avoid food with seeds because they may block the neck of the diverticulum and cause pain. The patient should also avoid laxatives and enemas and increase dietary fiber.

19   Answer b

Major complications of diverticular disease include obstruction, perforation, and bleeding. Hematemesis is not a major complication of diverticular disease. Perforations may lead to abscess formation and peritonitis. Erosion into the blood vessel may lead to rectal bleeding.

20   Answer b

Peptic ulcer disease is associated with aspirin use. It is more common in men, and there is no correlation with seasons.

21   Answer a

The physical exam for ascites reveals dullness shifting to the more dependent side. Rebound tenderness and RLQ tenderness may be associated with appendicitis.

22   Answer b

A hepatic bruit suggests liver carcinoma.

23   Answer a

With IBS there is not an increased incidence in men; rather there is a 2:1 ratio for women. IBS is characterized by chronic constipation, pencil-like pasty stools, and chronic abdominal pain.

24   Answer a

Megacolon is characterized by colonic distention. It is usually associated with chronic constipation rather than diarrhea, and is not associated with nausea, vomiting, or RUQ pain.

25 Answer d

Adynamic ileus usually does not require surgical intervention. The prognosis is good, it can be treated with decompression, and it may be medication induced.

26 Answer c

The treatment of choice of *C. difficile* pseudomembranous colitis is metronidazole. Vancomycin may by used but is given orally. Cefuroxime (Zinacef) may be one of the antibiotics that causes the condition. Diphenoxylate (Lomotil), an antidiarrheal drug, is not used because it may hamper the elimination of the *C. difficile* toxins.

27 Answer b

The next intervention in a patient who continues with diarrhea after 7 days of treatment for *C. difficile* is to start the patient on oral vancomycin. Oral and intravenous metronidazole are equally effective in treating *C. difficile*. If the symptoms persist, along with fever, leukocytosis, and bloody diarrhea, a colonoscopy may be indicated.

28 Answer c

Loperamide is contraindicated for patients with *C. difficile* colitis because it may cause toxic megacolon.

29 Answer d

Diagnostic tests that may be used in management of a bile duct leak after a cholecystectomy include abdominal ultrasound, abdominal CT scan, and hepatobiliary scans.

30 Answer d

The gold standard for assessment of patients with chronic hepatitis is a liver biopsy.

31 Answer d

With hepatitis C, the liver function tests are not normal. Most persons with hepatitis C will have elevated ALT levels. Hepatitis C may be transmitted by contaminated supplies used in body piercing or by sexual contact, and the acute phase may be accompanied by anorexia and fatigue.

32 Answer b

The hallmark symptom of acute pancreatitis is LUQ abdominal pain, which is present in approximately 90% of patients.

33 Answer a

The most important laboratory value in the diagnosis of pancreatitis is serum amylase.

34 Answer b

The management of a patient admitted with acute pancreatitis includes having the patient take nothing by mouth (NPO) and initiating total parental nutrition to decrease the pancreatic enzymes and allow the bowel to rest. Surgical consultation and peritoneal lavage may be necessary if there is necrotizing pancreatitis. Pain control is usually achieved with intravenous meperidine (Demerol) because it has the least spasmodic effect on the sphincter of Oddi.

35 Answer d

Small-bowel obstruction may lead to reverse peristalsis, which may lead to malnutrition. Also the increase in abdominal pressure created with a small-bowel obstruction may lead to diaphragmatic pressure and atelectasis.

36 Answer d

Clinical findings of large-bowel obstruction include all of the following except pneumonia. Findings consistent with large-bowel obstruction include abdominal distention, and the obstruction may lead to bowel perforation with resultant peritonitis and sepsis. Pneumonia may be associated with small-bowel obstruction secondary to diaphragmatic elevation.

37 Answer a

The most common mode of transmission of *G. lamblia* is water.

38 Answer b

The medication used to treat giardiasis is metronidazole (Flagyl) 250 mg 3 times a day for a week. It has an efficacy of 80%.

39 Answer b

Volvulus of the intestines most frequently involves the sigmoid flexure.

40 Answer d

The most likely diagnosis for the patient described is carcinoid syndrome, especially the associated vasomotor symptoms.

41 Answer d

The classic triad of symptoms associated with AAA are hypotension, pulsatile abdominal mass, and low back pain. Hypertension is not a symptom associated with the classic triad.

42 Answer b

The initial step in the management of the patient described is to obtain blood and wound cultures and to start a broad-spectrum antibiotic. Additional measures would be to notify the vascular surgeon and to obtain a chest x-ray and abdominal ultrasound, but the cultures should be obtained and antibiotic started first.

43 Answer b

Aortic graft infections require surgery to definitively treat the infection. Antibiotics alone will usually not eradicate the infection; graft infections may occur at any time, not just late in the course; and most graft infections are caused by staphylococcus.

44 Answer b

Ultrasound screening for AAA should be done for the 60-year-old man with hypertension. Risk factors for AAA include male sex, age 60 years or older, and a history of smoking and hypertension.

45 Answer d

The most common causes of pancreatic disease are alcoholism, gallbladder disease, and prescription medication use.

46 Answer d

The initial presentation of IBS commonly occurs in young adults ages 15 to 40 years.

47 Answer c

IBS is commonly associated with microcytic anemia.

48 Answer a

The next plan of care for the patient described would be to obtain a stat surgical consultation and start broad-spectrum antibiotics. You suspect that the patient has perforated the bowel, and you want to prevent peritonitis.

49 Answer d

Potential complications of jejunoileal bypass include diarrhea, malabsorption, and bile salt deficiency.

50 Answer b

Elderly patients with appendicitis usually present with perforation. The mortality in this group can approach 50% secondary to the delay in diagnosis. The incidence is approximately 10%, and patients seldom have the classic RLQ abdominal pain.

51 Answer d

Risk factors for peptic ulcer disease include cigarette smoking, use of aspirin, and intake of alcohol.

52 Answer d

Eating food will relieve the pain and discomfort. Duodenal ulcers are equally prevalent in men and women, and are not associated with malignancy and weight loss.

53 Answer c

H. pylori infection is diagnosed by gastric biopsy. It is more common in adulthood and may be correlated with adenocarcinoma. Serologic tests may show a false negative, especially if the person has taken antibiotics or omeprazole (Prilosec).

54 Answer a

The treatment of *H. pylori* infection does not include the use of antacids. Peptic ulcer disease not related to *H. pylori* infection may be treated with a trial of antacids. Treatment of *H. pylori* infection does include antibiotics, proton pump inhibitors, and H2-antagonists.

55 Answer d

The most likely diagnosis for the patient described is GERD.

56 Answer b

The most likely diagnosis for the patient described is pancreatic cancer. Pancreatic cancer may present with persistent abdominal pain and weight loss. Physical exam findings may include jaundice, hepatomegaly, palpable gallbladder, periumbilical lymph nodes, splenomegaly, and a LUQ bruit.

57 Answer b

The most common presenting complaint in peptic ulcer disease is dyspepsia; it is present in approximately 90% of patients. Less common symptoms may include vomiting, anorexia, and fatigue.

58 Answer d

The abnormality seen in severe diarrhea is metabolic acidosis. As diarrhea persists, there is loss of bowel water, potassium, calcium, and hydrogen ions.

59 Answer c

The most common viral organism that causes diarrhea in the United States is rotavirus. *Giardia* is a parasite and often causes diarrhea in day-care centers. Adenovirus may cause diarrhea, and cytomegalovirus usually does not cause diarrhea in nonimmunocompromised hosts.

60 Answer a

The average incubation period with hepatitis A is 30 days, not 3 months. It can be diagnosed with IgM anti-HAV; it causes an elevation of AST, and mortality is rare.

61 Answer d

The plan of care for the health-care worker described should be to give HBIG and hepatitis B vaccine. The HBIG provides immediate, high-level passively acquired anti-hepatitis B immunity, whereas the hepatitis vaccine offers lasting immunity.

62 Answer b

The most likely diagnosis for the patient described is lead poisoning. The history of being homeless and sleeping in abandoned buildings would give him access to cracked paint. Lead poisoning may have a similar clinical picture to intestinal obstruction, and may be associated with muscle aching and neuropathies.

63 Answer a

The marker indicative of acute hepatitis A infection is hepatitis A IgM positive.

64 Answer b

You should advise the patient described that she can receive a hepatitis A vaccination, but that she is not protected. If traveling to an area where hepatitis A is common, she would have to have received her first dose 4 weeks prior to exposure to be protected. Immunoconversion usually occurs with three injections at 1, 6, and 12 months.

65 Answer b

The incubation period for hepatitis B may extend from 6 weeks to 6 months; it is not 10 days. Hepatitis B is common in health-care workers and may be associated with arthralgia and fatigue. There may be a chronic carrier state.

66 Answer a

Hepatitis C is the most common chronic blood-borne infection in the United States. It has been associated with injection drug use and organ transplantation; however, there have been no reported cases of transmission via maternal breast milk.

67 Answer d

The differential diagnosis for the patient described includes diverticulosis, colonic arterial venous malformations (AVMs), and upper GI bleeding. Hemorrhoids are usually not associated with the degree of bleeding that the patient is experiencing.

68 Answer b

The immediate plan of care for the patient described is to draw blood for a hemoglobin and hematocrit, and to start IV fluids. A hemoglobin and hematocrit should be done to ascertain the degree of anemia. The patient is orthostatic secondary to blood and volume loss and should have volume resuscitation. When the bleeding stops, a colonoscopy may be performed to aid in the diagnosis. There is no role for an abdominal CT scan, and a barium enema may interfere with subsequent testing.

69 Answer d

The most common cause of acute lower GI bleeding is diverticulosis, which accounts for 40% of the cases. Hemorrhoids and colonic carcinoma are the leading causes of chronic lower GI bleeding. Angiodysplasias are the second most common cause of acute lower GI bleeding.

70 Answer d

Mallory-Weiss tears are caused by forceful retching, are a cause of upper GI bleeding, and are mucosal lacerations near the GE junction.

71 Answer d

Causes of acute liver injury include exposure to toxins such as acetaminophen (Tylenol), infections such as hepatitis, and ischemia.

72 Answer a

Alcoholic liver disease is usually associated with elevated AST.

73 Answer d

The most likely diagnosis for the patient described is IBS. The patient is young and has had bouts of diarrhea alternating with constipation. Pain relief after defecation is often associated with IBS.

74 Answer d

Treatment of IBS does not include narcotics. Narcotics would decrease peristalsis, which may lead to constipation, bloating, and pain. Treatment of IBS does include the use of tricyclic antidepressants and antispasmodics, as well as increased fiber in the diet.

75 Answer c

Rome criteria for diagnosing IBS include bouts of alternating diarrhea and constipation. Other criteria include abdominal pain anywhere in the abdomen, pain relief with defecation, and abdominal bloating. The presence of weight loss, anemia, and nocturnal pain may imply pathology.

76 Answer d

Salmonella is not a cause of malabsorption. Causes of malabsorption include pancreatic insufficiency, diseases of the small intestine such as celiac sprue, and bacteria overgrowth.

77 Answer b

Acute diarrhea is characterized by diarrhea that lasts less than 6 weeks. Approximately 90% of the causes of acute diarrhea are viral in nature.

78 Answer d

Analgesics, calcium channel blockers, and diuretics may all cause constipation.

79 Answer a

The initial plan of care for the patient described is to obtain a more detailed history. There is a suspicion for colon cancer in this patient because he has a new onset of constipation and weight loss. You should check the stool for occult blood and perhaps refer to a gastroenterologist for a colonoscopy, but you need more information first.

80 Answer a

Treatment for constipation does not include a low-fiber diet; rather, it usually includes increasing dietary fiber in the diet.

81 Answer a

Causes of secretory diarrhea include ulcerative colitis. Other causes include Crohn's disease, colon cancer, and villous adenomas.

82 Answer d

Abdominal pain with coughing suggests peritoneal inflammation.

83 Answer b

The most common cause of a protuberant abdomen is abdominal fat.

84 Answer a

Hypoactive bowel sounds may be associated with an ileus. Diarrhea and early intestinal obstruction will produce hyperactive bowel sounds. Abdominal tumors may have no effect on bowel sounds unless there is an obstruction.

85 Answer d

An enlarged, irregular liver suggests hepatic malignancy.

References

Dunphy, L: Management Guidelines for Adult Nurse Practitioners. FA Davis, Philadelphia, 1999.

Goroll, A, et al: Primary Care Medicine Office Evaluation and Management of the Adult Patient, 4th ed. Lippincott Williams & Wilkins, Philadelphia, 2000.

Loayza, T: Hepatitis C. J Am Acad Nurs Practit. 11(9):407–412, September 1999.

Solomon, MJ, and Schnitzler, M: Cancer and inflammatory bowel disease: Bias, epidemiology, surveillance and treatment. World J Surg 22:352–358, 1998.

Tyrell, A: Abdominal aortic aneurysm: Diagnosis, treatment and implications for advanced practice nursing. J Am Acad Nurs Practit 11(9):397–401, September 1999.

Uphold, C, and Graham, M: Clinical Guidelines in Adult Health, 2nd ed. Barmarrae Books, Gainesville, Florida, 1999.

Voderholzer, WA, et al: Clinical response to dietary fiber treatment of chronic constipation. Am J Gastroenterol 92 (1):95–98, 1997.

9

Hematology and Oncology Problems

1 The laboratory test used to diagnose iron-deficiency anemia is the:

a serum hemoglobin.
b reticulocyte count.
c ferritin level.
d peripheral smear.

2 A 45-year-old postmenopausal woman has been diagnosed with iron-deficiency anemia and given iron supplementation. What should be the duration of the iron replacement therapy?

a 1 month
b 2 weeks
c 4 to 6 months
d 2 months

3 Side effects associated with intravenous iron therapy include:

a hives.
b anaphylaxis.
c hypotension.
d all of the above.

4 The most common cause(s) of megaloblastic anemia is(are):

a chronic liver disease and alcoholism.
b cobalamin and folate deficiency.
c chronic renal failure.
d cigarette smoking.

5 A 60-year-old woman 1 month after a partial gastrectomy may be expected to have:

a hemolytic anemia.
b pernicious anemia.
c aplastic anemia
d iron-deficiency anemia.

6 The Schilling test is used to diagnose:

a pernicious anemia
b aplastic anemia.
c iron-deficiency anemia.
d sickle cell anemia.

7 A patient who has had a myocardial infarction (MI) is diagnosed with an elevated homocysteine level. What is the treatment?

a Vitamin C
b Vitamin E
c Folate
d Pyridoxine

8 The most common cause of thrombocytopenia is:

a heparin.
b idiopathic thrombocytopenia purpura (ITP).
c sepsis.
d leukemia.

9 Treatment options for patients diagnosed with ITP include:

a steroids.
b intravenous immunoglobulin (IVIG).
c splenectomy.
d all of the above.

10 A patient diagnosed with ITP is scheduled for a splenectomy. Which immunization should be given 2 weeks prior to the procedure?

a Influenza vaccine
b Pneumococcal vaccine
c Hepatitis B vaccine
d None of the above

11 *Treatment modalities for chronic ITP include all of the following* **EXCEPT:**

a platelet transfusion.
b steroids.
c splenectomy.
d intravenous immunoglobulin.

12 *A 55-year-old man is having a routine physical examination. The nurse practitioner palpates a left supraclavicular node, which is mobile and nontender. What is the most likely etiology of this finding?*

a This is a normal finding.
b Thyroid malignancy.
c Viral infection.
d Thoracic or upper gastrointestinal (GI) malignancy.

13 *A 35-year-old woman is diagnosed with hypochromic microcytic anemia. Differential diagnosis for hypochromic microcytic anemia includes all of the following* **EXCEPT:**

a thalassemia.
b thiamine deficiency.
c iron deficiency.
d chronic blood loss.

14 *A 40-year-old woman is diagnosed with aplastic anemia and is scheduled to have a bone marrow transplant from one of her siblings. What is the most likely complication of this procedure?*

a Renal failure
b Graft-versus-host disease
c Sepsis
d Death

15 *A 30-year-old woman is diagnosed with iron-deficiency anemia. You would expect a:*

a high serum iron level, low serum ferritin level, and a decrease in total iron-binding capacity (TIBC).
b low serum iron level, low serum ferritin level, and an increase in TIBC.
c normal serum iron level and a decreased serum ferritin level.
d low serum iron level, normal serum ferritin level, and a decrease in TIBC.

16 *Risk factors associated with breast carcinoma include:*

a early onset of menarche.
b multiple pregnancies.
c early onset of menopause.
d all of the above.

17 *The most common type of lung carcinoma in the United States is:*

a adenocarcinoma.
b metastatic cancer to the lungs.
c small-cell carcinoma.
d squamous cell carcinoma.

18 *A 40-year-old man of Italian descent is being evaluated for a hypochromic microcytic anemia. Laboratory tests reveal a hemoglobin of 10.2, white blood cell count of 8000, platelet count of 300,000, and reticulocyte count of 6%. What is the most likely diagnosis?*

a Iron-deficiency anemia
b Anemia of chronic disease
c Sickle cell anemia
d Thalassemia minor

19 *Infectious mononucleosis is caused by:*

a herpes simplex.
b Epstein-Barr virus (EBV).
c human papillomavirus (HPV).
d cytomegalovirus (CMV).

20 *Complications of infectious mononucleosis in the acute phase include:*

a Bell's palsy.
b pericarditis.
c encephalitis.
d all of the above.

21 *A 70-year-old woman is diagnosed with folic acid deficiency anemia. Which of the following statements concerning folic acid deficiency anemia is true?*

a Folic acid deficiency anemia is associated with inadequate dietary intake.
b Folic acid deficiency anemia is a microcytic anemia.
c Folic acid deficiency is most common in younger persons.
d Folic acid deficiency is not associated with alcoholism.

22 *A 50-year-old man is being treated with chemotherapy for Hodgkin's disease. During the treatment, his neutrophil count has fallen to 800/mm^3 and he is scheduled to receive granulocyte colony-stimulating factor (G-CSF). How long should the therapy be continued?*

a 2 to 3 days.
b 7 to 10 days.
c 1 month.
d G-CSF is contraindicated in Hodgkin's lymphoma.

23 *A 60-year-old man is scheduled for induction therapy for treatment of acute leukemia. All of the following statements concerning induction therapy are true* **EXCEPT:**

a it is intended to accomplish complete remission.
b it is usually started on an outpatient basis.

c it is very toxic.
d it is initial therapy in treatment of leukemia.

24 *A 30-year-old man has a diagnosis of sickle cell disease. What is the most prevalent symptom?*

a Pain
b Epistaxis
c Urinary retention
d Diarrhea

Questions 25–27 refer to the following scenario:

A 50-year-old man is seen in the emergency department. He has a 5-day history of vomiting bright red blood at least twice a day and a 2-day history of black stools. He denies any history of bleeding. Past medical history is significant for type 2 diabetes and arthritis. He takes two to four aspirins daily for the pain associated with arthritis. He also has a history of alcohol use and drinks 8 to 10 beers daily. On physical exam, he is pale with icteric scleras, poor skin turgor, and ecchymotic areas on his upper torso and thigh area. The heart and lung exam is normal. Abdominal exam reveals no tenderness to palpation; the liver span is 16 cm in the right mid-clavicular line. The initial laboratory data reveals: hemoglobin, 7.0 g/dL; hematocrit, 20%; platelet count, 75,000/mm³; aspartate aminotransferase (AST), 120 mU/mL; total bilirubin, 4.0 mg/dL; prothrombin time (PT), 18.0; international normalized ratio (INR), 2.0; partial prothrombin time (PTT), 50.

25 *What blood products would you give to this patient?*

a Fresh frozen plasma and red blood cells.
b Fresh frozen plasma and cryoprecipitate.
c Red blood cells and platelets.
d Fresh frozen plasma and platelets.

26 *What factor in this patient's history may be contributing to the thrombocytopenia?*

a Type 2 diabetes
b Use of aspirin
c History of arthritis
d History of alcohol consumption

27 *What other treatment may be used to treat the bleeding in this patient?*

a Administration of vitamin K
b Splenectomy
c Use of dopamine
d Infusion of cryoprecipitate

28 *The risk factor(s) for colon cancer include:*

a a high-fat diet.
b inflammatory bowel disease.

c a low-fiber diet.
d all of the above.

29 *Symptoms of polycythemia vera are:*

a headache and malaise.
b fever and chills.
c nausea and vomiting.
d dizziness and syncope.

30 *A 40-year-old man with a diagnosis of hemophilia is seen in the emergency department with an arm injury suffered while playing touch football. Which blood product would you order?*

a Fresh frozen plasma
b Packed red blood cells
c Platelets
d Cryoprecipitate

31 *The electrolyte abnormalities that may be associated with massive blood transfusions are:*

a hypocalcemia and hyperkalemia.
b hypocalcemia and hypomagnesemia.
c hypokalemia and hypercalcemia.
d hyperkalemia and hypercalcemia.

32 *A 50-year-old woman with a history of non-Hodgkin's lymphoma develops superior vena cava syndrome. Symptoms of superior vena cava syndrome include:*

a a sense of fullness in the head.
b facial puffiness.
c dyspnea.
d all of the above.

33 *Which cancer is associated with superior vena cava syndrome?*

a Thyroid cancer
b Small-cell lung cancer
c Leukemia
d Gastric cancer

34 *Which diagnostic modality should you use to diagnose superior vena cava syndrome?*

a Chest x-ray
b Chest computed tomography (CT) scan
c Cardiac catheterization
d Cardiac echocardiogram

35 *A 45-year-old woman is diagnosed with cervical cancer. She has no past medical history. When you ask about her sexual history, she admits to multiple sexual partners. She is a nonsmoker and does not consume alcohol. She is not taking any medications and* has no previous history of sexually transmitted diseases. What is(are) her risk factor(s) for developing cervical cancer?

a Age
b Multiple sexual partners
c Nonsmoker
d All of the above

36 A 78-year-old man has a history of prostate cancer that was treated with radiation 4 years ago. He is seen in the emergency department with complaints of back pain that is worsened with lying down and coughing for the past week. Today, he notes weakness in his arms. What is the most likely diagnosis?

a Upper respiratory infection
b Acute back strain
c Spinal cord compression
d Malingering

37 Symptoms of spinal cord compression include:

a back pain.
b paralysis.
c loss of bowel and bladder control.
d all of above.

38 What is the preferred diagnostic tool to confirm spinal cord compression?

a Bone scan
b Myelogram
c Plain spine x-ray
d Magnetic resonance imaging (MRI) of the spine

39 All of the following statements concerning Hodgkin's disease are true EXCEPT:

a it may cause fever, night sweats, and weight loss.
b it is caused by EBV.
c it may occur at any age.
d it is more common in white patients.

40 A patient with atrial fibrillation is being treated with warfarin (Coumadin). What is the half-life of warfarin?

a 24 hours
b 36 to 42 hours
c 96 hours
d 72 to 96 hours

41 A 55-year-old man has just been diagnosed with chronic lymphocytic leukemia (CLL). You are explaining the diagnosis to the patient. Which of the following statements is true?

a CLL is a malignant proliferation of lymphocytes, which accumulate in the bone marrow, peripheral blood, lymph nodes, spleen, and liver.

b Radiation is not a treatment option.
c With radiation and chemotherapy, a cure may be obtained.
d The cause of CLL is related to viral infections.

42 A common symptom associated with CLL is:

a epistaxis.
b fatigue.
c back pain.
d a change in bowel habits.

43 Characteristics of lymph nodes palpated in patients with CLL include:

a fixed and hard.
b tender.
c mobile and nontender.
d fixed and tender.

44 Other hematologic abnormalities that may occur in patients with CLL include:

a anemia and thrombocytopenia.
b leukopenia.
c eosinophilia.
d polycythemia vera.

45 A patient with CLL is being treated with cyclophosphamide (Cytoxan). What is a common side effect associated with this medication?

a Decreased appetite
b Hemorrhagic cystitis
c Headache
d Hyperglycemia

46 A 35-year-old man has been diagnosed with acute lymphocytic leukemia (ALL). What laboratory findings support this diagnosis?

a Blast cells in the peripheral smear
b Anemia
c Thrombocytopenia
d All of the above

47 A patient with ALL has a white blood cell count greater than 100,000. You consult with the hematologist, and you discuss emergency measures to treat the elevated white blood cell count. What treatment options may be utilized?

a Plasmapheresis
b Leukapheresis and chemotherapy
c Bone marrow aspiration and irradiation
d G-CSF

48 The metabolic abnormality that may occur most commonly in patients being treated for ALL is:

a hyperuricemia.
b hypokalemia.

c hypercalcemia.
d hypocalcemia.

49 *Patients with ALL are at increased risk of developing renal failure. What risk factor(s) put the patient at risk?*

a Hyperuricemia
b Sepsis
c Drug toxicity
d All of the above

50 *A 50-year-old patient is currently receiving warfarin therapy for a history of pulmonary embolus 4 months ago. He is seen in the emergency department with complaints of epistaxis and bloody urine. Laboratory data reveal a PT of 55 and INR of 6.4. What is the treatment of choice for this patient?*

a Vitamin K
b Cryoprecipitate
c Platelet transfusion
d Fresh frozen plasma

51 *A 30-year-old woman in her third trimester of pregnancy presents with hypertension and hemolytic anemia. What is her diagnosis?*

a Hemolytic anemia with elevated liver enzymes and low platelets (HELLP) syndrome
b Hemolytic uremic syndrome
c Thrombotic thrombocytopenia purpura
d Idiopathic thrombocytopenia

52 *A 60-year-old man with polycythemia vera has a phlebotomy every 2 months. Complications of polycythemia vera include:*

a hemorrhage.
b leukemic transformation.
c thrombosis.
d all of the above.

53 *Which of the statements concerning thalassemia is true?*

a It is more common in African-Americans.
b It is a disorder of hemoglobin synthesis.
c The mean corpuscular volume (MCV) is high.
d The red blood cell distribution width (RDW) is low.

54 *A 30-year-old man is diagnosed with a testicular mass. What is the treatment of choice for this patient?*

a Radiation
b Radical inguinal orchiectomy
c Chemotherapy
d Radium implants

55 *A patient with testicular cancer is undergoing a radical orchiectomy. What serum marker may be used to assess the presence of a tumor?*

a Prostrate-specific antigen (PSA)
b Alpha-fetoprotein (AFP)
c Carcinoembryonic antigen (CEA)
d CA 125

56 *As the acute care nurse practitioner, you are caring for a patient with a neutropenic fever. What is the definition of neutropenic fever?*

a Fever greater than 39.5° Celsius.
b Fever greater than 38.5° Celsius orally in a patient with an absolute neutrophil count less than 1000 mL.
c Fever greater than 37.5° Celsius for more than 2 days.
d Fever greater than 40° Celsius in a patient with an absolute neutrophil count less than 500 mL.

57 *Management of neutropenic fever includes all of the following* **EXCEPT:**

a pan culture including urine, blood, and sputum.
b empirical antibiotics.
c G-CSF.
d private room.

58 *A 60-year-old woman with metastatic breast cancer has been referred for hospice care. When explaining hospice care to the family, which of the statements best describes hospice care?*

a A coordinated, multidisciplinary program that is family and patient focused to support end-of-life care that provides a holistic approach
b A medical specialty that studies patients with advanced disease and limited prognosis
c A nurse-based program to treat terminally ill patients
d A plan of care for a patient with a life expectancy less than 6 months

59 *A 50-year-old woman is diagnosed with laryngeal cancer. What is the most common symptom associated with laryngeal cancer?*

a Hoarseness
b Dyspnea
c Dysphagia
d Chronic cough

60 *A 55-year-old man had a routine physical. Laboratory tests revealed an elevated PSA level. What is the normal PSA level?*

a Less than 10 ng/mL
b Less than 4.0 ng/mL
c 0 to 2 ng/mL
d 6 to 8 ng/mL

61 *A 55-year-old postmenopausal woman is being treated with enoxaparin sodium (Lovenox) for a deep vein thrombosis. All of the statements concerning Lovenox are correct* **EXCEPT:**

a   it can be given in twice-daily dosing.
b   thrombocytopenia is uncommon with its use.
c   its efficacy is monitored by PT.
d   some studies have shown it to be comparable to unfractionated heparin.

62 *A 70-year-old man is diagnosed with hemochromatosis. What is the most common presenting symptom?*

a   Abdominal pain
b   Shortness of breath
c   Bronzing of the skin
d   Lethargy

63 *In a patient with suspected hemochromatosis, which laboratory test should be ordered initially?*

a   Hepatic function test
b   Complete blood count
c   Transferrin saturation
d   Ferritin level

64 *Hemochromatosis is a disorder of abnormal iron metabolism. What other disease(s) may be associated with hemochromatosis?*

a   Congestive heart failure (CHF)
b   Diabetes mellitus
c   Hepatic cirrhosis
d   All of the above

65 *A 50-year-old man who has had an MI is receiving heparin. He has been hospitalized for the past 5 days on heparin therapy. His platelet count on admission was 200,000/mm³. On day 2 in the hospital the platelet count was 190,000/mm³. The platelet count was not checked on hospital days 3 and 4. Today his platelet count is 100,000/mm³. The activated partial thromboplastin time (APTT) is 60 seconds. Other medications consist of metoprolol tartrate (Lopressor) and isosorbide dinitrate (Isordil). He has no other previous health history. What is the most likely diagnosis?*

a   Heparin-induced thrombocytopenia
b   Idiopathic thrombocytopenia purpura
c   Disseminated intravascular coagulation
d   Von Willebrand's disease

66 *A 55-year-old woman is diagnosed with atrial fibrillation. She has no other health problems. Which of the following medications are recommended for long-term therapy to prevent thrombotic complications?*

a   Warfarin
b   Aspirin
c   Heparin
d   Protamine

67 *A 50-year-old man has had a stent placed in the left anterior descending coronary artery yesterday. All of the following medications are recommended in the care of this patient* **EXCEPT:**

a   dextran (Dextran).
b   ticlopidine hydrochloride (Ticlid).
c   warfarin (Coumadin).
d   aspirin.

68 *A 60-year-old man is diagnosed with von Willebrand's disease. Von Willebrand's disease is a deficiency of:*

a   factor V.
b   factor VIII.
c   factor IX.
d   factor II.

69 *Hematologic abnormalities associated with von Willebrand's disease include:*

a   anemia and leukocytosis.
b   prolongation of the bleeding time and APTT.
c   elevated PT.
d   thrombocytosis.

70 *A 55-year-old man with colorectal cancer is being treated with a fentanyl patch (Duragesic) for cancer pain. Which of the statements concerning the use of fentanyl patch is correct?*

a   Each fentanyl patch provides sustained drug release for 7 days.
b   After a fentanyl patch is removed, fentanyl continues to be released for 72 hours.
c   Fentanyl patches are ideal when rapid titration is needed.
d   Fentanyl patches are ideal for patients with cancer pain who have dysphagia.

71 *A 55-year-old woman with metastatic ovarian cancer is hospitalized for severe pain and found to have bony involvement of her cancer. She is receiving morphine via a patient-controlled analgesic system. She has been receiving a total of 20 mg of intravenous morphine daily for the past 3 days. What is the equivalent dose of oral morphine?*

a   20 mg
b   60 mg
c   120 mg
d   40 mg

72 *Which chemotherapeutic agent is commonly associated with peripheral neuropathy and neuropathic pain?*

a   Vincristine
b   Bleomycin
c   Methotrexate
d   5-fluorouracil (5-FU).

73 *Cancers associated with alcohol ingestion include:*

a esophagus and larynx.
b pancreas and stomach.
c pancreas and liver.
d liver and lung.

74 *Which of the following factors may help minimize one's risk of developing cancer?*

a Following a nutritious diet
b Avoiding hormones that may stimulate abnormal growth
c Minimizing exposure to ultraviolet light
d All of the above

75 *A 70-year-old man has hairy cell leukemia. What are the most common features of this disease?*

a Pancytopenia and hepatomegaly
b Thrombocytopenia and anemia
c Hirsutism and pancytopenia
d Pancytopenia, bone marrow infiltration, and splenomegaly

76 *A 55-year-old woman is suspected of having autoimmune hemolytic anemia. Which diagnostic test is used to confirm this diagnosis?*

a Antibody screen
b Hemoglobin
c Coombs test
d Mean corpuscular hemoglobin count (MCHC)

77 *Cervical cancer has been associated with:*

a EBV.
b human lymphotropic virus.
c herpes virus.
d HPV.

78 *A 65-year-old man has metastatic bone cancer with hypercalcemia. The serum calcium level is 14.0 mg/dL. What would be the most appropriate initial treatment regime?*

a Increased oral fluid intake.
b Normal saline alternating with D5W at a rate of 200 to 300 cc/h.
c Oral phosphates.
d Mithramycin.

79 *A patient receiving a blood transfusion reacts with a temperature of 103° Fahrenheit with complaints of chills, shortness of breath, and flank pain. As the acute care nurse practitioner, you suspect an acute hemolytic transfusion reaction. Which of the following may be used in the treatment of an acute hemolytic transfusion reaction?*

a Epinephrine
b Pepcid

c Sodium bicarbonate
d Calcium chloride

80 *The electrolyte abnormality that may be seen in patients who receive transfusion from stored blood is:*

a hypocalcemia.
b hypercalcemia.
c hypokalemia.
d hypomagnesemia.

81 *Which of the following physical exam findings suggests a bleeding diathesis?*

a Petechiae and ecchymosis
b Splinter hemorrhages
c Cherry angiomas
d Varicose veins in the lower leg

82 *A diagnosis of Hodgkin's disease is confirmed by:*

a the presence of generalized lymphadenopathy.
b a 6-month history of fatigue and weight loss.
c the presence of Reed-Sternberg cells in lymph node tissue.
d hemoglobin electrophoresis.

83 *Anemia of chronic disease is characterized by a:*

a decreased serum iron level and total iron-binding capacity and an increased serum ferritin level.
b Normal iron-binding capacity and an increased ferritin level.
c Normal serum iron and ferritin levels.
d Normal serum iron level and total iron-binding capacity.

84 *Multiple myeloma is associated with all of the following* **EXCEPT:**

a bone resorption.
b elevated alkaline phosphatase level.
c hypercalcemia.
d renal failure.

85 *Amyloidosis may affect:*

a the heart.
b the liver.
c the kidneys.
d all of the above.

Answers

1 Answer d
The peripheral smear should be used to diagnose iron-deficiency anemia. The peripheral smear will reveal hypochromia and microcytosis in the iron-deficient person.

Ferritin levels will correlate with body iron stores, but it is an acute phase reactant, and disorders such as chronic infections, liver disease, and malignancy may falsely elevate the ferritin level. The reticulocyte count and hemoglobin in iron-deficiency anemia is low, but it is not diagnostic.

2   Answer c

The proposed duration of iron-replacement therapy in a patient diagnosed with iron-deficiency anemia is 4 to 6 months.

3   Answer d

Side effects associated with intravenous iron therapy include hives, anaphylaxis, fever, seizures, chest pain, and hypotension.

4   Answer b

The most common causes of megaloblastic anemia are cobalamin (vitamin B12) and folate deficiencies. Chronic liver disease, alcoholism, chronic renal failure, and cigarette smoking may all cause macrocytic anemia.

5   Answer b

A patient who has had a partial gastrectomy may have pernicious anemia. Gastric surgery will cause malabsorption of cobalamin and pernicious anemia.

6   Answer a

The Schilling test measures the absorption of ingested radioactive cobalamin and is used to diagnose pernicious anemia.

7   Answer c

Elevated homocysteine levels have been associated with cardiovascular and thrombotic disease and are treated with 1 mg/d of folate.

8   Answer b

The most common cause of thrombocytopenia is ITP. ITP is an autoimmune bleeding diathesis characterized by development of antibodies to one's own platelets.

9   Answer d

Treatment options for patients diagnosed with ITP may initially include the use of steroids starting at 1 to 2 mg/kg per day for 2 to 3 weeks followed by a taper over 4 to 6 weeks. IVIG may also be used in patients who are refractory to steroids, who are actively bleeding, or in whom you want a rapid rise in platelet count. The platelet count will usually rise in 3 to 5 days in response to IVIG, but the response is transient and treatment may need to be repeated. IVIG is also costly. Splenectomy is effective and is reserved for refractory patients or for those who cannot tolerate steroids.

10   Answer b

A patient scheduled for a splenectomy should have a pneumococcal vaccine prior to the surgery.

11   Answer a

Treatment options for chronic ITP should not include platelet transfusion. Platelets that are transfused are consumed immediately by the reticuloendothelial system of the spleen and are not effective.

12   Answer d

Supraclavicular nodes are generally not palpated except in malignancy conditions. A left supraclavicular node may indicate a malignancy in the thoracic or upper GI areas.

13   Answer b

Hypochromic microcytic anemias are usually caused by disorders in which there are alterations in iron, globin, heme, or porphyrin metabolism. This is not seen in thiamine deficiency.

14   Answer b

The most likely complication after allogenic bone marrow transplant is graft-versus-host disease. This is caused by a reaction of the host tissue to the lymphoid donor cells.

15   Answer b

Iron deficiency would reveal a low serum iron level, a low serum ferritin level, and an increase in TIBC.

16   Answer a

Risk factors associated with breast carcinoma include early onset of menarche. Multiple pregnancies and early onset of menopause reduce the risk of breast cancer.

17   Answer a

The most common type of lung carcinoma in the United States is adenocarcinoma, accounting for approximately 40% of all cases.

18   Answer d

The most likely diagnosis is thalassemia minor. The patients are usually asymptomatic and will have hemoglobins in the range of 9 to 11 g/dL and elevated reticulocyte counts.

19   Answer b

Infectious mononucleosis is caused by EBV and is usually transmitted via kissing.

20   Answer d

Complications of infectious mononucleosis in the acute phase include Bell's palsy, pericarditis, myocarditis, encephalitis, Guillain-Barré syndrome, and pneumonia.

21   Answer a

Folic acid deficiency anemia is associated with inadequate dietary intake of folate and should be treated with 1 mg of folate per day. Folic acid deficiency anemia is a macrocytic anemia and is seen in elderly persons and alcoholics.

22   Answer b

G-CSF therapy should be continued for 7 to 10 days or until the neutrophil count has exceeded 1500/mm³. G-CSF may prove to be less effective after the patient has developed neutropenia. Guidelines for the use of G-CSF include a history of febrile or prolonged neutropenia, advanced malignancy, extensive chemotherapy, and pre-existing neutropenia.

23   Answer b

Induction therapy for the treatment of acute leukemia, the initial phase of treatment, intends to accomplish complete remission with no symptoms, normal blood counts, and absence of leukemia in the bone marrow. It is toxic and is administered in the hospital setting.

24   Answer a

The most prevalent symptom reported in patients with sickle cell disease is pain. The pain is thought to be from sludging of red cells and infarction. The sickled cells increase the blood viscosity, which leads to small vessel occlusion, pain, and organ infarction.

25 Answer a

The blood products you would give to this patient are fresh frozen plasma (to correct the PT and PTT) and red blood cells (to correct anemia). Cryoprecipitate may be given if the fibrinogen level is low.

26 Answer d

The factor in this patient's history that may be contributing to thrombocytopenia is the history of alcoholism consumption, which may lead to bone marrow suppression and folate deficiency.

27 Answer a

Another treatment option for this patient is the administration of vitamin K. This patient has a history of alcohol use and is at risk for malnutrition and vitamin K depletion. Splenectomy and cryoprecipitate are not indicated based on the information given. Dopamine may be used in the bleeding patient for blood pressure support, but it is not indicated based on the presented information.

28 Answer d

Risk factors for development of colon cancer include a high-fat and low-fiber diet, inflammatory bowel disease, colonic polyps, and family history.

29 Answer a

Symptoms of polycythemia vera are headache and malaise. The symptoms are usually reflective of vascular congestion caused by the blood viscosity.

30 Answer d

The blood product that should be administered is cryoprecipitate. In patients with hemophilia, there is a deficiency of factor VIII.

31 Answer a

Massive blood transfusion may lead to hypocalcemia and hyperkalemia. Citrate, a preservative used in blood-bank blood, causes hypocalcemia by binding with calcium and producing an acidosis. Hyperkalemia may ensue secondary to the red blood cell life span.

32 Answer d

Symptoms of superior vena cava syndrome include a sense of fullness in the head, facial puffiness, dyspnea, cough, and arm edema.

33 Answer b

The cancer associated with superior vena cava syndrome is small-cell lung cancer. Other tumors that may be associated are non-Hodgkin's lymphoma, Hodgkin's disease, and other mediastinal tumors.

34 Answer b

The diagnostic modality that should be utilized to diagnose superior vena cava syndrome is the chest CT scan. Chest CT scan will enable you to define the anatomy in the area and define the mass.

35 Answer b

The risk factor for developing cervical cancer in this patient is multiple sexual partners. Other risk factors that have been associated with cervical cancer are smoking, first coitus at an early age, and HPV.

36 Answer c

The most likely diagnosis is spinal cord compression. Spinal cord compression may occur as a result of metastatic cancer from the prostate, breast, and lung. Symptoms commonly associated with spinal cord compression are back pain that is worsened with lying down and with Valsalva maneuvers. It may progress to weakness.

37 Answer d

Symptoms of spinal cord compression include back pain, weakness or sensory loss in the extremities, paralysis, and loss of bowel and bladder control.

38 Answer d

The preferred diagnostic tool to confirm spinal cord compression is MRI of the spine.

39 Answer b

The cause of Hodgkin's disease is unknown, but it has been associated in some studies with EBV. It may occur at any age and is more common in whites. The presentation of Hodgkin's disease may be constitutional symptoms of weight loss, fever, and night sweats.

40 Answer b

The half-life of warfarin (Coumadin) is 36 to 42 hours.

41 Answer a

CLL is malignant proliferation of lymphocytes, which may accumulate in the bone marrow, peripheral blood, lymph nodes, spleen, and liver. The cause of CLL is unknown, and in patients older than age 50 years, it is usually not curable. Treatment options for CLL include radiation, chemotherapy, and bone marrow transplantation.

42 Answer b

Common symptoms associated with CLL include fatigue, malaise, easy bruisability, and lymph node enlargement.

43 Answer c

Lymph nodes palpated in patients with CLL are mobile and nontender. The cervical, supraclavicular, and axillary nodes are the most commonly involved.

44 Answer a

Other hematologic abnormalities that may occur in patients with CLL include anemia and thrombocytopenia. The reason for anemia is thought to be secondary to bone marrow infiltration of the lymphocytes leading to destruction of red cells. The thrombocytopenia may relate to sequestration in the spleen.

45 Answer b

A common side effect associated with cyclophosphamide (Cytoxan) is hemorrhagic cystitis. Cytoxan is an alkylating agent and may be used in combination with steroids initially to treat CLL.

46 Answer d

Laboratory findings in patients with ALL are blast cells in the peripheral smear, anemia, and thrombocytopenia. The white blood cell count is elevated in approximately 50% of patients at the time of diagnosis.

47 Answer b

Treatment options that may be utilized in patients with ALL who have white blood counts greater than 100,000 are leukapheresis and chemotherapy. Leukocytosis of this magnitude is considered an oncologic emergency.

48 Answer a

The metabolic abnormality most commonly observed in patients being treated for ALL is hyperuricemia. Hyperuricemia may develop secondary to the rapid lysis of blast cells, which may lead to renal insufficiency.

49 Answer d

The risk factors that put the patient with ALL at risk of developing renal failure are hyperuricemia, sepsis, drug toxicity, dehydration, base line renal insufficiency, and renal infiltration.

50 Answer d

The treatment of choice in a patient with elevated INR and bleeding, in whom you suspect warfarin toxicity, is fresh frozen plasma. If the patient is not bleeding, vitamin K could be utilized. Once treated with vitamin K, it may be difficult to attain proper anticoagulation. Platelet transfusions and cryoprecipitate have no role for this patient.

51 Answer a

HELLP syndrome is observed in pregnant patients in either the second or third trimester and is marked by pre-eclampsia, hemolytic anemia, elevated liver enzymes, and low platelet count.

52 Answer d

Complications of polycythemia vera include hemorrhage, thrombosis, and leukemia transformation. The most common complication associated with polycythemia vera is thrombosis and may occur in the splenic and hepatic veins.

53 Answer b

Thalassemia is a disorder of hemoglobin synthesis, which may be a minor disease to a more severe disease. It is more common in persons of Mediterranean descent. The MCV is usually low, and the RDW may be normal to high.

54 Answer b

The treatment of choice in a patient with a testicular mass is radical inguinal orchiectomy.

55 Answer b

The serum marker that should be used to assess the presence of a tumor in a patient with testicular mass is AFP. CEA may be elevated in gastric and lung cancers. PSA may be elevated in prostate cancer. CA 125 may be elevated in ovarian cancer but is a very nonspecific marker.

56 Answer b

Neutropenic fever is a temperature greater than 38.5° Celsius orally in a patient with an absolute neutrophil count less than 1000 mL.

57 Answer c

Management of neutropenic fever comprises pan culture to include urine, blood, and sputum; removal of all lines; and administration of empirical antibiotics with aminoglycides, cephalosporins, or quinolones. The patient should be placed in a private room and strict handwashing should be mandated. G-CSF should not be used in the setting of neutropenic fever.

58 Answer a

Hospice care is a coordinated and multidisciplinary program that is family and patient focused to support end-of-life care. The care is an integrated holistic focus that encompasses psychological, cultural, spiritual, and quality-of-life needs.

59 Answer a

The most common and earliest symptom associated with laryngeal cancer is hoarseness. Symptoms of dyspnea may occur with airway obstruction. Dysphagia and cough may be associated with extralaryngeal involvement.

60 Answer b

The normal PSA is less than 4.0 ng/mL.

61 Answer c

There is no laboratory test to monitor Lovenox; heparin is monitored by PTT. Lovenox is a low-molecular-weight heparin and has fewer propensities to bind plasma proteins and endothelial cells. It has a long half-life and is given in twice-daily dosing, and in some research studies has been shown to be comparable to unfractionated heparin.

62 Answer d

The most common presenting symptom in patients with hemochromatosis is lethargy; it is usually present in 90% of patients at the time of presentation. Abdominal pain, reflecting involvement of the pancreas and liver, is also a common symptom. Bronzing of the skin may occur. Shortness of breath may imply CHF.

63 Answer c

In a patient with suspected hemochromatosis, a transferrin saturation should be ordered. The normal level is less than 50%. Sensitivity of the transferrin saturation is approximately 96%.

64 Answer d

Other disease states that may be associated with hemochromatosis are CHF, diabetes mellitus, and hepatic cirrhosis.

65 Answer a

The most likely diagnosis is heparin-induced thrombocytopenia (HIT). HIT usually develops after a second exposure to heparin and is manifest with a decreasing platelet count on heparin therapy and potential thrombotic complications.

66 Answer b

The recommendation in a patient younger than age 65 with atrial fibrillation and no major risk factors is to give aspirin. If the patient has other major risk factors and is younger than age 65, warfarin therapy is recommended.

67 Answer a

The recommendations for care in the patient who has received a stent include the use of ticlopidine (Ticlid), warfarin (Coumadin), aspirin, heparin, and low-molecular-weight heparins. The use of dextran is not recommended.

68 Answer b

Von Willebrand's disease is an inherited disorder characterized by a low level of factor VIII.

69 Answer b

Hematologic abnormalities associated with von Willebrand's disease are prolongation of the bleeding time and APTT. The bleeding time is prolonged secondary to platelet dysfunction.

70 Answer d

Fentanyl (Duragesic) patches are ideal analgesia for cancer patients who have dysphagia. Each fentanyl patch provides sustained drug release for 72 hours and when removed continues to be released in the tissues for up to 24 hours. Fentanyl is not ideal when rapid titration is needed; therefore, the patient's pain regime may need to be augmented with short-acting analgesics.

71 Answer b

The equivalent dose of oral morphine would be 60 mg. The conversion ratio is 1 : 3. Long-acting oral morphine comes in 30-mg tablets, so the patient could be given one 30-mg tablet twice daily.

72 Answer a

The chemotherapeutic agent that is most commonly associated with peripheral neuropathy and pain is vincristine. The initial presentation of the neuropathy may be numbness and tingling in the fingers to progressive loss of deep-tendon reflexes.

73 Answer a

Esophagus and larynx cancers are associated with alcohol ingestion.

74 Answer d

It is impossible to minimize one's risk of developing cancer, but eating a well-balanced diet, avoiding excessive hormonal use, and minimizing exposure to ultraviolet light may lessen your chances.

75 Answer d

The most common features of hairy cell leukemia are pancytopenia, bone marrow infiltration, and splenomegaly.

76 Answer c

The diagnostic test used to confirm the diagnosis of autoimmune hemolytic anemia is the Coombs test, which is a direct antiglobulin test.

77 Answer d

Cervical cancer has been associated with HPV. EBV has been associated with Burkitt's lymphoma and Hodgkin's disease. Herpes virus has been associated with Kaposi's sarcoma. Human lymphotropic virus has been associated with leukemia.

78 Answer b

The initial treatment of hypercalcemia is to adequately hydrate the patient with normal saline alternating with D5W at rates of 200 to 300 cc/h. The patient should be closely monitored with evaluation of serum magnesium, phosphorus, potassium, and calcium levels. Other treatment modalities, which may be used to treat hypercalcemia chronically, include increasing oral fluid intake and giving oral phosphates and mithramycin.

79 Answer c

The treatment of an acute hemolytic transfusion reaction may include the use of sodium bicarbonate. Hemolytic transfusion reaction results in the destruction of red blood cells that may lead to renal failure. The use of sodium bicarbonate serves to alkalize the blood and prevent the sludging of hemoglobin in the renal tubules.

80 Answer a

The electrolyte abnormality that may be seen in patients who received stored blood-bank blood is hypocalcemia. Sodium citrate is usually added to stored blood, which binds to calcium and will produce hypocalcemia.

81 Answer a

Petechiae and ecchymosis are physical exam findings suggestive of a bleeding diathesis.

82 Answer c

A diagnosis of Hodgkin's disease is confirmed with the presence of Reed-Sternberg cells in lymph node tissue.

83 Answer a

Anemia of chronic disease is characterized by a serum iron level and TIBC, which is decreased, and an increased serum ferritin level.

84 Answer b

Multiple myeloma is associated with all of the following except elevated alkaline phosphatase. Despite bone loss, the alkaline phosphatase remains normal.

85 Answer d

Amyloidosis, which is an extracellular deposition of fibrous protein, may affect multiple body sites including the heart, liver, kidneys, skin, and GI tract.

Bibliography

Devita, VT, Hellman, S, and Rosenberg, SA: Cancer: Principles and Practice of Oncology, 6th ed. Lippincott Williams & Wilkins, Philadelphia, 2000.

Dunphy, L: Management Guidelines for Adult Nurse Practitioners. FA Davis, Philadelphia, 1999.

Goroll, A, et al: Primary Care Medicine Office Evaluation and Management of the Adult Patient, 4th ed. Lippincott Williams & Wilkins, Philadelphia, 2000.

Klaus, B, Grodesky, M: HIV in 2000: Historical perspectives and an outlook for the future. Nurs Practit 24:1, 103–109.

Levy, MH: Pharmacologic treatment of cancer pain. N Engl J Med 335: 1124–1132, 1996.

Stone, A, and Schumann, L: Update on hereditary hemochromatosis. The Clin Adv Nurs Practit 2(12):72–80, December 1999.

Yarbro, CH, et al: Cancer Nursing—Principles and Practice, 5th ed. Jones and Bartlett, Sudbury, 2000.

10

Immunology Problems

1 *The classes of antibodies include all of the following* **EXCEPT:**

a   IgA.
b   IgB.
c   IgM.
d   IgD.

2 *Which of the following antibodies are found primarily in secretions?*

a   IgA
b   IgD
c   IgG
d   IgM

3 *The virus responsible for shingles is:*

a   Herpes simplex.
b   Cytomegalovirus (CMV).
c   Varicella-zoster.
d   Poxvirus.

4 *The antiviral agent(s) used to treat CMV disease is(are):*

a   acyclovir (Zovirax).
b   ganciclovir (Cytovene).
c   trimethoprim sulfamethoxazole (Bactrim DS).
d   All of the above.

5 *Hepatitis E is transmitted via:*

a   blood transfusions.
b   intravenous drug users.
c   saliva.
d   the oral-fecal route.

6 *The most common opportunistic infection in patients with acquired immunodeficiency syndrome (AIDS) is:*

a   toxoplasmosis.
b   candidiasis.
c   cryptosporidiosis.
d   *Pneumocystis carinii.*

7 *The virus most commonly associated with the common cold is:*

a   adenovirus.
b   CMV.
c   rhinovirus.
d   respiratory syncytial virus (RSV).

8 *All of the statements concerning IgM are true* **EXCEPT:**

a   it comprises 10% of normal serum immunoglobulins.
b   it is the predominant early antibody.
c   it is able to pass through the placenta.
d   it is found on the surface of B cells.

9 *A history of profound fatigue, low-grade fever, and lymphadenopathy may be associated with:*

a   viral hepatitis.
b   human immunodeficiency virus (HIV) infection.
c   subacute bacterial endocarditis.
d   all of the above.

10 *Reed-Sternberg cells are associated with:*

a   Hodgkin's disease.
b   sickle cell anemia.
c   metastatic breast cancer.
d   multiple myeloma.

11 *A lung tumor staged as T3N2M0 is:*

a   carcinoma in situ.
b   a large lung tumor that has ipsilateral, mediastinal

lymph node involvement without distant metastases.

c a small lung tumor that has visceral pleural involvement.

d a small lung tumor with peribronchial nodal involvement.

12 *The treatment of choice for patients with stage IA or IIA Hodgkin's disease is:*

a radiation therapy.
b surgical resection.
c chemotherapy.
d gene therapy.

13 *Immunologic testing of renal transplant donors and recipients includes:*

a ABO compatibility testing.
b ABO and HLA compatibility testing.
c HLA compatibility testing.
d ABO and Rh testing.

14 *All of the following medications may be used to treat anaphylaxis* **EXCEPT:**

a Methylprednisolone succinate (Solumedrol).
b Epinephrine.
c Famotidine (Pepcid).
d Milrinone (Primacor).

15 *A normal lymph node:*

a contains a cortex.
b has no germinal center.
c contains low endothelial venules.
d has a tender center upon palpation.

16 *Cellular immunity is mediated by:*

a T cells.
b B cells.
c interleukin-2 (IL-2).
d tumor necrosis factor (TNF).

17 *Autoantibodies to basement membranes is seen in:*

a multiple sclerosis.
b myasthenia gravis.
c Hashimoto's thyroiditis.
d Goodpasture's syndrome.

18 *Ankylosing spondylitis is associated with which HLA antigen?*

a HLA-B17.
b HLA-B8.
c HLA-B27.
d HLA-DR4.

19 *A 50-year-old man develops angioedema after receiving enalapril (Vasotec) for treatment of hypertension. Angioedema is characterized by:*

a a maculopapular rash.
b involvement of the lips, tongue, eyelids, and dorsum of the hands and feet.
c pruritus.
d generalized edema for 7 to 10 days.

20 *Type 1 diabetes mellitus is associated with which HLA antigen?*

a HLA-DR4.
b HLA-B17.
c HLA-B27.
d HLA-DR3.

21 *A 25-year-old woman developed an allergic reaction to intravenous ampicillin. Which of the following statements concerning medication allergies is* **TRUE?**

a Women are less likely than men to develop allergic reactions to medications.
b Parenteral administration causes the most severe reactions.
c Genetic factors do not contribute to the metabolism of medications.
d Steroids should be given prior to the administration of a known drug allergen.

22 *Common findings in serum sickness include:*

a leukocytosis and lymphadenopathy.
b eosinophilia and a normal urinalysis.
c a nonpruritic skin rash.
d leukopenia.

23 *HIV infection is diagnosed by:*

a a positive enzyme-linked immunosorbent assay (ELISA).
b a positive Western blot assay.
c a clinical history of intravenous drug use or homosexuality.
d anemia and leukocytosis.

24 *Common adverse reactions associated with zidovudine (AZT) include:*

a bradycardia and complete heart block.
b bone marrow suppression and myalgias.
c diarrhea.
d viral pneumonia.

25 *A 30-year-old heterosexual man has been diagnosed with HIV infection. He has a CD4 count of 200 and an HIV RNA level of 12,000. He is asymptomatic and continues to work fulltime. What is your plan of care?*

a   Instruct the patient that no treatment is needed because of his asymptomatic state.
b   Start therapy with antiviral agents now.
c   Recheck the patient's CD4 count in 2 weeks.
d   Check the patient's viral load.

26   The diarrhea associated with HIV infection is usually caused by:

a   *Clostridium difficile.*
b   Cryptosporidium.
c   Salmonella.
d   Shigella.

27   IL-2 is clinically significant in that it:

a   increases IgE.
b   induces TNF release from the macrophages.
c   activates granulocytes.
d   increases T cell proliferation and activates B cells.

28   Which of the following is an autoimmune disorder?

a   Peptic ulcer disease
b   Asthma
c   Multiple sclerosis
d   Hashimoto's thyroiditis

29   Causes of generalized lymphadenopathy include:

a   infectious mononucleosis.
b   CMV infection.
c   serum sickness.
d   all of the above.

30   All of the statements concerning lymph node biopsy are true EXCEPT:

a   it may be diagnostic in 50% of patients.
b   it should be performed if the node has increased in size in an area associated with a high incidence of malignancy.
c   a 1-cm anterior cervical lymph node should always be biopsied.
d   it is a minor procedure.

31   Sickle cell disease is associated with:

a   a normal hemoglobin count.
b   microvascular occlusions.
c   normal growth and development.
d   rheumatoid arthritis.

32   A 30-year-old man with HIV infection is being followed in your practice. Which test is best used to evaluate disease progression?

a   Western blot assay
b   CD4 count
c   Viral load
d   Liver function testing

33   All of the statements concerning HIV infection are true EXCEPT:

a   female-to-male transmission is high.
b   50% of patients with untreated HIV infection will progress to developing acquired immune deficiency syndrome (AIDS) over a 10-year period.
c   candida esophagitis is an AIDS-defining illness.
d   AIDS dementia may occur in patients with CD4 counts less than 200.

34   The most common neoplasm associated with AIDS is:

a   Kaposi's sarcoma.
b   Hodgkin's disease.
c   breast cancer.
d   colorectal cancer.

35   Risk factors for HIV infection include a history of:

a   blood transfusion between 1980 and 1990.
b   cervical dysplasia.
c   intravenous drug use.
d   heterosexual relations.

36   Treatment for Mycobacterium avium complex associated with HIV infection includes the use of:

a   clarithromycin (Biaxin), ethambutol (Myambutol), and rifabutin (Mycobutin).
b   trimethoprim sulfamethoxazole.
c   acyclovir.
d   lamivudine (Epivir).

37   The most common viral infections in patients with HIV infection include:

a   herpes simplex.
b   herpes zoster.
c   CMV.
d   all of the above.

38   The most common pathogen associated with bacterial pneumonia in patients with HIV infection is:

a   *Staphylococcus aureus.*
b   *Streptococcus pneumoniae.*
c   *Klebsiella pneumoniae.*
d   Proteus.

39   A 50-year-old man with HIV infection also has a positive tuberculin skin test. What is the best approach for treating this patient?

a   Obtain a baseline chest x-ray and repeat the tuberculin skin test in 3 months.
b   Start isoniazid (Laniazid) therapy.
c   Start treatment with isoniazid, rifampin (Rifadin), and pyrazinamide.
d   Identify all of the patient's personal contacts within the past week.

40 *The most frequent symptom in women with early HIV infection is:*

a candidal vaginitis.
b dysphagia.
c weight loss.
d anorexia.

41 *What is the most immunologic defense in the lung?*

a Complement
b T cells
c Alveolar macrophages
d B cells

42 *Which of the following diseases is transmitted via mosquitoes?*

a Bubonic plaque
b Malaria
c Lyme disease
d Smallpox

43 *Which of the following viruses cause swelling in the parotid glands?*

a Parvovirus
b Herpes simplex virus (HSV)
c Epstein-Barr virus (EBV)
d CMV

44 *Rose-colored spots on the abdomen that blanche with pressure is consistent with:*

a typhoid fever.
b Serratia infection.
c West Nile fever.
d yellow fever.

45 *Which of the following respiratory viruses contain DNA?*

a Parvovirus
b Adenovirus
c RSV
d Influenza virus

46 *Negri bodies are pathognomonic of:*

a malaria.
b typhoid fever.
c tetanus.
d rabies.

47 *Molluscum contagiosum is caused by:*

a adenovirus.
b human papilloma virus (HPV).
c poxvirus.
d HSV type 2.

48 *All of the statements concerning cat-scratch disease are true EXCEPT:*

a it occurs more frequently in the fall and winter.
b splenomegaly is present.
c the prognosis is usually good.
d diagnosis is made by a skin test.

49 *All of the following are protozoan infections EXCEPT:*

a *Giardia lamblia.*
b toxoplasmosis.
c malaria.
d yellow fever.

50 *The classic triad of symptoms associated with yellow fever are:*

a fever, chills, and malaise.
b jaundice, fever, and weight loss.
c jaundice, hemorrhages, and albuminuria.
d jaundice, weight loss, and diarrhea.

51 *A disease that may be preventable by administering the toxoid vaccine is:*

a measles.
b chickenpox.
c hepatitis.
d tetanus.

52 *Target tissues for the herpes virus include all of the following EXCEPT:*

a the genitalia.
b the brain.
c the oral cavities.
d the kidneys.

53 *Immunization with the hepatitis B vaccine would concomitantly protect the patient from:*

a HIV infection.
b hepatitis C.
c hepatitis D.
d hepatitis A.

54 *A 35-year-old nurse has developed Rocky Mountain spotted fever. On physical exam, you note petechiae. She asks you why she has developed petechiae. What is the most likely explanation?*

a Platelet destruction and thrombocytopenia
b Suppression of fibrin synthesis
c Prolongation of the bleeding time
d Bone marrow suppression

55 *Most antibodies are synthesized in the:*

a liver.
b spleen.

c   lymph nodes.
d   thyroid.

56   *The universal blood type is:*

a   O−.
b   AB−.
c   AB+.
d   B+.

57   *Tzanck smears are positive in which of the following viral infections?*

a   HIV infection
b   HSV infection
c   EBV infection
d   HBV infection

58   *All of the statements concerning CMV infection are true* **EXCEPT:**

a   the virus may be transmitted during solid organ transplantation.
b   inclusion bodies are the histologic marker of infection.
c   disseminated CMV infection may affect the liver, brain, and lungs.
d   CMV is not transmitted perinatally.

59   *Donor transplantation from a different species is referred to as a(n):*

a   xenograft.
b   autograft.
c   allograft.
d   isograft.

60   *Donor transplantation from an individual to another who is genetically identical is referred to as a(n):*

a   allograft.
b   isograft.
c   autograft.
d   xenograft.

61   *A typical feature of systemic lupus erythematosus (SLE) is:*

a   hemolytic anemia.
b   abnormal IgM antibodies.
c   antibody to double-stranded DNA.
d   deposition of IgM and IgG antibodies in the synovia of joint fluid.

62   *The primary organ where T cells develop is the:*

a   liver.
b   spleen.
c   thymus.
d   heart.

63   *Bacteria that possess flexible cell envelopes with a corkscrew appearance are:*

a   bacilli.
b   streptococci.
c   spirochetes.
d   cocci.

64   *The transfer of bacterial DNA from one cell to another by means of a virus vehicle is referred to as:*

a   transfection.
b   transduction.
c   conversion.
d   conjugation.

65   *The etiologic agent responsible for chancroid is:*

a   *Haemophilus ducreyi.*
b   *Neisseria gonorrhoeae.*
c   *Streptococcus viridans.*
d   Enterococcus.

66   *Ingestion of infected milk may cause:*

a   *Yersinia pestis.*
b   brucellosis.
c   toxic shock syndrome.
d   *Helicobacter pylori.*

67   *Treatment of brucellosis may include:*

a   penicillin.
b   ciprofloxacin (Cipro).
c   doxycycline (Vibramycin) and rifampin.
d   vancomycin (Vancocin).

68   *All of the statements concerning* Escherichia coli *(*E. coli*) are true* **EXCEPT:**

a   it is a major cause of urinary tract infections.
b   it is a coliform organism.
c   it may produce enteric infections.
d   it is a spirochete.

69   *Manifestations of tertiary syphilis may include:*

a   aortitis and tabes dorsalis.
b   generalized skin rash.
c   chancre.
d   all of the above.

70   *The antibiotic of choice in the treatment of syphilis is:*

a   acyclovir.
b   penicillin.
c   rifampin.
d   trimethoprim sulfamethoxazole.

71 *A systemic reaction that may develop after the initial treatment for syphilis is:*

a cat-scratch fever.
b Jarisch-Herxheimer reaction.
c neurotoxicity.
d photosensitivity reaction.

72 *The causative agent of Lyme disease is:*

a *Treponema pallidum.*
b Mycobacterium.
c Borrelia.
d Spirillum.

73 *All of the statements concerning Lyme disease are true* **EXCEPT:**

a it is associated with migratory arthritis.
b it may cause complete heart block.
c the initial phase consists of a skin lesion—*erythema chronicum migrans.*
d the treatment of choice is erythromycin.

74 *Which of the following medications are used for treatment of systemic aspergillosis?*

a Metronidazole (Flagyl)
b Penicillins
c Amphotericin B (Amphotec)
d Dapsone

75 *The site of action for amphotericin B is:*

a RNA.
b plasma membrane.
c protein synthesis.
d the cytochrome P-450 system.

76 *Histoplasmosis:*

a is a fungal infection.
b is more prevalent in men.
c may be associated with soil disturbances.
d is all of the above.

77 *Pulmonary histoplasmosis may be treated with:*

a nystatin (Mycostatin).
b surgical resection.
c ketoconazole (Nizoral).
d all of the above.

78 *The route of infection for cryptococcus is:*

a blood.
b oral-fecal.
c inhalation.
d direct contact.

79 *The serologic marker for acute hepatitis A infection is:*

a anti-HAV IgM.
b anti-HCV.
c HB_sAg.
d IgG.

80 *Extrahepatic manifestations of hepatitis B viral infection may include:*

a arthralgias.
b glomerulonephritis.
c serum sickness.
d all of the above.

81 *All of the statements concerning rubella are true* **EXCEPT:**

a it is a double-stranded RNA virus.
b transmission is by droplet infection.
c it is associated with a 3-day rash and lymphadenopathy.
d it may be transmitted to the infant at birth.

82 *The most common coxsackievirus disease is:*

a cardiomyopathy.
b aseptic meningitis.
c hepatitis C.
d end-stage renal disease.

83 *Legionnaire's disease is:*

a a self-limiting disease.
b best treated with vancomycin.
c a severe respiratory infection.
d usually contracted via the water supply.

84 **Chlamydia trachomatis** *may cause:*

a rabies.
b inclusion conjunctivitis.
c Q fever.
d toxoplasmosis.

85 *Metronidazole is most effective against:*

a syphilis.
b Chlamydia.
c anaerobic bacteria.
d Staphylococcus.

Answers

1 Answer b
The classes of antibodies include IgA, IgG, IgD, IgE, and IgM. IgB is not a class of antibodies.

2   Answer a
IgA is found primarily in secretions and serves to protect the mucous membranes.

3   Answer c
The virus responsible for shingles is varicella-zoster virus. This virus is responsible for chickenpox early in life and shingles as a latent manifestation. HSV is responsible for oral ulcer and genital herpes. Poxvirus is responsible for smallpox. CMV may cause disseminated disease but is not responsible for shingles.

4   Answer b
The antiviral agent used to treat CMV is ganciclovir. Acyclovir is used to treat herpetic infections. Trimethoprim sulfamethoxazole is an antibiotic.

5   Answer d
Hepatitis E is transmitted via the oral-fecal route. It is usually seen in underdeveloped countries and transmitted via contaminated water.

6   Answer d
The most common opportunistic infection in patients with AIDS is *P. carinii,* which causes a pneumonia.

7   Answer c
Rhinovirus is the virus most commonly associated with the common cold.

8   Answer c
IgM comprises 10% of the normal serum immunoglobulins, is the predominant early antibody that fixes to complement, and is one of the two major immunoglobulins (in conjunction with IgD) found on the surface of B cells. IgG, not IgM, is the only class of immunoglobulins able to pass through the placenta.

9   Answer d
A history of profound fatigue, low-grade fever, and lymphadenopathy may be associated with viral hepatitis, HIV infection, and subacute bacterial endocarditis.

10   Answer a
Reed-Sternberg cells are associated with Hodgkin's disease.

11   Answer b
A lung tumor staged as T3N2M0 is a large lung tumor that has ipsilateral, mediastinal node involvement without distant metastases.

12   Answer a
The treatment of choice for patients with stage IA or IIA Hodgkin's disease is radiation therapy. Adjunctive chemotherapy may be used if the patient has a large mediastinal mass.

13   Answer b
Immunologic testing of renal transplant donors and recipients includes ABO and HLA compatibility testing.

14   Answer d
Anaphylaxis would not be treated with milrinone. Epinephrine and steroids are usually administered initially to reverse the effects of hypotension and bronchospasm. Famotidine, which is a histamine blocker, may decrease the vasodilatory response.

15   Answer c
A normal lymph node contains low endothelial venules, a germinal center, and primary follicles.

16   Answer a
Cellular immunity is mediated by T cells.

17   Answer d
Autoantibodies to basement membranes of the glomeruli and alveoli are seen in Goodpasture's syndrome.

18   Answer c
Ankylosing spondylitis is associated with HLA-B27.

19   Answer b
Angioedema is characterized by involvement of the lips, tongue, eyelids, and dorsum of the hands and feet. Angioedema does not usually involve a rash or pruritus, nor does the edema persist.

20   Answer a
Type 1 diabetes mellitus is associated with HLA-DR4.

21   Answer b
Medication allergies are more severe if the medication is administered parenterally. Many factors may contribute to allergic manifestations, including genetic metabolism of the medications. Unless desensitization is planned, a known drug allergen should not be administered. Women are affected by allergic reactions more commonly than men.

22   Answer a
Common findings in serum sickness include leukocytosis and lymphadenopathy, as well as circulating plasma cells, fever, urticaria, arthralgias, and albuminuria.

23   Answer b
HIV infection is diagnosed by a positive Western blot assay. ELISA is the initial test performed for HIV infection, and if positive, the diagnosis is confirmed by a positive Western blot assay. Patients at risk for HIV include those who are intravenous drug users and homosexual men; however, a clinical history is not specific for HIV.

24   Answer b
Common adverse reactions associated with zidovudine include bone marrow suppression and myalgias. Other reactions may include tremors, headaches, and seizures. Zidovudine has no cardiovascular or pulmonary effects. It has been associated with nausea and anorexia but not diarrhea.

25   Answer b
Your plan of care for the patient described is to start therapy with antiviral agents. The recommendation from the Centers for Disease Control and Prevention (CDC) for the patient with HIV infection is to start antiviral drug therapy if the patient has a CD4 count less than 500 and an HIV RNA level greater than 10,000.

26   Answer b
The diarrhea associated with HIV infection is usually caused by Cryptosporidium. Cryptosporidium usually affects the small bowel and causes massive diarrhea leading to dehydration.

27   Answer d
IL-2 is clinically significant in that it increases T cell proliferation and activates B cells.

28 Answer d

Hashimoto's thyroiditis is an autoimmune disorder and is the leading cause of multinodular goiter in the United States. This immunologically mediated process may lead to progressive loss of thyroid function and hypothyroidism. Peptic ulcer disease has been linked to infectious causes, but it is not an autoimmune disorder. Asthma is an inflammatory response, but sensitization plays an important role. Multiple sclerosis is a demyelinating disease of the central nervous system.

29 Answer d

Causes of generalized lymphadenopathy include infectious mononucleosis, CMV infection, and serum sickness. Other causes include HIV infection, syphilis, toxoplasmosis, non-Hodgkin's lymphoma, myeloid leukemia, rheumatoid arthritis, and SLE.

30 Answer c

A 1-cm lymph node may be a normal variant, and a biopsy should not be performed unless there is clinical suspicion. Lymph node biopsy is a minor procedure; and may be diagnostic in more than 50% of patients. Biopsy of a lymph node should be performed if the node has increased in size in an area associated with a high incidence of malignancy.

31 Answer b

Sickle cell disease is associated with microvascular occlusions that may lead to end-organ damage to the lungs, kidneys, bone, skin, and eyes. Sickle cell disease is associated with anemia secondary to shortened red blood cell survival, retardation of growth and development, and joint pain not associated with rheumatoid arthritis. Sickle cell crisis is characterized by joint pain secondary to the vaso-occlusive process and may be accompanied by noninflammatory effusions in the joint spaces.

32 Answer c

The best test to evaluate disease progression of HIV infection is a viral load. The viral load is the number of copies of the disease in a centimeter of blood. The viral load and CD4 count may be used in combination to monitor disease progression and response to treatments. Western blot assay is used to diagnose HIV. Liver function tests are taken at baseline in evaluation of HIV.

33 Answer a

The transmission of HIV infection is highest in men to women.

34 Answer a

The most common neoplasm associated with AIDS is Kaposi's sarcoma. Other neoplasms associated with AIDS include non-Hodgkin's lymphoma and cervical carcinoma.

35 Answer c

Risk factors for HIV infection include intravenous drug use, a history of blood transfusion between 1978 and 1985, multiple sexual partners, a history of sexually transmitted disease, prostitution, sex with prostitutes, and male homosexual relations.

36 Answer a

Treatment for *M. avium complex* may include clarithromycin, ethambutol, and rifabutin.

37 Answer d

The most common viral infections in patients with HIV infection include herpes simplex, herpes zoster, and CMV.

38 Answer b

The most common pathogen associated with bacterial pneumonia in patients with HIV infection is *S. pneumoniae*. Other pathogens that may occur include *H. influenzae* and *Moraxella catarrhalis*.

39 Answer c

The best approach for treating a patient with HIV infection and a positive tuberculin skin test is to start three-drug therapy with isoniazid, rifampin, and pyrazinamide. Investigation into the presence of extrapulmonary tuberculosis should also be pursued.

40 Answer a

The most frequent symptom in women with early HIV infection is candidal vaginitis. HPV may be seen also and contributes to the development of cervical warts and dysplasia.

41 Answer c

The most immunologic defense in the lung is alveolar macrophages.

42 Answer b

Malaria is transmitted via mosquitoes.

43 Answer a

Parvovirus causes swelling in the parotid glands, which is known as mumps.

44 Answer a

Typhoid fever is an acute systemic disease caused by *Salmonella typhi*. Common symptoms include malaise, fever, and headaches. The classic rash associated with typhoid fever includes rose-colored spots, usually 2 to 4 mm in size, located on the abdomen and upper thorax that blanche with pressure.

45 Answer b

The respiratory virus that contains DNA is adenovirus.

46 Answer d

Negri bodies are pathognomonic of rabies.

47 Answer c

M. contagiosum is an infectious disease of the skin and mucous membranes caused by poxvirus. The diagnosis can usually be made by the characteristic appearance of the lesions and is definitively made by electron microscopy.

48 Answer b

Cat-scratch fever is an infection characterized by generalized lymphadenitis following a scratch or close contact with a cat. Systemic symptoms are usually mild and may consist of headache, malaise, and fever. Many persons may be asymptomatic. Diagnosis is made by a skin test that will manifest as a 5- to 10-mm induration 24 to 48 hours after injection. Splenomegaly is not present.

49 Answer d

Yellow fever is caused by arbovirus and is not a protozoan infection. *G. lamblia*, toxoplasmosis, and malaria are all protozoan infections.

50 Answer c

The classic triad of symptoms associated with yellow fever comprises jaundice, hemorrhages, and albuminuria.

51   Answer d

A disease that may be preventable by administering the toxoid vaccine is tetanus.

52   Answer d

Target tissues for the herpes virus do not include the kidneys. Herpes may infect the genitalia, brain, and oral cavities.

53   Answer c

Immunization with the hepatitis B vaccine would concomitantly protect the patient from hepatitis D.

54   Answer a

The most likely explanation for the development of petechiae in patients with Rocky Mountain spotted fever is platelet destruction and thrombocytopenia.

55   Answer b

Most antibodies are synthesized in the spleen.

56   Answer a

The universal blood type is O−.

57   Answer b

Tzanck smears are positive in herpes simplex viral infection.

58   Answer d

CMV is not transmitted perinatally. CMV can be transmitted by primary infection of the pregnant woman, via infected cervical secretions at the time of delivery, and via infected breast milk. The virus may affect the liver, brain, and lungs, and can be transmitted during solid organ transplantation. The inclusion bodies are the histologic marker of infection.

59   Answer a

Donor transplantation from a different species is referred to as a xenograft.

60   Answer b

Donor transplantation from one individual to another who is genetically identical, such as in twins, is referred to as an isograft or a syngraft. An allograft is from one individual to another of the same species. An autograft is a graft from one area of the body to another in the same individual.

61   Answer c

A typical feature of SLE is the production of antibodies to double-stranded DNA.

62   Answer c

The primary organ where T cells develop is the thymus.

63   Answer c

Bacteria that possess flexible cell envelopes with a corkscrew appearance are spirochetes. Bacilli are rod-shaped bacteria. Cocci are spherical bacteria, whereas streptococci are arranged in chains.

64   Answer b

The transfer of bacterial DNA from one cell to another by means of a virus vehicle is referred to as transduction.

65   Answer a

The etiologic agent responsible for chancroid is *H. ducreyi.* Chancroid is an ulcerated, highly contagious lesion that is transmitted sexually.

66   Answer b

Ingestion of infected milk may cause brucellosis. Brucellosis is a disease found primarily in the genitourinary tract of domestic animals. It is prevalent in goats, cattle, and pigs, with the most common route of infection being infected milk, milk products, or meat.

67   Answer c

Treatment of brucellosis may include doxycycline and rifampin.

68   Answer d

E. coli is a coliform organism that may produce enteric infections, and it may be a cause of urinary tract infections. It is not a spirochete.

69   Answer a

Manifestations of tertiary syphilis usually involve the cardiovascular and central nervous systems. Cardiovascular manifestations may include aortitis and aortic regurgitation. Central nervous system manifestations may include meningitis, tabes dorsalis, generalized paresis, and mental deterioration.

70   Answer b

The antibiotic of choice in the treatment of syphilis is penicillin.

71   Answer b

A systemic reaction that may develop after the initial treatment for syphilis is Jarisch-Herxheimer reaction, which is characterized by headache, malaise, and fever.

72   Answer c

The causative agent of Lyme disease is *Borrelia burgdorferi,* which is a spirochete. *Treponema pallidum* and Spirillum are both spirochetes.

73   Answer c

Lyme disease is associated with migratory arthritis and may cause complete heart block. The initial phase of the disease consists of headaches, myalgias, stiff neck, and *erythema chronicum migrans.* The treatment of choice in Lyme disease is tetracycline, not erythromycin.

74   Answer c

Amphotericin B is the medication utilized to treat systemic aspergillosis.

75   Answer b

The site of action for amphotericin B is the plasma membrane. The drug interferes with the sterols in the fungal cell membrane, which affect membrane permeability.

76   Answer d

Histoplasmosis is a fungal infection that is more prevalent in men and may be associated with soil disturbance. The infection is also associated with roosting areas of birds.

77   Answer b

Pulmonary histoplasmosis may be treated with surgical resection. Other treatment may include the use of amphotericin B. Mycostatin and ketoconazole have no role in the treatment of histoplasmosis.

78   Answer c

The route of infection for cryptococcus is inhalation.

79 Answer a

The serologic marker for acute hepatitis A infection is anti-HAV IgM.

80 Answer d

Extrahepatic manifestations of hepatitis B viral infection may include arthralgias, arthritis, glomerulonephritis, serum sickness, and polyarteritis nodosa.

81 Answer a

Rubella is a single-stranded, not double-stranded, RNA virus. Transmission is by droplet infection, is associated with a 3-day rash and lymphadenopathy, and may be transmitted to the infant at birth.

82 Answer b

The most common Coxsackie virus disease is aseptic meningitis. Other disorders that may be associated with Coxsackie include pericarditis, myocarditis, respiratory infections, and diabetes mellitus.

83 Answer c

Legionnaire's disease is a severe respiratory infection and usually transmitted via air conditioner units.

84 Answer b

C. trachomatis may cause inclusion conjunctivitis.

85 Answer c

Metronidazole is most effective against anaerobic bacteria.

Bibliography

Ben-Efraim, S: Cancer Immunotherapy: Hopes and pitfalls: A review. Anticancer Res 16:3235–3240, 1996.

Buckley, RH, et al: The use of intravenous immunoglobulin in immunodeficiency diseases. N Eng J Med 325:100–117, 1991.

Chabner, BA, and Longo, DL: Cancer Chemotherapy and Biotherapy—Principles and Practice, 2nd ed. Lippincott Williams & Wilkins, Philadelphia, 1996.

Dunphy, L: Management Guidelines for Adult Nurse Practitioners. FA Davis, Philadelphia, 1999.

Goroll, A, et al: Primary Care Medicine Office Evaluation and Management of the Adult Patient, 4th ed. Lippincott Williams & Wilkins, Philadelphia, 2000.

11

Musculoskeletal Problems

1 *Bony enlargement in the proximal interphalangeal joints is called:*

a gout.
b Heberden's nodes.
c Bouchard's nodes.
d acromegaly.

2 *A 65-year-old woman has been diagnosed with osteoporosis. Which of the following are risk factors for the development of osteoporosis?*

a Inadequate calcium intake
b Smoking
c Small body statue
d All of the above

3 *The classic site for acute gout is the:*

a great toe.
b wrist.
c knee.
d ankle.

4 *A 75-year-old woman is suspected of having osteoarthritis of the hip. Which of the radiographic findings support the diagnosis?*

a Compression fracture of the femoral head
b Joint space narrowing in the hip
c Subluxation of the vertebral body
d Increased bone density

5 *Which portion of the shoulder may have a high incidence of degenerative arthritis?*

a Acromion
b Acromioclavicular joint
c Glenohumeral joint
d Coracoid process

6 *A palpable or even audible crunching or grating sound produced by movement of a joint is called:*

a crepitation.
b snap.
c rub.
d bruit.

7 *What normal musculoskeletal change(s) is(are) associated with aging?*

a Decreased range of motion
b Atrophy of the arms and legs
c Loss of height
d All of the above

8 *A 40-year-old woman is seen for complaints of swelling and tenderness (without erythema) of the wrist initially and then the ankle joints over the past 3 months. She also complains of decreased energy level and weight loss over the same time period. What is the most likely diagnosis?*

a Polymyalgia rheumatica
b Osteoarthritis
c Rheumatoid arthritis
d Acute gouty arthritis

9 *Which cranial nerve tests the motor aspect of the sternomastoid and trapezius muscles?*

a Cranial nerve V (trigeminal)
b Cranial nerve III (oculomotor)
c Cranial nerve VII (facial)
d Cranial nerve XI (spinal accessory)

10 *A 20-year-old man came to the emergency department after falling off his bicycle and thinks he has a sprained ankle. Which of the following findings support the diagnosis of a sprained ankle?*

a Eversion and dorsiflexion of the ankle produces pain

b Inversion and plantar flexion of the foot causes pain

c A bulging of fluid at the ankle

d The inability to bear weight on the ankle

11 *Swan neck deformities of the fingers may be seen in patients with:*

a chronic rheumatoid arthritis (RA).

b osteoarthritis.

c acute RA.

d acute tenosynovitis.

12 *A patient who has had lung surgery should be instructed to perform arm exercises to prevent which of the following complications?*

a Rotator cuff tear

b Adhesive capsulitis

c Medial epicondylitis

d Acromioclavicular arthritis

13 *Flattening of the lumbar curve, decreased spinal mobility, and lumbar muscle spasm may be associated with:*

a scoliosis.

b lumbar lordosis.

c a herniated lumbar disc.

d metastatic cancer.

14 *A 75-year-old woman has acute gout, and you are prescribing intravenous colchicine. Which side effects should be closely monitored in the older adults?*

a Diarrhea

b Syncope

c Bone marrow suppression

d Cardiac arrest

15 *The treatment of choice in a patient with acute crystalline-induced arthritis is:*

a bed rest.

b nonsteroidal anti-inflammatory drugs (NSAIDs).

c steroids.

d intravenous colchicine.

16 *A 45-year-old man has been diagnosed with Reiter's syndrome. What clinical manifestations are associated with Reiter's syndrome?*

a Genital infection, arthritis, and conjunctivitis

b Conjunctivitis, low-back pain, and fever

c Gout, urethritis, and night sweats

d Chills, diarrhea, and arthritis

17 *The therapeutic options for treating ankylosing spondylitis include:*

a surgery.

b patient education and physical therapy.

c NSAIDs only.

d surgery and physical therapy.

18 *A 35-year-old man is having a routine physical exam. He has no significant previous health history. He complains of low-back pain, relieved with exercise for the past 4 months. He states the pain is at its worst in the morning. What is the most likely diagnosis?*

a Sciatica

b Osteoarthritis

c Rheumatoid arthritis

d Ankylosing spondylitis

19 *Which of the following should be done to support a diagnosis of ankylosing spondylitis?*

a Further history

b Physical exam

c Radiograph of the pelvis

d All of the above

20 *What is the most common cause of death in patients with Duchenne's dystrophy?*

a Cardiomyopathy

b Seizures

c Pulmonary embolus

d Fractures

21 *A 30-year-old woman is seen for complaints of low-back pain after moving into her new home the past weekend. The pain is in her lower back and radiates down to the left thigh. What is the most likely diagnosis?*

a L5-S1 strain

b C5 strain

c L4-L5 strain

d T10 strain

22 *Which of the following therapies are not used to treat RA?*

a Steroids

b NSAIDs

c Antimalarials

d Antibiotics

Questions 23 and 24 refer to the following scenario:

A 25-year-old man is seen in the emergency department after suffering an injury while playing touch football. He describes a twisting of his left leg and a sharp pain at the anteromedial aspect of the left knee. He was unable to walk or straighten his knee after the incident and had to be taken off the field. Physical exam reveals swelling on the medial aspect of the left knee and excruciating anteromedial pain with passive extension of the knee.

23 *What is the most likely diagnosis?*

a Torn left medial meniscus
b Fractured patella
c Torn left medial collateral ligament
d Fractured tibia

24 *The treatment of choice for the patient is:*

a a full leg cast.
b heat and elevation.
c physical therapy.
d arthroscopic surgery.

25 *An 80-year-old woman is brought to the emergency department after falling down the steps and landing on her left hand. She is complaining of left wrist and hand pain. Physical exam reveals tenderness in the area of the left wrist and outward deformity of the wrist. The radial and brachial pulses are intact, as is sensation. What is the most likely diagnosis?*

a Fracture of the distal ulna
b Colles' fracture
c Carpal tunnel syndrome
d Dislocation of the ulnar head

26 *The treatment of choice for a Colles' fracture is:*

a internal fixation.
b external reduction and immobilization.
c ice and elevation.
d internal reduction and immobilization.

27 *All of the statements concerning Colles' fracture are true* **EXCEPT:**

a it is caused by a fall on an outstretched hand.
b it is associated with osteoporosis.
c it is more common in older men.
d it is a fracture of the distal radius.

28 *A malignant bone-forming tumor is:*

a osteochondroma.
b osteosarcoma.
c Paget's disease.
d osteoid osteoma.

29 *The most common malignant bone lesion is:*

a Ewing's sarcoma.
b metastatic carcinoma.
c multiple myeloma.
d osteosarcoma.

30 *A patient is suspected of having multiple myeloma. Which laboratory finding is associated with multiple myeloma?*

a Hypocalcemia
b Bence Jones protein in the urine
c Leukocytosis
d Hypokalemia

31 *What is the daily requirement of calcium in a postmenopausal woman?*

a 500 mg
b 1500 mg
c 1000 mg
d 2000 mg

32 *Causes of rickets include all of the following* **EXCEPT:**

a vitamin D deficiency.
b chronic renal insufficiency.
c hypophosphatasia.
d hypercalcemia.

33 *A 75 year-old woman had surgery to repair a left femur fracture 6 hours ago and has a long leg cast. You are called to evaluate her because of complaints of severe left leg pain and tingling in her foot despite intravenous morphine. Physical exam reveals diminished left pedal and posterior tibial pulses with sluggish capillary refill to the toenail beds. The left foot is edematous and cool, and lifting of the left leg produces excruciating pain. What is the most likely diagnosis?*

a Compartment syndrome
b Acute deep vein thrombosis
c Acute gout
d Postoperative infection

34 *The earliest sign of compartment syndrome is:*

a pain.
b pallor.
c paralysis.
d pulselessness.

35 *Which of the following are late signs associated with compartment syndrome?*

a Pain and pallor
b Pain and pulselessness
c Paralysis and pulselessness
d Pallor and paresthesias

36 *Common causes of compartment syndrome are:*

a arterial injury and fracture.
b deep-vein thrombosis and immobility.
c fracture and fat embolism.
d peripheral vascular disease and fracture.

37 *A 70-year-old woman is having a routine physical exam during admission to a nursing care facility. Her past medical history includes hypertension, gout, hypothyroidism, and osteoporosis. She complains of symmetrical skin tightening involving the hands and fingers for the past 3 to 4 months associated with cold intolerance of the hands. She also complains of a 20-lb weight loss over the past year and bilateral ankle swelling. Physical exam reveals normal vital signs. The skin has scattered facial and chest telangiectasias, skin tautness of the hands, and normal motor strength. What is the most likely diagnosis?*

a Reiter's syndrome
b RA
c Scleroderma
d Polymyalgia rheumatica

38 *Which of the following gastrointestinal (GI) complications may develop secondary to scleroderma?*

a Esophageal strictures
b Pancreatitis
c Cholelithiasis
d Peptic ulcer disease

39 *The CREST syndrome is associated with:*

a RA.
b Reiter's syndrome.
c systemic lupus erythematosus (SLE).
d scleroderma.

40 *A 50-year-old woman with RA is seen in the clinic. You are discussing with the patient other manifestations of the disease. Extra-articular manifestations of RA include:*

a renal failure.
b subcutaneous nodules and carpal tunnel syndrome.
c hypothyroidism.
d cardiomyopathy.

41 *According to the American College of Rheumatology, which of the following criteria must be fulfilled to diagnose RA?*

a Morning stiffness, arthritis of three areas lasting more than 6 weeks, and radiographic changes
b Morning stiffness and arthritis of hand joints lasting more than 2 weeks
c Positive rheumatoid factor and anemia
d Symmetric arthritis lasting more than 2 weeks and radiographic changes

42 *Which of the following rheumatic diseases may have significant skin findings?*

a Polymyalgia rheumatica
b Reiter's syndrome

c Osteoarthritis
d SLE

43 *Which of the following complications is associated with SLE?*

a Cerebritis
b Cardiomyopathy
c Hypertension
d Hypercalcemia

44 *Which of the following disorders may present with a polyarticular pattern?*

a Gonococcal arthritis
b Acute rheumatic fever
c Lyme disease
d All of the above

45 *The hallmark sign of hypertrophic pulmonary osteoarthropathy is:*

a cyanosis.
b edema.
c clubbing.
d pallor.

46 *All of the statements concerning SLE are true* **EXCEPT:**

a it is more common in men.
b its peak incidence is premenopausal.
c it is common among African-American women.
d it may lead to renal failure.

47 *A 30-year-old woman with a 4-month history of painful ankle, knee, and wrist joints comes to the clinic. She admits to swelling of the joint space and morning stiffness lasting approximately 2 hours. She has noted 3 months of extreme fatigue and two episodes of facial rash. Physical exam reveals a young woman in no acute distress. An erythematous rash is noted on her forehead and cheeks. Joint exam reveals swelling of the ankles and knees. You suspect SLE. What is the next step in your evaluation?*

a Order complement levels.
b Obtain a more detailed history and physical.
c Refer the patient to a rheumatologist.
d Order radiographs of the ankles, knees, and wrists.

48 *Which laboratory findings suggest a diagnosis of SLE?*

a Low complement levels and antibodies to double-stranded DNA
b Anemia and elevated erythrocyte sedimentation rate
c Leukocytosis
d Proteinuria and thrombocytopenia

49 A 40-year-old woman presents with complaints of bilateral swollen knees associated with painful ambulation for the past month. She denies trauma. You plan to aspirate one of the knees for fluid. Which of the synovial fluid findings are consistent with a diagnosis of RA?

a White blood cell count less than 100,000/mm^3
b Presence of ragocytes
c Positive culture findings
d Synovial fluid glucose level equal to that of the serum

50 All of the statements concerning ankylosing spondylitis are true **EXCEPT:**

a it is more common in men.
b it is associated with HLA-B27.
c the knee joints are most frequently affected.
d aortic insufficiency may be present.

51 Motor strength is graded on a scale of 0–5. What is a grade 2 muscle strength?

a Full strength.
b No muscle contraction.
c Muscle contraction occurs, but it is not sufficient to overcome gravity.
d Muscle contracts with little or no movement.

52 Golfer's elbow is:

a inflammation of the medial epicondyle.
b inflammation of the lateral epicondyle.
c associated with pain when extending the elbow against resistance.
d associated with carpal tunnel syndrome.

53 Heberden's nodes is usually seen in patients with:

a RA.
b scleroderma.
c osteoarthritis.
d ankylosing spondylitis.

54 A 40-year-old woman is seen in the emergency department with complaints of wrist pain after falling on the ice. Which of the following maneuvers assesses motor function of the ulnar nerve?

a Extending the wrist
b Extending the elbow
c Spreading the fingers
d Touching the fingers to the opposite hand

55 The most frequent portion of the **GI** tract to become involved in scleroderma is the:

a gallbladder.
b pancreas.
c duodenum.
d esophagus.

56 Treatment for patients with polymyalgia rheumatica may include:

a gold salts.
b quinine.
c steroids.
d aspirin therapy.

57 A 25-year-old woman is suspected of having polymyositis. What laboratory test would you expect to be abnormal?

a Complete blood cell count (CBC)
b Calcium level
c Creatine kinase level
d Phosphorus level

58 Differential diagnosis of a patient with proximal muscle weakness and fatigue includes:

a hypothyroidism.
b polymyositis.
c RA
d All of the above

59 Which of the following arthritic conditions is associated with diarrhea?

a Reiter's syndrome
b Scleroderma
c SLE
d Fibromyalgia

60 Treatment for fibromyalgia includes:

a NSAIDs, amitriptyline (Elavil), and aerobic exercises.
b heat and NSAIDs.
c steroids.
d bedrest and NSAIDs.

61 All of the statements concerning Paget's disease are true **EXCEPT:**

a most patients are asymptomatic.
b treatments may include calcitonin.
c effective treatment results in an increase in serum alkaline phosphatase levels.
d the most common sites of involvement are the spine, pelvis, skull, femur, and tibia.

62 A 60-year-old man with known Paget's disease is seen for a 24-hour history of leg weakness and the inability to control bowels. What should be your priority for care in this patient?

a Check alkaline phosphatase level.
b Start calcitonin.
c Obtain a prompt neurosurgery consultation.
d Obtain pelvic radiographs.

63 *The use of calcitonin for Paget's disease causes a(n):*

a decrease in osteoclastic resorption.
b decrease in inflammation in the bones.
c increase in bone resorption.
d decrease in vitamin D stores.

64 *The most common cause of generalized musculoskeletal pain in women between the ages of 20 and 55 is:*

a fibromyalgia.
b arthritis.
c SLE.
d osteoporosis.

65 *A 65-year-old carpenter is seen for complaints of pain in the right shoulder, particularly at night, and he has been unable to sleep on his right side because of the pain. He states that the symptoms have been present for the past 10 days and denies injury to the shoulder. Physical exam reveals pain over the right deltoid area and radiation to the right upper arm with pain on abduction of the arm. What is the most likely diagnosis?*

a RA
b Osteoarthritis
c Polymyalgia rheumatica
d Rotator cuff tendinitis

66 *Which diagnostic modality is preferred in the evaluation of a patient with chronic shoulder pain?*

a Magnetic resonance imaging (MRI)
b Ultrasound
c Radiograph
d Bone scan

67 *Differential diagnosis of shoulder pain should include which of the following?*

a Myocardial ischemia
b Gallbladder disease
c Disc herniation
d All of the above

68 *Pain on palpation and crepitation over the acromioclavicular joint may indicate:*

a RA.
b a shoulder fracture.
c impingement of the rotator cuff.
d a frozen shoulder.

69 *The rheumatoid factor is positive:*

a 100% of the time in RA.
b in patients with gout.
c in only RA.
d in approximately 20% of patients with juvenile RA.

70 *Patients with ankylosing spondylitis may have concurrent:*

a mitral valve prolapse.
b aortic insufficiency.
c mitral stenosis.
d aortic stenosis.

71 *The major cause(s) of hip fractures in young adults is(are):*

a falls and trauma.
b osteomyelitis.
c arthritis.
d avascular necrosis.

72 *A 50-year-old patient with an anterior hip dislocation after a motor vehicle accident should be closely monitored for which of the following early complications?*

a Bleeding
b Injury to the femoral artery and nerve
c Lower extremity edema
d Aseptic necrosis

73 *A 75-year-old woman is 1 year after total hip replacement (THR). Which position should she be told to avoid to minimize posterior location of the THR?*

a Extension of the knee
b Flexion of the hip
c External rotation of the hip
d Flexion of the knee

74 *The most common organism that may cause infection in the patient with a THR is:*

a *Escherichia coli.*
b *Staphylococcus aureus.*
c Pseudomonas.
d Candida.

75 *Differential diagnosis of low-back pain includes:*

a a herniated disc.
b tuberculosis.
c ovarian cysts.
d all of the above.

76 *A 40-year-old woman was treated for 2 weeks with heat and NSAIDs for complaints of neck and upper back pain. She now states she awakened this morning with the inability to move her neck and says she has weakness in her arms. Physical exam findings reveal decreased sensation in the index finger, weakness of the deltoid and biceps muscles, and pain upon movement of neck to the left. She denies trauma or previous history of similar symptoms. What is the most likely diagnosis?*

a   C5-C6 herniated disc
b   C7 herniated disc
c   C6 herniated disc
d   C8 herniated disc

77   *What is the most common arthritis involving the elbow?*

a   Osteoarthritis
b   RA
c   Traumatic arthritis
d   Gouty arthritis

78   *The first step in evaluating an elbow injury is:*

a   to perform a physical exam of the elbow.
b   to order an x-ray of the joint.
c   to obtain a thorough history.
d   to obtain a computed tomography (CT) scan of the elbow.

79   *Treatment for multiple myeloma includes:*

a   chemotherapy.
b   surgery.
c   radiation.
d   all of the above.

80   *What is the most likely cause of an acute monoarthritis in an elderly patient hospitalized for exacerbation of congestive heart failure (CHF)?*

a   Gout
b   Lyme disease
c   Septic arthritis
d   RA

81   *Diagnostic studies that may be useful in the evaluation of monarthritic states include:*

a   a serum uric acid level.
b   a CBC.
c   a prothrombin time.
d   all of the above.

82   *HLA-B27 is positive in which of the following disorders?*

a   RA
b   Ankylosing spondylitis
c   Reiter's syndrome
d   Scleroderma

83   *A 45-year-old woman with erythema marginatum should be suspected of having:*

a   acute rheumatic fever.
b   hemochromatosis.
c   Lyme disease.
d   Reiter's syndrome.

84   *A 50-year-old man complains of low-back pain with weakness and pain in both legs. The pain is worsened with standing but is not present in the sitting position. What is the most likely diagnosis?*

a   Sciatica
b   L5 herniated disc
c   Spinal stenosis
d   Ankylosing spondylitis

85   *Which of the following is associated with avascular necrosis of the femoral head?*

a   Trauma
b   Steroid use
c   Sickle cell anemia
d   All of the above

Answers

1   Answer c
Bony enlargement in the proximal interphalangeal joints is called Bouchard's nodes, which are commonly seen in osteoarthritis. Gout usually is characterized by acute inflammation of the joint. Heberden's nodes are bony enlargements in the distal interphalangeal joints of the hands.

2   Answer d
Risk factors for the development of osteoporosis include inadequate calcium intake, smoking, and small statue persons with lower bone mass.

3   Answer a
The classic site for acute gout is the metatarsophalangeal (MTP) joint of the great toe. Gout may also occur in the wrist, knee, and ankle.

4   Answer b
Radiographic findings that support the diagnosis of osteoarthritis of the hip include joint space narrowing in the hip, usually the result of cartilage erosion. Other findings may include osteophyte formation secondary to synovial membrane stimulation, loose bodies secondary to degeneration of the osteochondral surface, and subchondral cysts secondary to extravasation of synovial fluid into the joint space.

5   Answer b
The portion of the shoulder with the highest incidence of degenerative arthritis is the acromioclavicular joint.

6   Answer a
A palpable or audible crunching or grating sound produced by movement of a joint is called crepitation.

7   Answer d
Normal physiologic musculoskeletal changes associated with aging include decreased range of motion, atrophy of the arms and legs, and loss of height.

8   Answer c
The most likely diagnosis in the patient described is RA. RA is a chronic inflammatory response in the synovial mem-

branes with degeneration of adjacent cartilage, bone, and ligaments. RA is a progressive process, which spreads to other joints while persisting in the initial joint, and is frequently accompanied by swelling and tenderness of the joints without erythema. Constitutional symptoms of fever, malaise, weight loss, and weakness may be associated with RA. Polymyalgia rheumatica is most often seen in women over age 50, commonly affects the muscles of the neck, shoulder, and upper arms, and is not associated with joint swelling. Osteoarthritis is usually not associated with constitutional symptoms. Acute gouty arthritis is less likely associated with the duration of symptoms and is usually confined to one joint.

9   Answer d

The cranial nerve that tests the motor aspect of the sternomastoid and trapezius muscles is cranial nerve XI, the spinal accessory nerve.

10   Answer b

The finding that supports the diagnosis of a sprained ankle is when inversion and plantar flexion of the foot causes pain. Soft-tissue swelling and the inability to bear weight on the ankle may be seen in ankle sprain, but neither is diagnostic.

11   Answer a

Swan-neck deformities of the fingers may be seen in patients with chronic RA. The swan-neck deformity is characterized by hyperextension of the proximal interphalangeal (PIP) joints with fixed flexion of the distal interphalangeal joints.

12   Answer b

A patient who has had lung surgery should be instructed to perform arm exercises to prevent adhesive capsulitis, which is a frozen shoulder. A frozen shoulder may develop because of limited movement of the arm and shoulder on the affected side. Rotator cuff tear and acromioclavicular arthritis is usually the result of injury. Medial epicondylitis is pain in the elbow following repetitive wrist flexion, as seen in pitchers.

13   Answer c

Flattening of the lumbar curve, decreased spinal mobility, and lumbar muscle spasm may be associated with a herniated lumbar disc.

14   Answer c

The side effect that should be closely monitored in the elderly patient receiving intravenous colchicine is bone marrow suppression. Diarrhea is an anticipated effect of the medication.

15   Answer b

The treatment of choice in a patient with acute crystalline-induced arthritis is to give NSAIDs. Other optimal treatment options may include aspiration of the joint fluid and instillation of steroids into the joint space.

16   Answer a

Reiter's syndrome is characterized by urogenital infection, arthritis, conjunctivitis, urethritis, and cutaneous lesions.

17   Answer b

The therapeutic options for treating ankylosing spondylitis are patient education, physical therapy, and the use of NSAIDs. There is no role for surgery in treating ankylosing spondylitis.

18   Answer d

The most likely diagnosis of the patient described is ankylosing spondylitis. Ankylosing spondylitis usually presents before the age of 40, has prolonged morning stiffness, improves with exercise, and may produce daily symptoms.

19   Answer d

History, physical exam, and a radiograph of the pelvis are done to support the diagnosis of ankylosing spondylitis. The x-ray will show evidence of bilateral sacroiliitis.

20   Answer a

The most common cause of death in patients with Duchenne's dystrophy is cardiomyopathy.

21   Answer a

The most likely diagnosis of the patient described is L5-S1 strain.

22   Answer d

Treatment of RA does not include antibiotics. It does include the use of steroids, NSAIDs, and antimalarials.

23   Answer a

The most likely diagnosis is a torn left medial meniscus. The history and presentation described in the scenario is classic for medial meniscus injuries, which are usually the result of a twisting injury. The knee will acutely swell, and the patient will be unable to fully extend the knee.

24   Answer d

The treatment of choice for the patient with a medial meniscus tear is arthroscopic surgery. Other treatment options may include ice and elevation, but arthroscopic surgery is the treatment of choice.

25   Answer b

The most likely diagnosis for the patient described is a Colles' fracture, which is a fracture of the distal radius. It is usually caused by a fall on the outstretched hand, and is associated with osteoporosis.

26   Answer b

The treatment of choice for a Colles' fracture is external reduction and immobilization. The external reduction is done under anesthesia.

27   Answer c

Colles' fracture is more common in elderly women, not men. It is caused by a fall on an outstretched hand, is associated with osteoporosis, and is a fracture of the distal radius.

28   Answer b

A malignant bone-forming tumor is osteosarcoma. Osteochondroma and osteoid osteoma are benign lesions. Paget's disease is characterized by deformity of the bone's external contour secondary to resorption of the bone.

29   Answer b

The most common malignant bone lesion is metastatic carcinoma.

30   Answer b

The laboratory finding associated with multiple myeloma is Bence Jones protein in the urine.

31   Answer b

The daily requirement of calcium in a postmenopausal woman is 1500 mg. The daily requirement for the lactating woman is 2000 mg. The daily requirement for an adolescent is 1000 mg and 500 mg for a young adult.

32 Answer d

Hypercalcemia is not a cause of rickets. Causes of rickets include vitamin D deficiency, chronic renal insufficiency, renal tubular insufficiency, and hypophosphatasia.

33 Answer a

The most likely diagnosis is compartment syndrome. The clinical history of recent casting of the extremity, pain, paresthesia, and diminution of pulses suggests compartment syndrome. Pain is usually the earliest sign of compartment syndrome.

34 Answer a

The earliest sign of compartment syndrome is pain.

35 Answer c

Late signs associated with compartment syndrome include paralysis and pulselessness. These signs may be associated with limb loss.

36 Answer a

Common causes of compartment syndrome are arterial injury and fracture. Other causes include soft-tissue injury, burns, and limb compression.

37 Answer c

The most likely diagnosis for the patient described is scleroderma, which is characterized by dermal fibrosis and may involve the lungs, heart, and kidneys.

38 Answer a

The GI complication that may develop secondary to scleroderma is esophageal strictures. Other GI complications that may develop include esophageal reflux and malabsorption.

39 Answer d

The CREST syndrome is a variant of scleroderma that includes calcinosis, Raynaud's phenomenon, esophageal dysfunction, sclerodactyly, and telangiectasias.

40 Answer b

Extra-articular manifestations of RA include subcutaneous nodules, carpal tunnel syndrome, interstitial lung disease, splenomegaly, and neutropenia.

41 Answer a

Diagnostic criteria for RA include morning stiffness, arthritis of at least three areas lasting more than 6 weeks, arthritis of hand joints lasting more than 6 weeks, symmetric arthritis lasting more than 6 weeks, serum rheumatoid factor, and radiographic changes. At least four of these criteria must be fulfilled to have a diagnosis of RA.

42 Answer d

The rheumatic disease that may have significant skin findings is SLE. There may be a malar or discoid rash.

43 Answer a

Cerebritis is a serious complication associated with SLE and may lead to visual loss.

44 Answer d

Gonococcal arthritis, acute rheumatic fever, and Lyme disease may all present with a polyarticular pattern.

45 Answer c

The hallmark sign of hypertrophic pulmonary osteoarthropathy is clubbing.

46 Answer a

SLE is more prevalent in African-American women in the premenopausal age group. SLE may lead to multi-organ involvement involving the kidneys, bone marrow, central nervous system, and heart.

47 Answer b

The next step in the evaluation of the patient described would be to obtain a more detailed history and physical. Further information to be obtained would include additional information on fatigue and its effects, family history, history of oral ulcerations, photosensitivity, seizures, history of anemias, and history of pleuritis or pericarditis. If a diagnosis of SLE is supported, the patient should be referred to a rheumatologist. Further diagnostic tests of complement levels and radiographs can be ordered after a more detailed history and physical.

48 Answer a

The laboratory findings of low complement levels, antibodies to double-stranded DNA, and proteinuria or hematuria support the diagnosis of SLE.

49 Answer b

The synovial fluid finding that is consistent with a diagnosis of RA is the presence of ragocytes, which are phagocytic cells with cytoplasmic inclusions. Other findings that may be seen in RA are white blood cell counts of 20,000 to 75,000 and a glucose level less than 50 gg/dL lower than that of the serum.

50 Answer c

Ankylosing spondylitis is more prevalent in men and is associated with HLA-B27. Extra-articular manifestations may include uveitis and aortic insufficiency. The sacroiliac joints, not the knee joints, are the most frequently affected.

51 Answer c

A grade 2 muscle strength means muscle contraction occurs, but it is not sufficient to overcome gravity.

52 Answer a

Golfer's elbow is inflammation of the medial epicondyle, and typically the patient will have pain when asked to lift the elbow with the palms facing upward.

53 Answer c

Heberden's nodes are usually seen in patients with osteoarthritis.

54 Answer c

Assessment of the motor function of the ulnar nerve is done by spreading the fingers.

55 Answer d

The most frequent portion of the GI tract to become involved in scleroderma is the esophagus. Approximately 50% of patients with scleroderma will have esophageal dysfunction with muscular atrophy and reflux.

56 Answer c

Treatment for patients with polymyalgia rheumatica may include steroids. Gold salts, quinine, and aspirin therapy may be used to treat RA.

57 Answer c

The laboratory test that you would expect to be abnormal in a patient with suspected polymyositis is the serum creatine kinase level, which indicates muscle breakdown that would occur in an acute inflammatory muscle disease.

58 Answer d

Differential diagnosis of the patient with proximal muscle weakness and fatigue includes hypothyroidism, polymyositis, and RA.

59 Answer a

The arthritic condition associated with diarrhea is Reiter's syndrome. The diarrhea may precede the arthritis by several weeks.

60 Answer a

Treatment for fibromyalgia includes a multifaceted approach consisting of NSAIDs, amitriptyline (Elavil), and aerobic exercises.

61 Answer c

All of the statements concerning Paget's disease are true except the statement that effective treatment results in an increase of serum alkaline phosphatase levels. Serum alkaline phosphatase levels should be monitored, and with treatment a decrease in this level should be seen. Most patients with Paget's disease are asymptomatic, and treatment regimens may include calcitonin, cytotoxic agents, and biphosphonates. Common sites of involvement of Paget's disease are the spine, pelvis, skull, femur, and tibia.

62 Answer c

The initial plan of care for the patient described is to obtain a prompt neurosurgical consultation. The patient is presenting with signs of spinal cord compression. Checking an alkaline phosphatase level, initiating calcitonin, and obtaining pelvic radiographs may all be helpful but are not the priority for this patient.

63 Answer a

The use of calcitonin for Paget's disease causes a decrease in osteoclastic resorption, thus leading to clinical improvement.

64 Answer a

The most common cause of generalized musculoskeletal pain in women between the ages of 20 and 55 is fibromyalgia.

65 Answer d

The most likely diagnosis for the patient described is rotator cuff tenditis, which is characterized by night pain, difficulty sleeping on the affected side, and pain on abduction of the arm. Rotator cuff injuries are more common in older adults and can occur with overuse of the shoulder in such activities as sports and carpentry. RA and polymyalgia rheumatica involving the shoulder is usually bilateral. Osteoarthritis of the shoulder is uncommon because the shoulder is not a weight-bearing joint. Osteoarthritis may result from a chronic rotator cuff tear.

66 Answer a

The preferred modality in evaluation of a patient with chronic shoulder pain is an MRI. An MRI may be useful in diagnosing rotator cuff lesions, osteoarthritis, glenohumeral instability, and subacromial impingement. Ultrasound may be an alternative to MRI for evaluation of rotator cuff tendinitis, subacromial bursitis, and rotator cuff tears. Ultrasound has its limitations and is not useful in the evaluation of the glenohumeral joint or the shoulder's stability and may miss small rotator cuff tears. Radiograph of the shoulder has limited benefit, but may be useful in identifying focal calcifications within the rotator cuff, joint space narrowing, and erosions in RA. Bone scan is not indicated unless you are assessing for evidence of metastatic disease.

67 Answer d

Differential diagnosis of shoulder pain should include myocardial ischemia, gallbladder disease, and disc herniation. All of these conditions may have referred shoulder pain.

68 Answer c

Pain on palpation and crepitation over the acromioclavicular joint may indicate an impingement of the rotator cuff. Atrophy of the muscles may be seen around the top and back of the shoulder if the process is long-standing.

69 Answer d

The rheumatoid factor is positive in approximately 20% of patients with juvenile RA.

70 Answer b

Patients with ankylosing spondylitis may have concurrent aortic insufficiency.

71 Answer a

The major causes of hip fractures in young adults are falls and trauma.

72 Answer b

A patient with an anterior hip dislocation should be closely monitored for injury to the femoral artery and nerve. Aseptic necrosis is a late complication that appears 2 years after hip dislocation.

73 Answer b

The patient who has had THR should be instructed to avoid flexion and internal rotation of the hip to prevent posterior dislocation of the THR prosthesis.

74 Answer b

The most common organism that may cause infection in the patient with a THR is *S. aureus.*

75 Answer d

Differential diagnosis of low-back pain includes herniated disc, tuberculosis, and ovarian cysts. The list of causes for low-back pain may include spinal disorders, trauma, GI disorders, vascular disease, malignancy, metabolic disorders, renal disease, and gynecologic disorders.

76 Answer a

The most likely diagnosis for the patient described is a C5-C6 herniated disc. The physical exam findings are consistent with a C5-C6 injury. C6 and C7 injuries will produce weakness of the triceps muscles and absent brachioradialis reflex. C8 injuries may exhibit a claw-hand deformity with weakness of the triceps muscles.

77 Answer b

The most common arthritis involving the elbow is RA.

78 Answer c

The first step in evaluating an elbow injury is to obtain a thorough history.

79 Answer d

Treatment for multiple myeloma includes chemotherapy, surgery of the impending fracture, and radiation.

80 Answer a

The most likely cause of an acute monoarthritis in an elderly patient hospitalized for exacerbation of CHF is gout. The patient admitted for CHF would require diuretics, which may exacerbate gouty symptoms.

81 Answer d

Diagnostic studies that may be useful in the evaluation of monarthritic states include a serum uric acid level, CBC, and prothrombin time. The CBC may reveal leukocytosis in a bacterial infection of the joint. The serum uric acid level may be normal or elevated in acute gout. Prothrombin time may be helpful when hemiarthrosis is suspected.

82 Answer b

HLA-B27 is positive in ankylosing spondylitis.

83 Answer a

A patient with *erythema marginatum* should be suspected of having acute rheumatic fever.

84 Answer c

The most likely diagnosis for the patient described is spinal stenosis. The clinical history is typical for spinal stenosis.

85 Answer d

Avascular necrosis of the femoral head is associated with trauma, steroid use, and sickle cell anemia.

Bibliography

Brandenburg, M, and Quick, G: Hand injuries: Fractures, dislocations, nailbed trauma, and bites. Consultant 40:2, 285–296, February 2000.

Canale, ST: Campbell's Operative Orthopedics, 9th ed. Harcourt, St. Louis, 1998.

Clark, S, and Odell, L: Fibromyalgia syndrome: Common, real and treatable. Clin Rev, 10:5, 57–76, May 2000.

Dunphy, L: Management Guidelines for Adult Nurse Practitioners. FA Davis, Philadelphia, 1999.

Goroll, A, et al: Primary Care Medicine Office Evaluation and Management of the Adult Patient, 4th ed. Lippincott Williams & Wilkins, Philadelphia, 2000.

Ruddy, S, et al: Textbook of Rheumatology, 6th ed. Philadelphia, Harcourt, 2000.

Puppione, A: Management strategies for older adults with osteoarthritis: How to promote and maintain function. J Am Acad Nurs Practit 11:4, 167–171, April 1999.

Schmitt, M: Osteoporosis: Focus on fractures. Patient Care Nurs Practit, 61–71, February 2000.

Woodhead, G, and Moss, M: Osteoporosis: Diagnosis and prevention. Nurs Practit 23:11, 18–35, November 1998.

12.
Head, Ear, Nose, and Throat Problems

1 *Roth spots may be associated with:*

a diabetes mellitus.
b bacterial endocarditis.
c hypertension.
d hypothyroidism.

2 *Consensual light reaction is pupillary:*

a constriction in the eye opposite to the one to which light is being directed.
b dilatation in the eye opposite to the one to which light is being directed.
c constriction in both eyes (the eye to which light is being directed, as well as the opposite eye).
d dilatation in both eyes (the eye to which light is being directed, as well as the opposite eye).

3 *Visual acuity is a test of:*

a peripheral vision.
b central vision.
c vision fields.
d nystagmus.

4 *Drooping of the upper eyelid is referred to as:*

a ptosis.
b hemianopsia.
c ectropion.
d dacryocystitis.

5 *The bacteria most commonly found in acute sinusitis are:*

a *Streptococcus pneumoniae* (*S. pneumoniae*) and *Escherichia coli* (*E. coli*).
b *S. pneumoniae* and *Haemophilus influenzae*.
c *Staphylococcus aureus* and *H. influenzae*.
d *Pseudomonas* and *E. coli*.

6 *A 50-year-old woman presents with complaints of nasal congestion, cough, a fever of 101°F, and tenderness over the frontal sinuses of 10 days' duration. You suspect acute bacterial sinusitis. What should be included in your initial treatment plan?*

a Fluid restriction and antibiotics
b Antibiotics only
c Antibiotics and decongestants
d Nasal lavage and fluid restriction

7 *Potential complications of sinusitis include:*

a central nervous system (CNS) infections.
b deafness.
c transient ischemic attack (TIA).
d esophageal fistula.

8 *Which ophthalmic finding is consistent with cataracts?*

a A cloudy view of the optic nerve and retinal vessels
b A high cup-to-disc ratio
c Papilledema
d Retinal vein occlusion

9 *One of the most common causes of visual impairment in adults is:*

a retinal detachment.
b optic neuritis.
c retinal vein occlusion.
d macular degeneration.

10 *All of the following statements concerning macular degeneration are true* **EXCEPT:**

a it usually occurs in patients over age 50.
b it may progress to permanent visual loss.

c it can be cured with laser treatment.
d initially, there may be no visual changes.

11 *Risk factors for open-angle glaucoma include all of the following* **EXCEPT:**

a diabetes.
b family history of glaucoma.
c hyperlipidemia.
d age over 40 years.

12 *How often should a 55-year-old woman with type 2 diabetes be screened for glaucoma?*

a Every year
b Every 5 years
c Every 2 years
d Every 6 months

13 *The most common cause of visual loss in adolescents and young adults is:*

a retinopathy.
b ocular trauma.
c retinal tears.
d optic neuritis.

14 *A 70-year-old woman presents with complaints of severe left eye pain with loss of vision for the past 4 hours. The exam reveals a dilated left pupil, which is nonreactive to light, and conjunctiva erythema. The patient's past medical history includes type 2 diabetes, hypertension, and iron-deficiency anemia. Her current medications include metformin (Glucophage), metoprolol (Lopressor), and aspirin. What is the most likely diagnosis?*

a Acute closed-angle glaucoma
b Conjunctivitis
c Retinal tear
d Keratitis

15 *Treatment for acute closed-angle glaucoma should include:*

a warm soaks to the eye.
b eye rest.
c prompt referral to an ophthalmologist.
d topical steroids.

16 *A 25-year-old woman swimmer has developed rupture of the tympanic membrane. What instructions should be given?*

a Continue with your usual swimming routine.
b Insert eardrops three times a day.
c Place earplugs in the ears during swimming or showering.
d No special precautions need to be taken.

17 *Which of the following conditions is associated with uveitis?*

a Ankylosing spondylitis
b Diabetes mellitus
c Hyperthyroidism
d Rheumatic fever

18 *A 65-year-old woman has a 50-year history of hypertension. What are the features of hypertensive retinopathy?*

a Roth spots
b Cotton-wool spots
c Poorly visualized optic disc
d Conjunctival hemorrhage

19 *Which of the following medications may be associated with hearing loss?*

a Metoprolol
b Furosemide (Lasix)
c Heparin
d Famotidine (Pepcid)

20 *Acoustic neuromas are characterized by all of the following* **EXCEPT:**

a tinnitus.
b dizziness.
c speech impairment.
d conductive hearing loss.

21 *A 40-year-old man has acquired immunodeficiency syndrome (AIDS). Which of the following ocular disorders may be associated with AIDS?*

a Cytomegalovirus (CMV) retinitis
b Allergic conjunctivitis
c Diplopia
d Acute closed-angle glaucoma

22 *The most common form(s) of hearing loss in the elderly patient is (are):*

a sensorineural hearing loss.
b conductive hearing loss.
c mixed hearing loss.
d all of the above.

23 *The proper technique for performing the Rinne test is to place a vibrating tuning fork on the:*

a middle of the skull, and then ask the patient if the tone is audible.
b mastoid process, and then ask the patient to acknowledge when the sound is no longer audible.
c middle of the skull, and then ask the patient to acknowledge when the sound is no longer audible.
d mastoid process, and then ask the patient if the tone is audible.

24 *All of the following statements concerning tinnitus are true* **EXCEPT:**

a   acetazolamide (Diamox) may cause tinnitus.
b   patients with tinnitus should be advised to avoid loud noises and alcohol use.
c   most cases of tinnitus are unilateral.
d   patients with severe forms of tinnitus should be referred to an otolaryngologist.

25 *A patient presents with sudden bilateral hearing loss. As the ACNP, what should be your initial plan of care?*

a   Order an audiogram.
b   Order a magnetic resonance imaging (MRI) of the skull.
c   Obtain a detailed history and physical exam.
d   Order a complete blood cell count (CBC) and serum electrolyte profile.

26 *A 40-year-old woman is diagnosed with acute otitis media. She has no known health problems and no medication allergies. She is prescribed amoxicillin (Amoxil) for 10 days. She notifies you after 3 days of treatment that she continues to have otalgia, a fever of 101°F, and a sore throat. What would be your next plan of care?*

a   Instruct the patient to continue the amoxicillin for the 10-day course.
b   Discontinue the amoxicillin, and place the patient on a more broad-spectrum antibiotic, such as levofloxacin (Levaquin).
c   Refer the patient to an otolaryngologist.
d   Have the patient return for re-evaluation.

27 *Classic presenting symptoms associated with acute otitis media include:*

a   otalgia, fever, and hearing loss.
b   fever and discharge in the external canal.
c   hearing loss and otorrhea.
d   fever and cough.

28 *Treatment of otitis externa includes:*

a   prompt referral to an otolaryngologist.
b   parenteral antibiotics.
c   antibiotic eardrops.
d   oral antibiotics.

29 *Signs and symptoms associated with frontal sinusitis include:*

a   pain and tenderness over the cheeks.
b   pain and tenderness over the lower forehead.
c   pain and tenderness over the nose.
d   referred tooth and hard-palate pain.

30 *Risk factors associated with the development of sinusitis include:*

a   nasal polyps.
b   nasal piercing.
c   migraine headaches.
d   sensorineural hearing loss.

31 *A 25-year-old woman with suspected ethmoid sinusitis has not responded to an antibiotic and decongestant regimen. Which diagnostic test should be ordered?*

a   Sinus x-ray
b   Computed tomography (CT) scan of the sinuses
c   Ultrasound of the sinuses
d   Nasal cultures

32 *Infectious mononucleosis is caused by:*

a   Epstein-Barr virus (EBV).
b   Chlamydia.
c   CMV.
d   Herpes zoster.

33 *The most common symptom associated with EBV is:*

a   fever.
b   headache.
c   fatigue.
d   sore throat.

34 *A 20-year-old college student is seen for complaints of sore throat, temperature of 100°F, fatigue, and headache for the past 2 weeks. Physical exam reveals a young woman in no acute distress with a temperature of 99.5°F, pulse of 100, respiratory rate of 16, and blood pressure of 110/60. Petechiae are noted on the hard-palate and tonsillar exudates. Anterior and posterior cervical adenopathy is also noted. Cardiac and respiratory exam is normal. Abdominal exam reveals tenderness in the right upper quadrant, a liver span of 13 cm, and no splenomegaly. What is the most likely diagnosis?*

a   Oral candidiasis
b   EBV
c   Peritonsillar abscess
d   Herpes pharyngitis

35 *Pharyngeal candidiasis is usually treated with:*

a   oral mycostatin (Nystatin) suspension (100,000 U/mL).
b   intravenous amphotericin (Amphocin).
c   penicillin.
d   acyclovir (Zovirax).

36 *The primary symptom associated with temporomandibular joint (TMJ) dysfunction is:*

a   dysphagia.
b   hoarseness.
c   unilateral jaw or facial pain.
d   diplopia.

37 *The organism most responsible for epiglottitis in the adult is:*

a   *Streptococcus.*
b   *S. aureus.*
c   *Chlamydia trachomatis.*
d   *H. influenzae* type B.

38 *A 70-year-old woman is seen for complaints of hoarseness for 2 months, an unexplained 10-lb weight loss, and dysphagia. What should be your initial plan of care?*

a   Order a prompt referral to an ENT specialist.
b   Instruct the patient to rest her voice.
c   Obtain a throat culture.
d   Order a CT scan of the head and neck.

39 *The treatment of choice for acute streptococcal pharyngitis (ASP) is:*

a   500 mg of penicillin V three times a day for 10 days.
b   trimethoprim sulfamethoxazole (Bactrim DS) twice daily for 7 days.
c   600 mg of clindamycin (Cleocin) twice daily for 10 days.
d   500 mg of amoxicillin/clavulanate (Augmentin) three times a day for 10 days.

40 *Potential complications of ASP include:*

a   rheumatoid arthritis (RA).
b   rheumatic fever.
c   cardiomyopathy.
d   renal calculi.

41 *A 55-year-old man has a history of chronic otitis media with at least six ear infections yearly. What is the most serious complication associated with chronic otitis media?*

a   sensorineural hearing loss.
b   cholesteatomas.
c   mastoiditis.
d   antibiotic resistance.

42 *A tonic pupil that fails to constrict in response to accommodation and light is referred to as:*

a   Horner's syndrome.
b   Adie's syndrome.
c   Argyll Robertson pupil.
d   ptosis.

43 *Yellowish fatty deposits localized over the eyelids are:*

a   styes.
b   xanthelasmas.
c   cataracts.
d   floaters.

44 *Arcus senilis is:*

a   a lipid deposit in the cornea.
b   edema of the bulbar conjunctiva.
c   an abnormal finding in elderly patients.
d   a subconjunctival hemorrhage.

45 *The most common cause of bilateral exophthalmos in the adult is:*

a   Horner's syndrome.
b   Graves' disease.
c   Myasthenia gravis.
d   none of the above; it is a normal variant.

46 *A 45-year-old man is undergoing physical exam in preparation for cholecystectomy. He is noted to have nystagmus. Nystagmus may be indicative of:*

a   cerebellar dysfunction.
b   early cataracts.
c   thyroid disease.
d   nothing; it is a normal variant.

47 *Blue sclerae may be associated with:*

a   osteogenesis imperfecta.
b   aplastic anemia.
c   hyperthyroidism.
d   diabetes.

48 *A 25-year-old man is involved in a motor cycle accident and is seen in the emergency department with facial swelling and a suspected blow-out fracture of the orbit. Which of the following symptoms would you expect the patient to exhibit?*

a   Blindness of the eye on the affected side
b   Diplopia when looking upward
c   Ptosis
d   Exophthalmos

49 *Which of the following conditions may be associated with loss of the red reflex?*

a   Hypertension.
b   Diabetes
c   Retinal detachment
d   Glaucoma

50 *Treatment of retinal detachment includes:*

a   eye rest.
b   prompt referral to an ophthalmologist.
c   Neo-Synephrine ophthalmic drops.
d   acetazolamide.

51 *Which of the following may be indicative of acute closed-angle glaucoma?*

a   Diplopia
b   Unilateral visual loss

c Appearance of halos in vision
d Blurred vision

52 *Symptoms associated with retinal detachment include:*

a floaters and flashes of light.
b eye pain and tearing of the eye.
c diplopia.
d loss of peripheral vision.

53 *A 70-year-old man is seen for complaints of red eye for the past week. All of the following should be considered in the differential diagnosis of red eye* **EXCEPT:**

a glaucoma.
b conjunctivitis.
c corneal abrasion.
d macular degeneration.

54 *A 20-year-old woman is brought to the emergency department after she is ejected from her car when it hits a tree. The point of most impact was her head. She is awake and alert, but you suspect a basilar skull fracture. Symptoms of a basilar skull fracture include:*

a loss of consciousness.
b Battle sign.
c projectile vomiting.
d hearing loss.

55 *The timeframe for the development of the Battle sign after a basilar skull fracture is usually:*

a 1 to 2 hours.
b 24 hours.
c 48 hours.
d 6 hours.

56 *Lack of mobility of the tympanic membrane on pneumatic inflation may indicate:*

a rupture of the tympanic membrane.
b acute otitis media.
c blockage of the eustachian tube.
d all of the above.

57 *A 25-year-old man is seen for suspected otitis externa. Which of the following physical findings is consistent with otitis externa?*

a Pain with movement of the tragus
b Bulging of the tympanic membrane
c Earlobe creases
d Loss of the cone of light reflex

58 *Which of the following ophthalmic problems does not present with pain?*

a Keratitis
b Acute glaucoma

c Iridocyclitis
d Conjunctivitis

59 *Causes of nasal obstruction include:*

a nasal polyps.
b septal deviation.
c foreign bodies.
d all of the above.

60 *A 35-year-old woman is seen for a routine physical exam. She is noted to have hairy leukoplakia. All of the statements concerning hairy leukoplakia are true* **EXCEPT:**

a the painless plaques may be located on the lateral aspects of the tongue and inner mucosa of the cheeks.
b it may be scraped off the lateral aspects of the tongue.
c it may be associated with immunocompromised states.
d it consists of painless plaques with hairlike projections.

61 *Cheilosis may be associated with:*

a folate deficiency.
b thiamine deficiency.
c iron-deficiency anemia.
d all of the above.

62 *Halitosis may be associated with:*

a periodontal disease.
b chronic sinusitis.
c peritonsillar abscess.
d all of the above.

63 *Ludwig's angina is:*

a a form of angina pectoris.
b an acute cellulitis in the submandibular salivary gland area.
c an inflammation of the parotid glands.
d associated with tracheobronchitis.

64 *Physical manifestations of Ludwig's angina may include:*

a dorsal deviation of the tongue.
b tenderness below the angle of the jaw.
c drooling.
d all of the above.

65 *A 55-year-old man is seen for painful unilateral swelling over the parotid glands. The most likely diagnosis is:*

a a parotid duct stone.
b a parotid tumor.
c human immunodeficiency virus (HIV) infection.
d lymphoma.

66 *Sjogren's syndrome is characterized by:*

a dry eyes and a dry mouth.
b clubbing.
c unilateral salivary gland swelling.
d anorexia.

67 *Xerostomia is:*

a loss of taste.
b loss of smell.
c dry mouth.
d altered perception of taste.

68 *The painless ulcer(s) of primary syphilis is (are):*

a a canker.
b a chancre.
c a ranula.
d Koplik's spots.

69 *Koplik's spots may be seen with:*

a rubeola.
b adenovirus.
c ECHO virus.
d all of the above.

70 *The presence of a thyroid bruit may indicate:*

a hypothyroidism.
b a normal variant.
c carotid artery disease.
d Graves' disease.

71 *A 60-year-old male smoker presents with complaints of a nonhealing ulcer on his tongue for the past 3 weeks. He states that the ulcer is painless. What should be your next step in evaluation of this ulcer?*

a Instruct the patient that oral ulcers may take up to 8 weeks to heal.
b Refer the patient for biopsy.
c Instruct the patient to discontinue smoking, telling him the ulcer will then heal.
d Tell the patient to return in 3 weeks if the ulcer has not healed.

72 *A 75-year-old man presents with a complaint of loss of taste. After obtaining a thorough history and physical exam, what should be your next step?*

a Obtain a CT scan of the head.
b Have the patient discriminate the tastes of table salt, sugar, and lemon juice.
c Refer the patient for a tongue biopsy.
d None of the above.

73 *A papillary lesion involving the uvula and anterior tonsillar pillar is:*

a hairy leukoplakia.
b squamous papilloma.
c torus palatinus.
d melanoma.

74 *Geographic tongue consists of:*

a white plaques on the base of the tongue.
b a painless ulcer on the lateral aspect of the tongue.
c loss and regrowth of papillae leading to red patches on the tongue.
d white hairy plaques over the entire tongue.

75 *A chalazion is:*

a more common in children.
b a mass on the eyelids with inflammation of the upper or lower eyelid.
c more prevalent in women.
d a painful mass with inflammation of the meibomian gland.

76 *Differential diagnosis for chalazion includes:*

a a foreign body.
b blepharitis.
c sebaceous cell carcinoma.
d all of the above.

77 *A 40-year-old man is seen in the emergency department with epistaxis for the past 2 hours, which he has not been able to control with manual pressure. Vital signs are stable. The patient has no known health problems. Use of continued pressure and an ice pack stops the bleeding. What should be part of the patient's discharge instructions from the emergency department?*

a Advise the patient to avoid blowing his nose or sneezing for at least 12 hours.
b Prescribe antibiotics and provide patient instructions.
c Advise the patient to avoid using products containing acetaminophen (Tylenol).
d Advise the patient to avoid pinching his nose.

78 *All of the following statements concerning Ménière's disease are true* **EXCEPT:**

a it is characterized by tinnitus and progressive hearing loss.
b it is more prevalent in women.
c it occurs more commonly between the ages of 30 to 60 years.
d it is treated with calcium channel blockers.

79 *Risk factors that may be associated with oral cancers include all of the following* **EXCEPT:**

a poor dentition.
b tobacco use.

c HIV infection.
d hyperthyroidism.

80 *Auditory acuity is assessed by checking cranial nerve:*

a VIII.
b V.
c II.
d III.

81 *The average age of onset of temporal arteritis is age:*

a 50 years.
b 25 years.
c 70 years.
d 40 years.

82 *The common cold is best treated with:*

a steroids.
b decongestants and rest.
c influenza vaccine.
d antibiotics.

83 *Allergic conjunctivitis may be associated with:*

a tearing.
b pruritus.
c erythema.
d all of the above.

84 *Night blindness may be secondary to a deficiency of vitamin:*

a D.
b A.
c C.
d E.

85 *Initial treatment of acute central retinal artery occlusion may include:*

a antibiotics.
b intravenous acetazolamide.
c acetaminophen.
d high doses of steroids.

Answers

1 Answer b

Roth spots, which are superficial hemorrhages with a white center, may be associated with bacterial endocarditis. Deep retinal hemorrhages are seen in diabetes mellitus. Retinal hemorrhages may be seen in severe hypertension, along with occlusion of the retinal vein and papilledema.

2 Answer c

Consensual light reaction is pupillary constriction in both eyes (the eye to which light is being directed and concomitant constriction of the opposite eye).

3 Answer b

Visual acuity is a test of central vision.

4 Answer a

Ptosis is drooping of the upper eyelid. Ptosis may be seen in myasthenia gravis, Horner's syndrome, or damage to the oculomotor nerve. Hemianopsia is loss of vision in a defined field. Ectropion is outward turning of the eyelid margin. Dacryocystitis is inflammation of the lacrimal sac; there may also be swelling between the lower eyelid and nose.

5 Answer b

The bacteria most commonly found in acute sinusitis are *S. pneumoniae, H. influenzae,* and *M. catarrhalis.*

6 Answer c

The initial treatment plan for a patient with suspected acute bacterial sinusitis includes antibiotics and decongestants. The antibiotics help to eradicate the pathogens responsible for rhinosinusitis. The decongestants serve to open and drain the sinuses. Patients should also be instructed to increase fluid intake to six to eight glasses a day.

7 Answer a

Potential complications of sinusitis, particularly in the untreated patient, include CNS infections such as meningitis. The sinus infection may destroy adjacent bony structures or dissect into the orbit and brain, thus causing meningitis.

8 Answer a

The ophthalmic finding consistent with cataracts is a cloudy view of the optic nerve and retinal vessels associated with a loss of brightness of the red reflex. A high cup-to-disc ratio may be seen in open-angle glaucoma. Optic disc blurring may be seen with papilledema and retinal vein occlusion.

9 Answer d

One of the most common causes of visual impairment in adults is macular degeneration. Other common causes include cataracts and chronic glaucoma.

10 Answer c

The patient with macular degeneration cannot be cured with laser treatment, but the vision may be helped if there is macular degeneration associated with neovascularization.

11 Answer c

Risk factors for open-angle glaucoma include diabetes, family history of glaucoma, age over 40 years, and myopia. Hyperlipidemia is not a risk factor for glaucoma.

12 Answer a

A patient with diabetes who is older than 40 years should be screened every year for glaucoma.

13 Answer b

The most common cause of visual loss in adolescents and young adults is ocular trauma.

14 Answer a

The most likely diagnosis for the patient described is acute closed-angle glaucoma. Conjunctivitis may or may not produce visual changes. Retinal tears and keratitis may produce visual blurring, but not complete visual loss.

15   Answer c

Treatment for acute closed-angle glaucoma should include prompt referral to an ophthalmologist.

16   Answer c

The instructions that should be given to a patient who has developed rupture of the tympanic membrane is to place earplugs in the ears during swimming or showering to avoid getting water in the ear.

17   Answer a

Ankylosing spondylitis is associated with uveitis.

18   Answer b

Features of hypertensive retinopathy include cotton-wool spots, arteriovenous nicking, copper-wire appearance, and papilledema.

19   Answer b

Furosemide is a diuretic that may be associated with hearing loss and tinnitus. Beta blockers such as metoprolol may be associated with tinnitus, but not hearing loss. Heparin and famotidine have not been associated with hearing loss.

20   Answer d

Acoustic neuromas may involve the fifth, seventh, and eighth cranial nerves. Involvement of these nerves may produce tinnitus, dizziness, speech impairment, and sensorineural hearing loss. They do not produce conductive hearing loss.

21   Answer a

CMV retinitis may be associated with AIDS. Complications associated with the retina are found in more than 50% of patients with AIDS.

22   Answer a

The most common form of hearing loss in the elderly is sensorineural hearing loss. This may be the result of exposure to loud noises, causing damage to the cochlea or eighth cranial nerve.

23   Answer b

The proper technique for performing the Rinne test is to place a vibrating tuning fork on the mastoid process, and to then ask the patient to acknowledge when the sound is no longer audible.

24   Answer c

Tinnitus is usually bilateral, not unilateral. Tinnitus may be caused by numerous medications, such as diuretics, beta blockers, antihistamines, narcotics, nonsteroidal anti-inflammatory drugs, aspirin therapy, angiotensin-converting enzyme inhibitors, and anesthetics. Patients with severe forms of tinnitus should be referred to an otolaryngologist, an audiologist, and in some cases a neurologist.

25   Answer c

The initial plan of care for a patient with sudden bilateral hearing loss is to obtain a detailed history and physical exam. Based on the history and physical exam findings, other testing may be indicated, for example, blood work, an audiogram, and an MRI.

26   Answer d

The patient with acute otitis media whose symptoms continue on antibiotic therapy for 3 or more days should be seen and re-evaluated. Based on the re-evaluation, the patient may be placed on a broader-spectrum antibiotic.

27   Answer a

The classic presenting symptoms associated with acute otitis media include otalgia, fever, and hearing loss. Fever and discharge in the external canal are associated with otitis externa. Hearing loss and otorrhea are associated with chronic otitis media. Fever and cough may be associated with an upper respiratory tract infection.

28   Answer c

Treatment of otitis externa includes topical application of antibiotic eardrops.

29   Answer b

Signs and symptoms associated with frontal sinusitis include pain and tenderness over the lower forehead, with purulent drainage from the middle meatus of the nasal turbinates. Pain and tenderness over the cheeks with referred tooth and hard-palate pain may be associated with maxillary sinusitis. Pain and tenderness over the nose may be associated with ethmoid sinusitis.

30   Answer a

Risk factors associated with the development of sinusitis include nasal polyps, deviated septum, foreign bodies, and trauma. Nasal piercing, migraine headaches, and sensorineural hearing loss have not been identified with development of sinusitis.

31   Answer b

The diagnostic test that should be ordered for a patient with suspected ethmoid sinusitis is a CT scan of the sinuses. The ethmoid sinuses are not usually well visualized with plain sinus x-rays. Ultrasound has a lower sensitivity than x-ray, and nasal cultures are not reliable.

32   Answer a

Infectious mononucleosis is caused by EBV.

33   Answer d

The most common symptom associated with EBV is sore throat. Other symptoms include fever, headache, and malaise.

34   Answer b

The most likely diagnosis is EBV, which is common in college students and is associated with fever, headache, generalized malaise, and fatigue. Physical findings in EBV usually include tonsillar exudates, palate petechiae, adenopathy, splenomegaly, and hepatomegaly, all of which are seen with this patient. Oral candidiasis is usually associated with a white, cheesy exudate in the oral mucosa. Peritonsillar abscess usually presents with a grayish white exudate on the tonsils with febrile illness and bacteremia. Herpes pharyngitis usually involves small vesicles seen in the pharynx and buccal mucosa.

35   Answer a

Pharyngeal candidiasis is usually treated with oral nystatin suspension swish and swallow. There is no role for intravenous amphotericin or antibiotics. Acyclovir may be used to treat herpetic infections.

36 Answer c

The primary symptom associated with TMJ dysfunction is unilateral jaw or facial pain.

37 Answer d

The organism most responsible for epiglottitis in the adult is *H. influenzae* type b.

38 Answer a

The initial plan of care should be a prompt referral to an ENT specialist. A 2-month history of hoarseness with associated weight loss and dysphagia should raise suspicion for malignancy and should be evaluated promptly.

39 Answer a

The treatment of choice for ASP is 500 mg of penicillin V three times a day for 10 days. Studies have shown that cephalosporins may also be comparable to penicillin in the treatment of ASP. The treatment course should be at least 10 days.

40 Answer b

A potential complication of ASP is the development of rheumatic fever. Other complications may include glomerulonephritis, peritonsillar and retropharyngeal abscesses, and suppurative otitis media.

41 Answer b

The most serious complication associated with chronic otitis media is the development of cholesteatomas, which may cause destruction of the stapes and malleus and lead to conductive hearing loss. The development of cholesteatomas may also cause facial nerve paresis and meningitis.

42 Answer b

A tonic pupil that fails to constrict in response to accommodation and light is referred to as Adie's pupil. Argyll Robertson pupil refers to a pupil that constricts in response to accommodation but not in response to light. Ptosis is drooping of the eyelid. Horner's syndrome is a drooping of the upper eyelid and constriction of the pupil on the affected side.

43 Answer b

Yellowish fatty deposits localized over the eyelids are xanthelasmas.

44 Answer a

Arcus senilis is a lipid deposition in the cornea and is a normal finding in elderly patients.

45 Answer b

The most common cause of bilateral exophthalmos in the adult is Grave's disease.

46 Answer a

Nystagmus may be indicative of cerebellar dysfunction.

47 Answer a

Blue sclerae may be associated with osteogenesis imperfecta. They may also be associated with iron-deficiency anemia, Marfan's syndrome, and hypoparathyroidism. Blue sclerae may be a normal variant in the newborn.

48 Answer b

The symptom you would expect in the patient with a blow-out fracture of the orbit is diplopia when looking upward.

49 Answer c

Retinal detachment may be associated with loss of the red reflex. Cataracts may cause an abnormal red reflex.

50 Answer a

Treatment of retinal detachment includes prompt referral to an ophthalmologist. Retinal detachment may lead to loss of vision and is a medical emergency.

51 Answer c

The appearance of halos in vision may be indicative of acute closed-angle glaucoma. The appearance of halos is thought to be secondary to corneal edema.

52 Answer a

Symptoms associated with retinal detachment include floaters and flashes of light in the visual field.

53 Answer d

The differential diagnosis of red eye includes glaucoma, conjunctivitis, and corneal abrasion. Red eye is not a manifestation of macular degeneration.

54 Answer b

The symptoms of a basilar skull fracture include Battle's sign: periorbital ecchymoses, rhinorrhea, and otorrhea.

55 Answer c

The timeframe for the development of the Battle's sign after a basilar skull fracture is usually 48 hours.

56 Answer d

Lack of mobility of the tympanic membrane on pneumatic inflation may indicate a rupture of the tympanic membrane, acute otitis media, blockage of the eustachian tube, and dense adhesions in the middle ear.

57 Answer a

The physical finding consistent with otitis externa is pain with movement of the tragus. The bulging of the tympanic membrane and the loss of the cone of light reflex may be seen in otitis media. Earlobe creases may be a normal finding and have been correlated to patients with coronary artery disease.

58 Answer d

Conjunctivitis usually does not present with eye pain.

59 Answer d

Causes of nasal obstruction include nasal polyps, septal deviation, foreign bodies, and nasal mucosal edema.

60 Answer b

Hairy leukoplakia is the presence of multiple white, painless plaques with hairlike projections usually located on the lateral aspects of the tongue and the inner mucosa of the cheeks. Hairy leukoplakia may be associated with immunocompromised states. The white plaques may not be scraped off. If the plaques may be scraped off, consider a differential diagnosis of thrush.

61 Answer d

Cheilosis, which is a reddening and cracking of one or both angles of the mouth, may be associated with folate deficiency, thiamine deficiency, and iron-deficiency anemia.

62 Answer d

Halitosis may be associated with various disorders including periodontal disease, chronic sinusitis, and peritonsillar abscess.

63 Answer b

Ludwig's angina is an acute cellulitis in the submandibular salivary gland area, in close proximity to the mylohyoid muscle.

64 Answer d

Physical manifestations of Ludwig's angina may include tenderness and induration below the angle of the jaw associated with dorsal deviation of the tongue, drooling, and mouth edema.

65 Answer a

The most likely diagnosis for a patient who presents with painful unilateral swelling over the parotid gland is a parotid duct stone. A parotid tumor, HIV infection, and lymphoma will usually present with painless bilateral swelling.

66 Answer a

Sjogren's syndrome is an autoimmune disorder characterized by infiltration of the salivary and lacrimal glands. It is associated with dry eyes and a dry mouth.

67 Answer c

Xerostomia is dry mouth and is associated with Sjogren's syndrome.

68 Answer b

The painless ulcer of primary syphilis is a chancre. A canker is a painful, benign aphthous ulcer. A ranula is a unilateral painful, fluctuant nodule in the floor of the mouth. Koplik's spots are white macules on the buccal mucosa, and are seen with early rubeola.

69 Answer d

Koplik's spots may be seen with rubeola, adenovirus, and ECHO virus.

70 Answer d

The presence of a thyroid bruit may indicate Grave's disease. A thyroid bruit indicates that there is increased vascularity of the thyroid gland.

71 Answer b

The patient who presents with a painless, nonhealing tongue ulcer of 3 weeks' duration should be referred for biopsy. A nonhealing ulcer may be highly suspicious for squamous cell carcinoma.

72 Answer b

The initial evaluation of the complaint of loss of taste should be to have the patient discriminate among the tastes of table salt, sugar, and a bitter taste of lemon juice. If the patient is able to discern these tastes, the sense of taste is intact.

73 Answer b

A papillary lesion involving the uvula and the anterior tonsillar is a squamous papilloma, which is usually benign. Hairy leukoplakia are white painless lesions on the lateral aspects of the tongue. Torus palatinus is a benign bony enlargement that occurs on the hard palate. Melanoma is a malignancy that may present as an oral lesion.

74 Answer c

Geographic tongue is loss and regrowth of the tongue papillae leading to red patches on the tongue.

75 Answer b

A chalazion is a painless mass on the eyelids, resulting from inflammation of a meibomian gland of the upper or lower eyelid. A chalazion may occur at any age and occurs equally in men and women.

76 Answer d

Differential diagnosis for chalazion includes foreign body, blepharitis, and sebaceous cell carcinoma.

77 Answer a

The discharge instructions for a patient with epistaxis should include advising the patient to avoid blowing his nose or sneezing for at least 12 hours to prevent dislodging protective blood clots.

78 Answer d

Ménière's disease is a peripheral sensory disorder of both the labyrinth and the cochlea. It is characterized by tinnitus, progressive hearing loss, and is more prevalent in women. It commonly occurs between the ages of 30 and 60 years. Treatment of Ménière's disease includes the use of antimuscarinics, anticholinergics, and vestibulosuppressive histamine blockers. Calcium channel blockers are not used.

79 Answer d

Hyperthyroidism is not a risk factor for oral cancers. Risk factors may include poor dentition, tobacco use, HIV infection, nutrition deficiencies, oral trauma, and exposure to wood dust.

80 Answer a

Auditory acuity is assessed by checking cranial nerve VIII.

81 Answer c

The average age of onset of temporal arteritis is 70 years.

82 Answer b

The common cold is best treated with decongestants and rest.

83 Answer d

Allergic conjunctivitis may be associated with tearing, pruritus, and erythema.

84 Answer b

Night blindness may be secondary to a deficiency of vitamin A.

85 Answer b

Initial treatment of acute central retinal artery occlusion may include the use of intravenous acetazolamide, which will decrease the production of aqueous humor and lower intraocular pressure.

Bibliography

Fitzgerald, M: Acute otitis media in an era of drug resistance: Implications for NP practice. Supplement to Nurse Practitioner 24:10, 10–16, October, 1999.

Goroll, A, et al: Primary Care Medicine Office Evaluation and Management of the Adult Patient, 4th ed. Lippincott Williams & Wilkins, Philadelphia, 2000.

Kaliner, M: Sinusitis Disease Management Guide. PDR 2000, 1st ed. Medical Economics Company, Montvale, NJ, 2000.

Lee, KJ: Essential Otolaryngology-Head and Neck Surgery, 6th ed. Appleton & Lange, Norwalk, Conn., 1995.

Prisco, M: Evaluating neck masses. Nurse Practitioner 25:4, 30–49, April 2000.

Rosa, S: Primary care management of otitis externa. Nurse Practitioner 23:6, 125–133, June 1998.

Tiggs, B: Acute otitis media and pneumococcal resistance: Making judicious management decisions. Nurse Practitioner 25:1, 69–79, January 2000.

COMMON PROBLEMS IN ACUTE CARE

13

Fever

Questions 1–5 refer to the following scenario:

A 25-year-old woman is seen in the emergency department with complaints of fever, malaise, headache, myalgias, diarrhea, and vomiting for the past 2 days. She denies any other health problems. Her current medications include a multivitamin and an oral contraceptive. Allergies include penicillin. She is currently having her menstrual cycle and wears tampons. Physical exam reveals an ill-appearing woman with a temperature of 103°F, a pulse of 130, a respiratory rate of 24, and blood pressure of 90/60. Neurologic exam reveals a lethargic woman who is easily arousable. HEENT exam is normal with no nuchal rigidity. Lung exam is normal, and heart tones are regular without murmurs or rubs. Abdominal exam reveals bloating without tenderness, poor skin turgor, and a macular rash on the upper torso. The mucous membranes are dry and erythematous. Laboratory findings reveal an elevated white blood cell count of 20,000/mm³ with 10% bands, a hemoglobin of 12.5, a platelet count of 90,000, a blood urea nitrogen (BUN) level of 40, and creatinine value of 2.4. Urinalysis reveals a large amount of blood with 10–20 white blood cells.

1 *What is the most likely diagnosis?*

a Lyme disease
b Rocky mountain spotted fever
c Scarlet fever
d Toxic shock syndrome

2 *Which laboratory test is diagnostic of the most likely diagnosis?*

a Complete blood cell count
b Elevated erythrocyte sedimentation rate (ESR)
c Hyperalbuminuria
d None of the above

3 *Which of the following are diagnostic of the most likely diagnosis?*

a Fever, rash, hypotension, thrombocytopenia, and desquamation

b Tampon use
c Hypotension only
d Oral contraceptive and tampon use

4 *What is the organism responsible for the most likely diagnosis?*

a *Streptococcus pneumoniae*
b *Staphylococcus aureus*
c *Streptococcus bovis*
d *Escherichia coli*

5 *What is the antibiotic of choice in the patient described?*

a Penicillin
b Vancomycin (Vancocin)
c None
d Amoxicillin/clavulanic acid (Augmentin)

6 *The most common cause of fever is:*

a an autoimmune disorder.
b cancer.
c trauma.
d an infection.

7 *All of the statements concerning drug-related fever are true* **EXCEPT:**

a there may be an associated rash.
b there may be associated eosinophilia.
c aspirin is the most common medication linked to drug-related fever.
d the fever usually begins 7 to 10 days after initiation of treatment.

8 *The most common causes of fever of unknown origin (FUO) are:*

a infection and malignancy.
b medication and infection.
c malingering and infection.
d collagen vascular diseases and infection.

9 *FUO is defined as a fever more than:*

a 100°F for 30 consecutive days without obvious cause.
b 102°F for 14 consecutive days.
c 100.9°F for 21 days, without a known diagnosis after 1 week of evaluation in the hospital.
d 102°F for 30 consecutive days without evidence of infection.

10 *The most common cause of fever in a patient in the intensive care unit is:*

a medication related.
b infection.
c an autoimmune disorder.
d atelectasis.

11 *Fever with associated bradycardia is correlated with:*

a malaria.
b typhoid fever.
c herpes encephalitis.
d catheter-related sepsis.

Questions 12–18 refer to the following scenario:

A 55-year-old man is admitted to the hospital with a history of temperature greater than 102°F for the past week which has been associated with chills, fatigue, anorexia, and shortness of breath. The patient's past medical history is significant for hypertension, type 2 diabetes, and aortic stenosis. He had a human aortic valve replacement 2 months ago. Medications include 80 mg of aspirin daily, and 10 mg of Vasotec twice daily. Physical exam reveals an ill-appearing man with a temperature of 101.5°F, a pulse of 120, a respiratory rate of 16, and blood pressure of 100/70. HEENT exam is normal. Chest exam reveals bibasilar crackles. The sternal incision scar is well healed. Cardiac exam reveals a normal first heart sound, a diastolic murmur 2/6 at the left sternal border, with positive third and fourth sounds. His abdomen is soft without hepatomegaly or tenderness. The extremities reveal no edema; however, erythematous, nonpainful lesions are noted on the soles of his feet.

12 *What should be your initial step in the evaluation of this patient?*

a Order blood cultures.
b Arrange for a stat cardiac catheterization.
c Arrange for a cardiology consultation, and order an echocardiogram.
d Start intravenous antibiotics.

13 *The patient has a macular, erythematous, and nonpainful lesion on the soles of his feet. What is this physical finding?*

a Roth spots.
b Osler's nodes.

c Splinter hemorrhages.
d Janeway lesions.

14 *What is the most likely diagnosis for the patient described?*

a Prosthetic valve endocarditis
b Pneumonia
c Pericarditis
d Congestive heart failure (CHF)

15 *Physical findings consistent with CHF include:*

a crackles and a third heart sound.
b a fourth heart sound and absence of hepatomegaly.
c tachycardia and Janeway lesions.
d fever and tachycardia.

16 *Which of the following laboratory abnormalities may be associated with the most likely diagnosis for the patient described?*

a Anemia
b Low serum complement
c Leukocytosis
d All of the above

17 *Which of the following organisms are difficult to isolate in a culture?*

a *Staphylococcus*
b *Streptococcus*
c *Enterococcus*
d *Haemophilus*

18 *The most common cause of prosthetic valve endocarditis is:*

a coagulase-negative Staphylococci.
b *Streptococcus viridans.*
c *Staphylococcus aureus.*
d aspergillosis.

19 *All of the statements concerning factitious fever are true* **EXCEPT:**

a it is more common in women.
b it is more common in health-care professionals.
c there is an absence of chills or tachycardia with temperatures above 106°F.
d the patient always presents with chills along with a low-grade fever.

20 *A 25-year-old woman scheduled for elective cholecystectomy informs you that her mother and sister developed malignant hyperthermia during surgical procedures that they had. What would be your next plan of action?*

a Reassure the patient that she will not likely have a problem.
b Notify the anesthesiologist and the surgeon.

c Have the surgery postponed and pretreat the patient with dantrolene (Dantrium) for 5 days.
d Have staff nurses check the patient's baseline temperature prior to her going to the operating room.

21 Which of the following laboratory abnormalities may be seen in malignant hyperthermia?

a Elevated creatine kinase
b Hypokalemia
c Hypocalcemia
d Metabolic alkalosis

22 A 40-year-old man has been admitted to the hospital for evaluation of fever. He has a history of fever with a temperature to 101°F for the past week without evidence of infection. He has had a fever every day at 8 PM for the last 3 nights. What time should blood cultures be drawn for greatest yield in this patient?

a At the onset of the fever
b Any time
c One hour before the anticipated fever
d Two hours after the temperature returns to normal

23 The mechanism of action(s) for amphotericin B (Amphocin) is (are):

a impairment of bacterial DNA synthesis.
b inhibition of cell wall synthesis.
c disruption of membrane barrier function.
d all of the above.

24 Pustular lesions at the site of a cat scratch along with associated with fever, malaise, and lymphadenopathy (cat-scratch disease) is most likely caused by:

a spirochete.
b gram-negative bacillus.
c cytomegalovirus (CMV).
d a fungus.

25 A 40-year-old man is seen for complaints of dry cough, fatigue, shortness of breath, and fever. Physical exam reveals an ill-appearing man with a temperature of 100.5°F, a pulse of 100, a respiratory rate of 24, and blood pressure of 100/70. He has anterior cervical and inguinal adenopathy. His spleen is enlarged. He is bisexual. His chest x-ray shows bilateral infiltrates. His arterial blood gas reveals a PO_2 of 50 on room air. His human immunodeficiency virus (HIV) serology is positive. The most likely diagnosis is:

a Bacterial pneumonia.
b aspergillosis.
c Epstein-Barr virus.
d Pneumocystis carinii pneumonia (PCP).

Questions 26–28 refer to the following scenario:

A 30-year-old male athlete is participating in a bicycle race for a local charity. After riding 50 miles in 100° temperatures, he is brought to the emergency department after collapsing at the end of the race. His vital signs include a temperature of 103°F orally, a pulse of 112, and blood pressure of 110/55. He is unarousable. His past medical history is significant for hypertension and he is taking triamterene/hydrochlorothiazide (Dyazide) once daily.

26 What is the most likely diagnosis?

a Heat cramps
b Heatstroke
c Hyperventilation syndrome
d Heat exhaustion

27 Treatment for the patient includes:

a oral electrolyte replacement.
b lowering the body temperature.
c vigorous fluid replacement.
d institution of cardiopulmonary bypass.

28 Risk factors for the development of the most likely diagnosis in this patient include:

a high environmental temperatures.
b being an athlete.
c a history of diuretic use.
d all of the above.

29 A fever is defined as a temperature greater than:

a 102°F rectally.
b 100.4°F rectally.
c 99.5°F orally.
d 98°F axillary.

30 Which of the following patients with a fever should be referred for hospitalization?

a Patients with disorientation associated with fever
b Patients with enlarged lymph nodes
c Patients with suspected bronchitis
d Patients with fever for the past 2 days without other constitutional symptoms

31 Treatment of fever in the adult may include:

a use of acetaminophen (Tylenol).
b use of aspirin.
c sponging.
d all of the above.

Questions 32–34 refer to the following scenario:

A 70-year-old man had a colon resection for colorectal carcinoma 4 days ago. You are notified by the staff nurse that the patient has a temperature of 101.5°F.

Other vital signs are a pulse of 88, a respiratory rate of 18, blood pressure of 130/78, and pulse oximetry of 90% on room air that improves with deep breathing to 94%. The patient is without complaints. The lungs are diminished at both bases and the heart tones are normal. The abdominal incision is clean without drainage, and there is no abdominal tenderness.

32 What is the most likely cause of the patient's fever?

a Pneumonia
b Pulmonary embolus
c Atelectasis
d Abdominal abscess

33 What would be your initial plan of care for this patient?

a Start antibiotics.
b Obtain a chest x-ray and blood cultures.
c Order a chest computed tomography (CT) scan.
d Start intravenous heparin.

34 What other interventions should be ordered for this patient?

a Coughing and deep-breathing exercises
b Oxygen therapy
c An abdominal binder for the incision
d Lower-extremity Doppler evaluation

35 The most common cause of bacterial pneumonia in the adult is:

a *Mycoplasma.*
b *Pneumococcus.*
c *Haemophilus.*
d *Legionella.*

36 A 60-year-old man with a 2-month history of fever occurring every 2 to 3 days along with weight loss and fatigue is seen in the clinic. The patient's HIV infection status is negative, and he has no other health history. Differentials for this patient should include:

a pneumonia.
b lymphoma.
c temporal arteritis.
d rheumatic fever.

37 The surgical procedure that has the highest incidence of wound infection is:

a joint surgery.
b coronary artery bypass grafting.
c cholecystectomy.
d colon resection.

Answers

1 Answer d
The most likely diagnosis for the patient described is toxic shock syndrome. The history of current menstruation, tampon use, and macular rash along with a septic-appearing picture makes toxic shock syndrome the most likely diagnosis.

2 Answer d
Toxic shock syndrome is a clinical diagnosis made on the basis of defined criteria. No specific laboratory test is diagnostic. The patient may have positive blood cultures.

3 Answer a
As defined by the Centers for Disease Control and Prevention (CDC), to be diagnosed with toxic shock syndrome, six clinical criteria must be met: (1) temperature of 102°F or greater; (2) diffuse macular rash; (3) desquamation, (4) hypotension; (5) multisystem involvement; and (6) negative blood, throat, or cerebrospinal fluid cultures. Multisystem involvement must have three of the following: (1) vomiting or diarrhea, (2) myalgias, (3) elevated creatine kinase level, (4) mucous membrane erythema, (5) BUN/creatinine levels elevated two times over normal, (6) liver enzymes two times normal levels, (7) platelet count less than $100,000/mm^3$, and (8) disorientation with focal neurologic deficits.

4 Answer b
The organism most likely responsible for toxic shock syndrome is *S. aureus.*

5 Answer b
The antibiotic of choice in the patient described is vancomycin. The patient is allergic to penicillin, so penicillin and amoxicillin/clavulanate are contraindicated.

6 Answer d
The most common cause of fever is an infection.

7 Answer c
Penicillin and its derivatives, not aspirin, are the most common medications linked to drug-related fever. Drug-related fever may occur 7 to 10 days after the initiation of treatment, and there may be an associated rash and eosinophilia on peripheral smear.

8 Answer a
The most common causes of FUO are infection and malignancy, which account for approximately 60% of causes.

9 Answer c
FUO is defined as a fever more than 100.9°F for 21 days, without a known diagnosis after 1 week of evaluation in the hospital.

10 Answer b
The most common cause of fever in the patient in intensive care is infection. Infection sources may include pneumonia, those related to urinary or gastrointestinal systems, or those related to intravenous catheters.

11 Answer b
Fever associated with bradycardia is usually correlated with typhoid fever or drug-related fever.

12 Answer a

The initial evaluation of the patient described is to order blood cultures. A cardiology consultation, echocardiogram, and institution of antibiotics may be done, but the immediate step is to obtain blood cultures. A stat cardiac catheterization is not indicated based on the information provided.

13 Answer d

The lesions on the sole of the patient's feet are Janeway lesions. Janeway lesions are macular, blanched, erythematous, and nonpainful lesions found on the palms of the hands and the soles of the feet. Roth spots are exudative, edematous hemorrhagic lesions on the retina. Osler's nodes are painful nodules found on the fingers and toes. Splinter hemorrhages are nonblanching, linear, reddish brown lesions found under the nail bed.

14 Answer a

The most likely diagnosis for the patient described is prosthetic valve endocarditis. This diagnosis is supported by the history of recent heart valve replacement, fever, murmur of aortic insufficiency, CHF, and Janeway lesions on the soles of his feet. The patient has CHF, but it is secondary to prosthetic valve endocarditis.

15 Answer a

Physical findings consistent with CHF include crackles and a third heart sound (ventricular gallop).

16 Answer d

Prosthetic valve endocarditis may be associated with anemia, leukocytosis, and low serum complement levels. Destruction of red blood cells with hemolysis may occur secondary to valve destruction. A low serum complement level may be an indicator of immune-mediated glomerular disease. Leukocytosis may be present, but the white blood cell count may be normal.

17 Answer d

Haemophilus is difficult to isolate in culture, and can take from 7 to 21 days to isolate.

18 Answer a

The most common cause of prosthetic valve endocarditis is coagulase-negative staphylococci.

19 Answer d

Factitious fever is the purposeful false elevation in temperature by the patient. This happens more commonly in women and health-care professionals. The motive may be malingering. Suspicion for this phenomenon should occur if the patient reports an excessive fever without systemic symptoms.

20 Answer b

The next plan of action for the patient described would be to notify the anesthesiologist and surgeon of the family history of malignant hyperthermia. Surgery would proceed with the precautions of avoiding anesthetic agents that release calcium from the membrane of the muscle-cell sarcoplasmic reticulum. If possible, the surgery should be done under spinal or epidural anesthesia. Dantrolene may be given preoperatively.

21 Answer a

An elevated creatine kinase level may be seen in malignant hyperthermia. Other laboratory abnormalities that may develop include myoglobinuria, hyperkalemia, and metabolic acidosis.

22 Answer c

The likelihood of obtaining a positive blood culture increases if it is obtained 1 hour before the anticipated fever.

23 Answer c

The mechanism of action for amphotericin B is disruption of the membrane barrier function. Amphotericin B is a polyene antibiotic that binds to the cytoplasmic cellular membrane. The ability of an organism to bind amphotericin B depends on the presence of ergosterol in the cytoplasmic membrane. Bacterial cell walls contain no sterols and are not affected by amphotericin B.

24 Answer b

Cat-scratch disease is caused by gram-negative bacillus.

25 Answer d

The most likely diagnosis is *P. carinii* pneumonia (PCP). The chest x-ray findings and relative hypoxemia are consistent with PCP, which is an AIDS-defining illness. The generalized adenopathy and enlarged spleen may be seen in HIV-positive persons.

26 Answer b

The most likely diagnosis for the patient described is heatstroke. Heatstroke is usually associated with elevated temperature, neurologic symptoms, and absence of sweating.

27 Answer b

Treatment for the patient described includes aggressive lowering of the body temperature, which may be achieved with hypothermia blankets and ice packs to the groin and axillae. Other methods of lowering the temperature may include gastric lavage and enemas, and iced water peritoneal dialysis. The patient has lost consciousness, so oral electrolyte replacement would not be an option. Vigorous fluid replacement may result in pulmonary edema. Cardiopulmonary bypass may be implemented in patients with hypothermia to aid in warming.

28 Answer d

Risk factors for the development of heatstroke include high environmental temperatures and humidity; being an athlete, laborer, or military recruit; and use of diuretics, antidepressants, and phenothiazines.

29 Answer b

A fever is defined as a temperature greater than 100.4° rectally, 100°F orally, or 99°F axillary.

30 Answer a

The patient with disorientation associated with fever should be hospitalized to rule out possible CNS infection or meningitis. Enlarged lymph nodes may signify a viral infection that does not require hospitalization. Suspected bronchitis and fever without constitutional symptoms can be evaluated on an outpatient basis.

31 Answer d

Treatment of fever in the adult may include the use of acetaminophen, aspirin, and sponging. Aspirin has been associated with Reye's syndrome in children.

32 Answer c

The most likely cause of the patient's fever is atelectasis. The temperature is low grade, the patient has diminished breath sounds, and pulse oximetry improves with deep breathing.

The patient is not toxic. There is no information to support the diagnosis of abdominal abscess or pulmonary embolus. The improvement in pulse oximetry when the patient is deep breathing makes pneumonia less likely.

33 Answer b

The initial plan of care for the patient described would be to obtain a chest x-ray and blood cultures. After obtaining the chest x-ray and blood cultures, antibiotics could be started, but this patient does not appear toxic. There is no indication for a chest CT scan or the institution of intravenous heparin.

34 Answer a

Other interventions that should be ordered for the patient described include coughing and deep-breathing exercises. The patient has atelectasis and would benefit from this intervention as well as incentive spirometry and increased activity level.

35 Answer b

The most common cause of bacterial pneumonia in the adult is *Pneumococcus*.

36 Answer b

The most likely diagnosis for a patient with a 2-month history of fever, weight loss, and fatigue is lymphoma. Temporal arteritis is possible, but the patient has no visual symptoms. Pneumonia is possible, but the 2-month history makes it less likely. There is no data to support rheumatic fever as a cause of this patient's problem.

37 Answer d

The surgical procedure with the highest incidence of wound infection is colon resection.

Bibliography

Goroll, A, et al: Primary Care Medicine Office Evaluation and Management of the Adult Patient, 4th ed. Lippincott Williams & Wilkins, Philadelphia, 2000.

Hirschmann, JV: Fever of unknown origin in adults. Clin Infect Dis 24:291–302, 1997.

Kingston, ME: Skin clues in the diagnosis of life-threatening infections. Rev Infect Dis 8:1–11, 1996.

Mandell, GL, et al: Principles and Practice of Infectious Disease, 5th ed. Churchill Livingstone, New York, 2000.

Nathanson, N, and Alexander, ER: Infectious disease epidemiology. Am J Epidemiol 144 (suppl 8):S34–S38, 1996.

14

Pain

1 *A 40-year-old woman diagnosed with sarcoma is complaining of constant pain. As the ACNP you recognize this as:*

a visceral pain.
b psychogenic pain.
c somatic pain.
d neuropathic pain.

Questions 2–4 refer to the following scenario:

A 55-year-old man had a thoracotomy for squamous cell lung cancer 2 months ago. The tumor was totally resected, and all nodes were negative. He is seen in the office with complaints of burning, stabbing pain at the site of the incision and has been unable to sleep since the surgery because of the pain. He is employed as a butcher in a local store and has been unable to work because of the pain. He is taking two tablets of acetaminophen with codeine (Tylenol No. 3) twice a day and 600 mg of ibuprofen (Motrin) three times a day.

2 *Which type of pain is this patient experiencing?*

a Neuropathic pain
b Somatic pain
c Central pain
d Visceral pain

3 *What treatment options should be explored with this patient?*

a Start intravenous morphine via a patient-controlled analgesia (PCA) pump at home.
b Continue with the acetaminophen with codeine and ibuprofen.
c Consider use of intercostal blocks with steroids.
d Stop the patient's medications and prescribe amitriptyline (Elavil) alone.

4 *Anticonvulsants may help to control this patient's pain by:*

a blocking the reuptake of monoamines.
b decreasing the perception of pain.
c decreasing the inflammatory response at the site of pain.
d stabilizing nerve membrane firing.

5 *Which of the following factors may alter pain perception?*

a Anxiety
b Depression
c Fear
d All of the above

6 *A 50-year-old woman with metastatic breast cancer has chronic pain. What are the characteristics of an ideal analgesic for her?*

a An agent with a rapid onset of action and a long half-life
b An agent to which tolerance develops quickly
c An agent with a rapid onset of action and a short half-life
d An agent that can be administered orally

7 *Which of the medications is the preferred first option for cancer pain?*

a Morphine
b Meperidine (Demerol)
c Methadone (Dolophine)
d Amitriptyline

8 *Which of the following is an antagonist to morphine?*

a Pentazocine (Talwin)
b Hydromorphone (Dilaudid)

c Meperidine
d Naloxone (Narcan)

9 *A 65-year-old man underwent left hip surgery 5 hours ago, and you are asked to evaluate him because his increasing pain is not relieved by morphine. The patient has no other known health problems. Upon reviewing his records, you find that the patient has been in the recovery room for the past 3 hours and received 4 mg of morphine intravenously 2 hours ago. Vital signs are stable, and the patient is complaining of pain in his left hip. What is your plan of action?*

a Instruct the nurse to give hydromorphone because the patient is not responding to morphine.
b Order 4 mg of morphine intravenously now, and start a morphine PCA pump.
c Order 4 mg of morphine intravenously every 2 hours.
d Order 15 mg of morphine sustained-released tablets every 12 hours.

10 *Which of the following neurotransmitters plays a role in pain transmission?*

a Acetylcholine
b Dopamine (Intropin)
c Serotonin
d All of the above

11 *All of the statements concerning acute pain are true EXCEPT:*

a it is generally of short duration.
b it may arise from injury to body parts.
c it usually is associated with bradycardia.
d it usually is associated with surgical procedures.

12 *Which of the following nonsteroidal anti-inflammatory drugs (NSAIDs) may be used as an alternative to morphine for acute postsurgical pain?*

a Indomethacin (Indocin)
b Naproxen (Naprosyn)
c Ibuprofen
d Ketorolac (Toradol)

Questions 13–16 refer to the following scenario:

A 50-year-old man with type 2 diabetes and hypertension is brought to the emergency department with complaints of scrotal pain and swelling for the past 48 hours, along with associated fever, and right lower extremity pain. He has no other medical or surgical history. The patient is on an oral agent for his diabetes. Vital signs are temperature of 102°F orally, pulse of 120, respiratory rate of 20, and blood pressure of 110/70 mm Hg. The scrotal area is edematous, erythematic, and tender with an ulceration on the right anterior scrotal wall with a foul odor. There is crepitus of the scrotum. The testicles and penis are nontender to touch and without drainage. The right midthigh has a 5-cm ulceration with foul smelling drainage and surrounding erythema. Laboratory data reveal a white blood cell count of 18,000/mm^3 with 10 bands and hemoglobin of 7.0. Serum glucose is 250.

13 *What is the most likely diagnosis?*

a Undescended testicle
b Testicular torsion
c Epididymitis
d Fournier's gangrene

14 *What comorbid condition is commonly associated with the above condition?*

a Hypertension
b Peripheral vascular disease
c Diabetes mellitus.
d Colorectal carcinoma

15 *The most common aerobic pathogen associated with this disorder is:*

a *Escherichia coli (E. coli).*
b *Staphylococcus.*
c *Streptococcus.*
d *Klebsiella.*

16 *Definitive treatment of the above condition is:*

a the use of broad-spectrum antibiotics.
b emergency surgical intervention.
c the use of broad-spectrum antibiotics and warm soaks.
d the use of broad-spectrum antibiotics and the placement of an indwelling urinary catheter.

17 *An 18-year-old college student is seen at the walk-in clinic with complaints of painful urination and vaginal itching. Examination reveals inflammation involving the vagina and urethra. Cervical smear reveals flagellated organisms. What is the most likely diagnosis?*

a Chlamydial infection
b *Trichomoniasis*
c Syphilis
d *Candida* vaginitis

18 *All of the statements concerning postconcussion headache are true EXCEPT:*

a it is the leading cause of headaches.
b it is characterized by a chronic headache.
c it is usually associated with neck pain.
d it may be associated with depression.

19 *Acute compartment syndrome occurs most often in the:*

a wrist and thigh.
b forearm and leg.
c foot and ankle.
d hand.

20 *A 45-year-old woman had abdominal aortic aneurysm repair surgery 2 days ago and now complains of pain in her right calf. Examination of the extremity reveals asymmetric swelling in the right leg, tenderness in the right calf, no erythema, and a positive Homans' sign. The patient's current medications include 5000 units of heparin subcutaneously every 12 hours, 81 mg of aspirin daily, and 50 mg of metoprolol (Lopressor) twice daily. What is the most likely diagnosis?*

a Acute gouty arthritis
b Deep-vein thrombosis of the right leg
c Myositis
d Tibia fracture

21 *Which of the following nerves supply the adductors of the thigh?*

a Sciatic nerve
b Lateral femoral cutaneous nerve
c Obturator nerve
d Saphenous nerve

22 *A 70-year-old woman undergoes a total knee replacement under epidural anesthesia. She is receiving postoperative epidural analgesia. On postoperative day 1, you are called to evaluate her because she is complaining of lower bilateral extremity weakness and has sensory changes. Your plan of action should include:*

a ordering a magnetic resonance imaging (MRI) study.
b reassuring the patient that this is a normal event with epidural analgesia.
c notifying the anesthesia department about removal of the catheter.
d ordering an x-ray of the knee.

23 *Trigeminal neuralgia is:*

a characterized by a dull, aching pain.
b may be treated definitively with intravenous steroids.
c characterized by sharp pain in the neck.
d characterized by sharp pain in the face.

24 *Which of the following findings is consistent with an anterior hip dislocation?*

a Rotated and abducted leg
b Internal rotation
c Adduction
d Flexed and shortened leg

Questions 25–30 refer to the following scenario:

A 25-year-old man is admitted from the emergency department to your nurse practitioner service with complaints of fever, neck pain, and swelling for the past 7 days. He had his wisdom teeth removed a week ago on the right side and has been on penicillin. He reports difficulty handling secretions, and has been unable to eat for the past 3 days. He has no prior medical or surgical history and no known drug allergies. Current medications consist of 500 mg of penicillin every 6 hours. Physical exam reveals an ill-appearing man, sitting on the side of the bed with constant drooling from the mouth. Vital signs are a temperature of 103°F, heart rate of 120, respiratory rate of 24, and blood pressure of 90/60 mm Hg. Head and neck exam reveals extensive swelling of the right jaw with erythema, tenderness, and palpable fluctuation. The patient is unable to open his mouth fully because of the edema. There is no evidence of stridor. The anterior cervical lymph nodes on the right are enlarged. The heart, lung, and abdominal exam are normal. Skin turgor is poor.

25 *What should be this patient's initial plan of care?*

a Evaluate the airway.
b Order a computed tomography (CT) scan of the head and neck.
c Order an x-ray of the mandible.
d Order an oral rinse.

26 *What is the most likely diagnosis of this patient?*

a Sinusitis
b Otitis externa
c Ludwig's angina
d Parotitis

27 *Classic signs of the above condition include:*

a nuchal rigidity.
b gangrene with serosanguinous fluid.
c pneumonia.
d mediastinitis.

28 *The organism most commonly responsible for the condition is:*

a *Streptococcus viridans.*
b *Staphylococcus aureus.*
c *Staphylococcus epidermis.*
d *Candida albicans.*

29 *The most serious complication of the above condition is:*

a bacteremia.
b asphyxiation.
c carotid artery infection.
d empyema.

30 *Definitive treatment of the condition on page 145 should include:*

a surgical drainage, antibiotics, and possible tracheostomy.
b tracheostomy and surgical drainage.
c antibiotics only.
d consultation with an infectious disease specialist.

Questions 31–33 refer to the following scenario:

A 30-year-old nurse is seen for complaints of severe, sharp pain in the right index finger for the past 3 days. She states that this is a recurrent problem and denies any trauma to the finger. She has fluid-filled vesicles on the side of her finger.

31 *What is the most likely diagnosis?*

a Ganglion
b Wart
c Herpetic whitlow
d Bacterial infection of the finger

32 *How would you confirm the diagnosis?*

a Order an x-ray of the finger.
b Obtain a Tzanck smear.
c Perform a Wood's ray examination.
d Obtain a complete blood cell count.

33 *Treatment of the condition includes:*

a administration of oral antibiotics.
b use of acyclovir (Zovirax), cool compresses, and analgesics.
c hand rest.
d surgical removal.

34 *Which of the following may contribute to pain in the cancer patient?*

a Direct tumor invasion
b Postradiation therapy
c Various procedures
d All of the above

35 *Psychogenic pain:*

a is unrelieved by standard treatment regimens.
b may be caused by tumor involvement in solid organs.
c is described as a constant, gnawing pain.
d is described as a shock-like sensation.

36 *A patient is receiving oral morphine for cancer pain. He admits to breakthrough pain. What is breakthrough pain?*

a Pain that the patient experiences right before the next scheduled dose of analgesic

b The transient increase in pain to a greater intensity than baseline
c Severe pain
d A period of time when there is no pain

37 *A 55-year-old woman with metastatic lung cancer has chronic pain. She is taking 5 mg of oxycodone (Percocet), 2 tablets every 4 hours. You want to switch her to morphine orally. What is the equivalent dose?*

a 30 mg of morphine sulfate (MS Contin) twice daily.
b 30 mg of MS Contin daily.
c 45 mg of MS Contin twice daily.
d 15 mg of MS Contin twice daily.

Answers

1   Answer c

The constant pain of a sarcoma represents somatic pain. Somatic pain usually involves bone and muscle and is described as a constant, aching, gnawing discomfort.

2   Answer a

This patient is experiencing neuropathic pain. Neuropathic pain is usually caused by disruption of peripheral or central neural pathways. This type of pain can be seen in postsurgical patients with such procedures as thoracotomies, mastectomies, or radial neck surgeries.

3   Answer c

The treatment option that should be explored with this patient is the use of intercostal blocks with steroids. The patient should be referred to a pain specialist for consideration of the intercostal block. Other options that could be explored include the use of opioids, such as long-acting morphine tablets or a fentanyl (Duragesic) patch along with adjunctive therapy with amitriptyline or anticonvulsants. The use of amitriptyline alone will not alleviate the pain.

4   Answer d

Anticonvulsants help to control pain by stabilizing the nerve membrane firing, with subsequent reduction of pain perception and transmission.

5   Answer d

Pain perception may be altered by many factors including anxiety, depression, fear, anger, isolation, and the degree to which the pain interferes with the person's activities of daily living.

6   Answer c

The characteristics of the ideal agent for cancer pain include one that has rapid onset of action, a short half-life, and strong analgesic potency, and allows the patient to be lucid.

7   Answer a

The preferred first-option medication for cancer pain is morphine. Meperidine is generally avoided because of its low potency and propensity for toxic metabolite accumulation leading to central nervous system (CNS) side effects. Methadone has a long half-life and is difficult to titrate. Amitriptyline may be used as an adjunct to pain but not by itself.

8   Answer d

The antagonist to morphine is naloxone.

9   Answer b

The plan of action for the patient described would be to order 4 mg of morphine intravenously now, and then start a morphine PCA pump. This patient has not received adequate analgesia. Morphine sustained release tablets are not appropriate in the management of acute surgical pain.

10   Answer d

The neurotransmitters that play a role in pain transmission are acetylcholine, dopamine, norepinephrine, and serotonin.

11   Answer c

Acute pain is generally of short duration, may arise from injury to body parts, and is associated with surgical procedures. Acute pain is associated with stimulation of the sympathetic nervous system that results in tachycardia, hypertension, tachypnea, and diaphoresis. Acute pain is not associated with bradycardia.

12   Answer d

Ketorolac may be used as an alternative to morphine for acute postsurgical pain. It has fewer CNS side effects and the same analgesic effects as morphine. Ketorolac may be given intravenously as well as intramuscularly. Indomethacin, naproxen, and ibuprofen are only available in oral forms.

13   Answer d

The most likely diagnosis for the patient described is Fournier's gangrene. Fournier's gangrene is an uncommon, rapidly progressive infection of the genital, perineal, and perianal area with associated necrotizing fasciitis. The fasciitis may lead to thrombosis of small vessels and development of gangrene.

14   Answer c

The comorbid condition commonly associated with Fournier's gangrene is diabetes mellitus. Other factors that may contribute to this disease are alcoholism, advanced age, use of systemic steroids, malnutrition, and human immunodeficiency virus.

15   Answer a

The most common aerobic pathogen associated with this disorder is *E. coli,* with *Bacteroides* the most common anaerobic pathogens. Other aerobic pathogens include *Proteus, Enterococcus, Clostridium,* and *Streptococci.*

16   Answer b

The definitive treatment of Fournier's gangrene is emergency surgical intervention. The patient should also be started on broad-spectrum antibiotics to assist in treatment of this life-threatening problem. The mortality rate with this condition is greater than 50%.

17   Answer b

The most likely diagnosis is trichomoniasis. Trichomoniasis is a mobile flagellated protozoan infection that usually presents with vaginal discharge, dysuria, abdominal pain, and vaginal itching.

18   Answer a

Postconcussion headache is a chronic headache and is associated with trauma, neck pain, and depression. It is not the leading cause of headache. Tension-type headache is the leading cause of headache.

19   Answer b

Acute compartment syndrome occurs most often in the forearm and leg.

20   Answer b

The most likely diagnosis is deep-vein thrombosis. The symptoms of unilateral edema, calf tenderness, and positive Homans' sign are classic signs of deep-vein thrombosis.

21   Answer c

The obturator nerve supplies the adductors of the thigh.

22   Answer a

The plan of action for the patient described would be to order an MRI. Then based on the information obtained, a neurology or neurosurgery consultation may be needed. The epidural catheter could have moved and wrapped around the nerve root; therefore removal of the catheter may worsen the situation.

23   Answer d

Trigeminal neuralgia is characterized by a sharp pain in the face, in the maxillary portion of the trigeminal nerve. Definitive treatment of this condition is a neurolytic nerve block.

24   Answer a

An anterior hip dislocation is associated with a rotated and abducted leg. Posterior hip dislocation is associated with internal rotation, adduction of the leg with flexion, and shortening.

25   Answer a

The initial plan of care for the patient described would be to evaluate the airway. The patient has drooling of secretions and facial and neck edema, which may lead to compromise of the airway. An otolaryngologist should be notified for airway management.

26   Answer c

The most likely diagnosis for the patient described is Ludwig's angina. Ludwig's angina or necrotizing fasciitis is a cellulitis that may affect the submaxillary, sublingual, and submandibular spaces. It is usually due to a molar area infection or injury to the mouth floor.

27   Answer b

Classic signs of Ludwig's angina include gangrene with serosanguinous fluid, with little to no frank purulence. Other signs are involvement of more than one facial space, connective tissue, fasciae, and muscles. It is spread via fascial space continuity rather than lymphatics.

28   Answer a

The organism most commonly responsible for Ludwig's angina is *S. viridans,* which accounts for approximately 40% of the reported cases.

29   Answer b

The most serious complication associated with Ludwig's angina is asphyxiation.

30 Answer a

Definitive treatment of Ludwig's angina includes surgical drainage, antibiotics, and possible tracheotomy.

31 Answer c

The most likely diagnosis based on the clinical history is herpetic whitlow.

32 Answer b

Confirmation of the diagnosis could be made by Tzanck smear taken from the base of the vesicles or by a viral culture.

33 Answer b

Treatment of herpetic whitlow includes the use of acyclovir, cool compresses, and analgesics.

34 Answer d

Pain in the cancer patient may be secondary to direct tumor invasion, postradiation therapy, and various procedures.

35 Answer a

Psychogenic or central pain is unrelieved by standard treatment and cannot be explained organically.

36 Answer b

Breakthrough pain is the transient increase in pain to a greater intensity than baseline.

37 Answer a

The equivalent dose of morphine sulfate for this patient is 30 mg twice daily. The patient is taking 60 mg of oxycodone daily. The oxycodone to morphine conversion is 1:1.

Bibliography

Cherny, NI, and Foley, KM: Nonopioid and opioid analgesic: Pharmacotherapy of Cancer Pain. Hematol Oncol Clin N Am 10:79–102, 1996.

Goroll, A, et al: Primary Care Medicine Office Evaluation and Management of the Adult Patient, 4th ed. Lippincott Williams & Wilkins, Philadelphia, 2000.

Simmond, MA: Pharmacotherapeutic management of cancer pain: Current practice. Seminars in Oncology 24:1–16, 1997.

15

Psychosocial Issues

1 *The most important risk factor for the development of major depression is:*

a substance abuse.
b family history of depression.
c the use of medications.
d personal past history of depression.

2 *A 35-year-old patient had a mastectomy for breast cancer 1 day ago and tells you on rounds that she wants to die. What is the most appropriate action?*

a Inform the patient that expressing a desire to die is inappropriate.
b Start antidepressant medications.
c Order a psychiatric consultation.
d Notify the patient's family.

3 *All of the statements concerning alcohol abuse are true* **EXCEPT:**

a it may occur in any age group.
b it is more prevalent in men.
c it is only a physiologic problem.
d it should be assessed for during health screenings.

4 *The most sensitive indicator of alcohol-induced hepatic damage is the:*

a γ-glutamyl transpeptidase (GGT) level.
b total bilirubin level.
c thiamine level.
d hemoglobin.

5 *A 25-year-old woman is admitted to the hospital after collapsing at home. She has a known history of anorexia nervosa. Which of the following is a DSM-IV criterion for anorexia?*

a Binge eating and inappropriate compensatory behavior occurring at least twice a week for 3 months

b Refusal to maintain body weight at or above 85% of normal weight for age and height
c Heavy menstrual blood flow in women of childbearing ages
d Suicidal ideations

6 *Which of the following medications may be helpful in treating the symptoms of anorexia nervosa?*

a Fluoxetine (Prozac) and low-dose lorazepam (Ativan) 30 minutes before a meal
b 1 mg of lorazepam every 6 hours
c 250 mg of disulfiram (Antabuse) daily
d 0.5 mg of risperidone (Risperdal) twice daily

7 *A 50-year-old male with a history of schizophrenia develops hand tremors and muscle rigidity. He is currently on haloperidol (Haldol). He should receive which of the following medications?*

a Lorazepam (Ativan)
b Chlorpromazine (Thorazine)
c Diazepam (Valium)
d Benztropine (Cogentin)

8 *A 40-year-old woman is seen at the clinic with complaints of insomnia and states that the FBI is following her and plans to kill her. The most appropriate response to this statement is:*

a "You sound upset, let's talk about it."
b "The FBI is not after you; that is absurd."
c "Let me call the FBI and find out more about this."
d "How long has the FBI been following you?"

9 *The normal serum lithium carbonate (Eskalith) level is:*

a 2–5 mEq/L.
b 0.6–1.0 mEq/L.
c 10–20 mEq/L.
d 5–10 mEq/L.

10 *Toxic side effects associated with lithium carbonate include:*

a   diabetes mellitus.
b   nausea.
c   congestive heart failure (CHF).
d   nephrogenic diabetes insipidus.

11 *All of the statements concerning obsessive-compulsive neurosis are true* **EXCEPT:**

a   it may be associated with depression.
b   failure to perform the compulsion produces depression.
c   it is a very uncommon condition occurring in less than 1% of psychiatric patients.
d   most obsessive-compulsive patients are first born or only children.

12 *A 65-year-old woman is on lithium carbonate (Eskalith) for manic-depressive disorder. Which of the statements is true in regard to lithium therapy?*

a   The elderly may require a lower dosage.
b   Lithium binds to plasma proteins.
c   The patient should be placed on twice-daily, rather than daily, dosing to prevent renal toxicity.
d   The polyuria associated with lithium may be treated with furosemide (Lasix).

13 *Tactile hallucinations may occur with all of the following* **EXCEPT:**

a   alcohol withdrawal.
b   schizophrenia.
c   cocaine withdrawal.
d   benzodiazepine withdrawal.

14 *Which of the following medications is used to treat opiate abuse?*

a   Lithium carbonate (Eskalith)
b   Loxapine (Loxitane)
c   Diltiazem (Cardizem)
d   Clonidine (Catapres)

15 *Electrolyte abnormalities associated with alcohol withdrawal include:*

a   hypermagnesemia.
b   hyperkalemia.
c   hyponatremia.
d   hypocalcemia.

16 *Which of the statements concerning rapid eye movement (REM) sleep is true?*

a   Sleep walking occurs during REM sleep.
b   Dreaming occurs only during REM sleep.
c   The use of benzodiazepines may increase the duration of REM sleep.
d   Monoamine oxidase inhibitors (MAOIs) reduce REM sleep.

17 *A 40-year-old male is diagnosed with schizophrenia. Which of the following statements concerning schizophrenia is(are) true?*

a   A lack of insight is a common feature.
b   Orientation is normal.
c   A common feature is a flat affect.
d   All of the above.

18 *A 25-year-old woman was raped 2 months ago and states she still feels traumatized. You refer her to a crisis intervention center. Objectives of crisis intervention centers include:*

a   ensuring that the patient can problem-solve.
b   assisting the person to gain a realistic perspective of the crisis.
c   helping the person remain composed.
d   encouraging adaptive behavior, mobilizing support persons, and identifying positive coping mechanisms.

19 *When assessing a patient with depression, what is most important to ascertain?*

a   Suicidal ideation
b   Family history of depression
c   Presence of delusions
d   History of previous depression

20 *Tricyclic antidepressants (TCAs) may take how long before clinical efficacy is obtained?*

a   48–72 hours
b   7 days
c   3 months
d   14–28 days

21 *A 35-year-old woman with complaints of palpitations, chest pain, and difficulty sleeping comes to the clinic. She also complains of a numb feeling all over, with tingling in the feet and hands. What is the most likely diagnosis?*

a   Mitral valve prolapse
b   Panic disorder
c   Supraventricular tachycardia
d   Hyperthyroidism

22 *Which of the following medications is effective in treating panic disorders?*

a   Imipramine hydrochloride (Tofranil)
b   Haloperidol
c   Sumatriptan (Imitrex)
d   Triazolam (Halcion)

23 *The CAGE questionnaire is used to assess for alcoholism. Which of the following questions is part of the CAGE questionnaire?*

a   Have people annoyed you by criticizing your drinking?

b Have you ever asked your family members not to drink around you?

c Have you ever had to wake up in the middle of the night for a drink?

d Have you lost a job because of alcohol intake?

24 *A 25-year-old male is diagnosed with generalized anxiety disorder. Which of the following needs to be considered in the differential diagnosis of a patient with generalized anxiety disorder?*

a Excessive caffeine intake
b Depression
c Mitral valve prolapse
d All of the above

25 *A woman with battered wife syndrome may present with:*

a a headache.
b suicidal behavior.
c depression.
d all of the above.

26 *Complications of bulimia nervosa include:*

a Mallory-Weiss syndrome.
b hyperkalemia.
c esophageal spasm.
d renal calculi.

27 *The most commonly abused drug among adolescents is:*

a marijuana.
b cocaine.
c benzodiazepines.
d alcohol.

28 *A 30-year-old woman had an 8-lb healthy baby 1 week ago. She comes to you, as the primary care provider, with complaints of tearfulness, fatigue, and depression since the delivery. She has no prior history of depression. What is the most likely diagnosis?*

a Adjustment disorder
b Postpartum anxiety
c Postpartum blues
d Manic-depressive disorder

29 *Treatment of postpartum blues should include:*

a benzodiazepines.
b lithium carbonate.
c hypnotics.
d reassurance and supportive care.

30 *Which of the following persons are at highest risk for suicide?*

a Persons with advanced cancer

b Women
c Persons having had solid organ transplantation
d Persons having had a stroke

31 *TCAs are contraindicated in which of the following patients?*

a A 40-year-old male with type 1 diabetes
b A 65-year-old woman with hypertension
c A 70-year-old woman with narrow-angle glaucoma
d A 60-year-old woman with renal insufficiency with a baseline creatinine value of 1.6.

32 *Sleep paralysis is:*

a a dreamlike visual hallucination at the transition between wakefulness and sleep.
b a sudden loss of skeletal muscle tone following excitement or fear.
c obstruction of the upper airway during sleep.
d a transitory inability to move or speak occurring at the transition between wakefulness and sleep.

33 *Acute psychosis may be defined by:*

a a dysfunction in the ability to process information.
b an inability to act upon reality.
c an inability to distinguish internal and external stimuli.
d all of the above.

34 *Medications linked to acute psychosis include:*

a insulin.
b prednisone.
c aspirin.
d calcium channel blockers.

35 *An 80-year-old man presents with acute psychosis. Which laboratory test(s) should be ordered?*

a Thyroid function tests
b Liver function tests
c Complete blood cell count
d All of the above

36 *A patient who presents with acute psychosis and fever should be ruled out for:*

a encephalitis.
b dementia.
c stroke.
d emotional disorder.

37 *The most common cause of psychosis and headache is:*

a an intracranial hemorrhage or tumor.
b hypoglycemia.
c meningitis.
d metabolic encephalopathy.

Answers

1 Answer d
The most important risk factor for the development of major depression is a personal past history of depression.

2 Answer c
The most appropriate action is to obtain a psychiatric consultation. The patient has expressed ideations. Appropriate reassurance is indicated.

3 Answer c
Alcohol abuse is a disorder that is characterized by physiologic and psychological components. It is thought that the physiologic aspects are related to the metabolism of alcohol, whereas the psychological aspects are thought to be related to underlying psychiatric conflict or disorder, stress, or a family history of alcohol abuse. Alcohol abuse may occur in any age group, is more prevalent in men, and should be assessed for during health screenings.

4 Answer a
The most sensitive indicator of alcohol-induced hepatic damage is the GGT level.

5 Answer b
One of the DSM-IV criteria for anorexia nervosa is the refusal to maintain body weight at or above 85% of normal weight for age and height. Other criteria include intense fear of gaining weight and undue influence of body shape or height on self-evaluation, denial of the seriousness of the problem, and amenorrhea or inability to have a menstrual cycle without hormonal manipulation. Binge eating and inappropriate compensatory behavior occurring at least twice a week for 3 months is consistent with bulimia nervosa.

6 Answer a
Pharmacologic treatment for anorexia may include the use of fluoxetine and low-dose lorazepam 30 minutes before a meal. Disulfiram is used to treat alcohol withdrawal, and risperidone is used for the treatment of psychosis.

7 Answer d
The patient is exhibiting hand tremors and muscle rigidity, which is consistent with extrapyramidal effects secondary to his use of haloperidol. Benztropine (Cogentin), which is an anticholinergic agent, should be used to reverse these symptoms.

8 Answer a
The most appropriate response to the patient described is to acknowledge her feelings and encourage her to verbalize more. Denying the patient's belief may prevent the establishment of an effective communication between you and the patient. Statements c and d ("Let me call the FBI and find out more about this," and "How long has the FBI been following you?") reinforce the patient's delusional ideas.

9 Answer b
The normal serum lithium carbonate level is 0.6–1.0 mEq/L.

10 Answer d
Toxic side effects associated with lithium carbonate include nephrogenic diabetes insipidus. The mechanism for this effect is thought to be related to interference with activity of the antidiuretic hormone on the renal tubules. Another toxic side effect is diffuse goiter.

11 Answer b
A patient with obsessive-compulsive neurosis experiences anxiety rather than depression if he or she is unable to perform the compulsive act. Obsessive-compulsive neurosis may be associated with depression and is a very uncommon condition occurring in less than 1% of psychiatric patients. Most obsessive-compulsive patients are first-born or only children.

12 Answer a
Lithium carbonate dosage in the elderly should be lowered. Lithium does not bind to plasma proteins and is excreted renally. The polyuria associated with lithium may be treated with amiloride (Midamor) rather than furosemide, which is a loop diuretic.

13 Answer c
Tactile hallucinations do not occur with cocaine withdrawal. They may occur with alcohol and benzodiazepine withdrawal and with schizophrenic patients.

14 Answer d
Clonidine, which is a central-acting agent, may be used to treat opiate abuse. Blood pressure should be monitored closely.

15 Answer c
Electrolyte abnormalities associated with alcohol withdrawal include hyponatremia, hypokalemia, and hypomagnesemia.

16 Answer d
REM sleep is reduced with the use of MAOIs.

17 Answer d
Schizophrenia may be characterized by a lack of insight and normal orientation, and a flat affect.

18 Answer d
Objectives of crisis intervention centers include encouraging adaptive behaviors, helping the person to identify support persons and eliciting their support, and identifying positive coping mechanisms.

19 Answer a
When assessing a patient with depression, it is most important to ascertain whether the person has suicidal ideations. Any suicidal ideations should be taken seriously.

20 Answer d
It is usually 14–28 days before clinical efficacy is achieved with patients taking TCAs.

21 Answer b
The most likely diagnosis for the patient described is panic disorder. Panic disorder is usually associated with symptoms of palpitations, chest pain, shortness of breath, numbness, tingling, and trembling. Physiologic conditions such as hyperthyroidism must be excluded.

22 Answer a
Imipramine is effective in treating panic disorders. Haloperidol is used for psychosis, sumatriptan is used to treat migraine headaches, and triazolam is used to treat insomnia.

23 Answer a

The CAGE questionnaire, which consists of four questions, is a screening tool for alcoholism. If the patient answers yes to two or more of the questions, more than likely a problem with alcohol exists. The four questions of the CAGE questionnaire are: Have you felt you ought to **c**ut down on your drinking? Have people **a**nnoyed you by criticizing your drinking? Have you felt bad or **g**uilty about your drinking? Have you ever had a drink first thing in the morning (**e**ye opener) to steady your nerves or get rid of a hangover?

24 Answer d

The differential diagnosis for generalized anxiety disorder should include consideration of depression, mitral valve prolapse, excessive caffeine intake, panic disorders, and hyperthyroidism.

25 Answer d

A woman with battered wife syndrome may present with any number of somatic complaints, including a headache, suicidal behavior, anxiety, and depression.

26 Answer a

Complications of bulimia nervosa include Mallory-Weiss syndrome. Other complications include dental cavities, hypokalemia, and callous formation on the hands.

27 Answer d

The most commonly abused drug among adolescents is alcohol.

28 Answer c

The most likely diagnosis for the patient described is postpartum blues. It is thought to be hormonally mediated, and may occur in over 50% of postpartum women. It is usually transient and resolves within a 2-week period. Symptoms of postpartum blues include fatigue, insomnia, poor concentration, crying spells, and depression.

29 Answer d

Treatment of postpartum blues should include reassurance and supportive care. The condition is usually transient, and there is no indication for pharmacologic intervention.

30 Answer a

The person at highest risk for suicide is the one with advanced cancer. Other groups that may be at increased risk include elderly males, those with substance abuse, and those with a defined suicide plan.

31 Answer c

TCAs are contraindicated in patients with narrow-angle glaucoma because of their anticholinergic effects.

32 Answer d

Sleep paralysis is a form of narcolepsy and is a transitory inability to move or speak, which occurs at the transition between wakefulness and sleep.

33 Answer d

Acute psychosis may be defined by a dysfunction in the ability to process information, with inability to act upon reality and discern internal and external stimuli.

34 Answer b

High doses of prednisone, a steroid, have been linked to acute psychosis. Other medications linked to psychosis include digoxin, TCAs, anticonvulsants, histamine blockers, beta blockers, amphetamines, benzodiazepines, and isoniazid (INH).

35 Answer d

Laboratory tests that should be ordered in an elderly patient who presents with acute psychosis include liver function tests, thyroid function tests, complete blood cell count, arterial blood gases, electrolytes, sedimentation rate, folate level, rapid plasma reagin (RPR), and a toxicology screen. A physiologic cause for the psychosis has to be investigated.

36 Answer a

A patient with acute psychosis and fever should be assessed for possible infectious causes, which may include meningitis, encephalitis, or bacteremia.

37 Answer a

The most common cause of psychosis and headache is an intracranial hemorrhage or tumor.

Bibliography

Goroll, A, et al: Primary Care Medicine Office Evaluation and Management of the Adult Patient, 4th ed. Lippincott Williams & Wilkins, Philadelphia, 2000.

Kendrick, T, and Tylee, A: The Prevention of Mental Illness in Primary Care. Cambridge University Press, Cambridge, England, 1996.

Kirmayer, LJ, and Robbins, JM: Somatization and the recognition of depression and anxiety in primary care. Am J Psychiatry 150: 734–41, 1993.

Nisenson, LG, et al: The nature and prevalence of anxiety disorders in primary care. Gen Hosp Psychiatry 20:21–28, 1998.

Ziedonis, D, and Brady, K: Dual diagnosis in primary care: Detecting and treating both the addiction and mental illness. Med Clin North Am 81:1017–1036, 1997.

16

Altered Mental State

1 A 50-year-old woman has had a craniotomy because of a subarachnoid hemorrhage. Which medication would be used to decrease vasospasm?

a Amlodipine (Norvasc)
b Digoxin (Lanoxin)
c Metoprolol (Lopressor)
d Warfarin (Coumadin)

2 A 30-year-old man is in the intensive care unit after suffering head trauma from a motorcycle accident. On physical exam he has horizontal diplopia. Which cranial nerve is affected?

a Cranial nerve III
b Cranial nerve IV
c Cranial nerve V
d Cranial nerve VI

3 The most common cause of dementia in the elderly is:

a polypharmacy.
b metabolic disorders.
c meningitis.
d Alzheimer's disease.

Questions 4–19 refer to the following scenario:

An 80-year-old man is admitted from the nursing home directly to the neurologic unit. According to his care providers, the patient was well until this morning, when he began complaining of headache, nausea, and chills. Over the past 2 hours he has become progressively lethargic and disoriented. His past medical history includes hypothyroidism, hypertension, and benign prostatic hypertrophy. He has no past surgical history. His current medications include levothyroxine (Synthroid), doxazosin mesylate (Cardura), and enalapril maleate (Vasotec). He is widowed and has lived in the nursing home for the past 2 years. He does not smoke and drinks red wine one to two times weekly, but no other alcohol. Vital signs reveal a temperature of 103°F, a pulse of 110, res-

piratory rate of 24, and blood pressure of 120/60 mm Hg. The patient's physical exam reveals the following: The patient is stuporous with nuchal rigidity. Fundoscopic exam reveals evidence of papilledema. Neck exam reveals no adenopathy nor jugular vein distention, a nonpalpable thyroid, and right carotid bruit. Cardiac exam reveals a 2/4 systolic ejection murmur at the second right intercostal space with radiation to the left sternal border and a positive S_4. Lung exam is normal. Abdominal exam reveals a distended bladder, but no tenderness. Motor exam finds the patient able to move all extremities randomly. There is no edema, and peripheral pulses are normal throughout. The skin exam reveals petechiae on the anterior chest, abdomen, and both upper extremities.

4 What is the most likely cause of this patient's change in mental status?

a Hypothyroidism
b Alcohol use
c Stroke
d Meningitis

5 Which of the following diagnostic studies should be done initially to further evaluate this patient?

a Computed tomography (CT) scan of the head
b Lumbar puncture (LP)
c Electroencephalogram (EEG)
d Myelogram

6 Which of the physical findings would help you determine the order of evaluation?

a Mental status
b Papilledema
c Heart murmur
d Fever

7 The patient had a CT scan of the head, which showed no evidence of mass, bleeding, or herniation. What should be the next intervention?

a Repeat the CT scan of the head with contrast.
b Obtain a magnetic resonance imaging (MRI) of the head.
c Perform an LP.
d Perform a carotid Doppler examination.

8 *Analysis of cerebrospinal fluid (CSF) can reveal:*

a a glucose content.
b a protein count.
c a white blood cell count.
d all of the above.

9 *Analysis of the CSF in a patient with meningitis normally reveals a:*

a low glucose level, high protein count, and normal white blood cell count.
b high glucose level, high protein count, and elevated white blood cell count.
c low glucose level, high protein count, and elevated white blood cell count.
d high glucose level, low protein count, and elevated white blood cell count.

10 *The neurologist informs you that the CSF is bloody. Which of the following may account for bloody CSF?*

a Hypertension
b Subarachnoid hemorrhage
c Meningococcal meningitis
d Epidural abscess

11 *Which of the following confirms subarachnoid hemorrhage as the cause of blood in the CSF?*

a The number of red blood cells present
b A positive bilirubin level on dipstick of the CSF.
c A drop in the hemoglobin
d Elevated protein level

12 *The most common complication of an LP is:*

a a subdural hematoma.
b osteomyelitis.
c bleeding at the puncture site.
d a headache.

13 *Which of the following physical findings support the diagnosis of meningitis in this patient?*

a Nuchal rigidity
b Petechiae
c Stuporous state
d Right carotid bruit

14 *Which of the following pathogens are most likely to be responsible for this patient's condition?*

a Pneumococcal meningitis
b *Haemophilus influenzae* meningitis

c *Pseudomonas* meningitis
d Meningococcal meningitis

15 *The antibiotic of choice for this patient is:*

a ampicillin and gentamicin (Unasyn).
b penicillin.
c nafcillin (Nallpen).
d ceftriaxone (Rocephin).

16 *Which of the following should also be considered in the differential diagnosis of meningococcal meningitis?*

a Tertiary syphilis
b Rocky mountain spotted fever
c Lyme disease
d Endocarditis

17 *The finding in this patient of a systolic ejection murmur indicates:*

a endocarditis.
b aortic sclerosis.
c mitral regurgitation.
d aortic regurgitation.

18 *The patient has an S_4 on physical examination. Which of the patient's conditions is most likely responsible for the S_4?*

a Hypertension
b Meningitis
c Hypothyroidism
d Advancing age

19 *Which of the following findings is not associated with meningitis?*

a Positive Romberg's sign
b Kernig's sign
c Nuchal rigidity
d Brudzinski sign

20 *Contacts of persons with meningococcal meningitis should be prescribed:*

a 500 mg of penicillin every 6 hours for 2 days.
b 500 mg of ciprofloxacin (Cipro) daily for 4 days.
c 1 tablet of trimethoprim sulfamethoxazole (Bactrim DS) twice daily for 1 week.
d 600 mg of rifampin (Rifadin) twice daily for 2 days.

Questions 21–28 refer to the following scenario:

A 60-year-old man with a history of hypertension and peripheral vascular disease had an abdominal aortic aneurysm repair 1 day ago. The staff nurse notifies you that the patient's speech is garbled, he is confused and is unable to move his left arm and leg. Vital signs are a temperature of 99°F, a pulse of 80, a respiratory rate of

24, and blood pressure of 160/90 mm Hg. The patient is on a cardiac monitor, and his rhythm has been normal sinus rhythm without arrhythmia.

21 What is the most likely cause of this patient's change in mental status?

a Hypertensive crisis
b Medication
c Stroke
d Electrolyte imbalance

22 Which of the following is a risk factor for stroke in this patient?

a Postoperative state
b Hypertension
c Age
d Presence of peripheral vascular disease

23 Which of the following should be part of the patient's initial plan of care?

a Obtaining a neurology consultation
b Lowering of the patient's blood pressure with nitroprusside (Nitropress)
c Obtaining an emergency MRI
d Performing an LP

24 The neurologist suspects a right middle cerebral infarct. If this is so, which of the physical findings may develop?

a Bradyarrhythmias.
b Left homonymous hemianopia.
c Right hemiplegia.
d Spasticity.

25 Left homonymous hemianopia indicates damage to the:

a Second cranial nerve.
b Sixth cranial nerve.
c Third cranial nerve.
d Fifth cranial nerve.

26 The patient becomes increasingly confused and his speech is more garbled. He is drooling and unable to handle oral secretions. What is the most appropriate intervention at this point?

a Initiate aspiration precautions and consider endotracheal intubation.
b Consult neurosurgery for an evaluation.
c Withhold all oral medications.
d Start intravenous heparin.

27 Which of the following tests should be ordered for the patient?

a Head magnetic resonance imaging (MRI).
b Head computed tomography (CT) scan.
c Electroencephalogram (EEG).
d Lumbar puncture (LP).

28 The patient progresses to a comatose state. The Glasgow Coma Scale measures:

a Pupillary and verbal responses.
b Pupillary and motor responses.
c Eye opening and pupillary reaction.
d Eye opening and motor and verbal responses.

29 Acquired immunodeficiency syndrome (AIDS) dementia complex is associated with a CD4 count of:

a 500.
b Less than 200.
c 200–500.
d More than 500.

30 AIDS dementia complex is characterized by all of the following **EXCEPT**:

a Memory loss.
b Depressed affect.
c Confusion.
d Paralysis.

31 The most common fungal infection of the central nervous system in patients who are positive for human immunodeficiency virus (HIV) is:

a Toxoplasmosis.
b Aspergillosis.
c Cryptococcus.
d Histoplasmosis.

32 Which of the following predisposes a patient to delirium?

a Advancing age.
b Head injury.
c History of substance abuse.
d All of the above.

33 All of the statements concerning coma are true **EXCEPT:**

a It is a depressed mental state.
b It may be the result of trauma.
c Renal failure will produce lethargy but not coma.
d Substance abuse may produce coma.

Questions 34–37 refer to the following scenario:

A 65-year-old man is found lying on the street and brought to the emergency department for evaluation. He is lethargic and unable to provide any history. His clothing is dirty and he appears unkempt. Vital signs are temperature 99°F, pulse 100, respiratory rate 22, and blood pressure 100/60 mm Hg.

34 *What diagnostic test(s) should be obtained on this patient?*

a Electroencephalogram (EEG).
b Lumbar puncture.
c Serum electrolytes and glucose levels.
d Head computed tomography (CT) scan.

35 *A prescription bottle for Percocet is found on the patient; you suspect narcotic ingestion. What is the treatment for narcotic overdose?*

a Activated charcoal.
b Naloxone (Narcan).
c Hemodialysis.
d Plasmapheresis.

36 *The patient's laboratory results reveal hypoglycemia. Treatment of hypoglycemia should include:*

a 2 liters of D5W solution at 125 cc/h.
b 1 ampule of D50W.
c 1 liter of D5W alternating with 1 liter of NS.
d None of the above.

37 *The patient starts to exhibit signs of increased intracranial pressure (ICP). He developed headaches, nausea, vomiting, diplopia, lethargy, bradycardia, and hypertension. What interventions should be instituted?*

a Administration of mannitol and intubation with hyperventilation.
b Administration of furosemide (Lasix) and naloxone (Narcan).
c Gastric lavage.
d Administration of mannitol only.

Answers

1 Answer a

Amlodipine (Norvasc) is a calcium channel blocker, which is used to treat vasospasm.

2 Answer d

Cranial nerve VI involvement, which may be caused by increased intracranial pressure, will result in horizontal diplopia.

3 Answer d

The most common cause of dementia in the elderly is Alzheimer's disease.

4 Answer d

The most likely cause of this patient's change in mental status is meningitis.

5 Answer a

This patient should have a head computed tomography (CT) scan performed initially to rule out a mass, herniation, shift of tissue, or obliteration of the central spinal fluid pathway.

6 Answer b

The presence of papilledema would help determine the order of evaluation of this patient. Papilledema would lead to the suspicion of an intracranial mass effect. If that were the case, a head computed tomography (CT) scan should be done first, before a lumbar puncture (LP).

7 Answer c

The next intervention for the patient described should be to perform a lumbar puncture (LP).

8 Answer d

Analysis of cerebrospinal fluid (CSF) can reveal a glucose count, protein count, and white blood cell count. Other studies performed from CS include cytologic testing, gram stain and culture, viral titers, and serologic testing for syphilis and Lyme disease.

9 Answer c

Analysis of the cerebrospinal fluid (CSF) in a patient with meningitis normally reveals a low glucose level, high protein count, and elevated white blood count with a predominance of neutrophils.

10 Answer b

Bloody cerebrospinal fluid (CSF) may result from a subarachnoid hemorrhage, or trauma during the lumbar puncture (LP) (spinal tap) procedure.

11 Answer b

A positive bilirubin on dipstick of the cerebrospinal fluid (CSF) confirms the diagnosis of a subarachnoid hemorrhage as the cause of blood in the CSF. The positive bilirubin suggests that blood has been present in the fluid for at least several hours, thus confirming subarachnoid bleeding rather than a traumatic lumbar puncture (LP). The opening pressure and the spinal fluid bilirubin count are elevated in subarachnoid hemorrhage, but are usually normal with a traumatic procedure.

12 Answer d

The most common complication post lumbar puncture (LP) is a headache. Subdural hematoma, osteomyelitis, and bleeding at the puncture site may occur post LP but are uncommon.

13 Answer a

The physical finding that supports the diagnosis of meningitis in this patient is the presence of nuchal rigidity. Common findings with meningitis include nuchal rigidity, Kernig's sign, and Brudzinski sign. Petechiae may imply infection, but are not diagnostic of meningitis. The stuporous state may be secondary to fever in this elderly man, but is not definitive for meningitis. The presence of a right carotid bruit implies atherosclerosis disease.

14 Answer d

The pathogen most likely to be responsible for this patient's condition is meningococcal meningitis. This diagnosis is supported by the rapid progression of the symptoms of fever, headache, nausea, and alteration in mental status. It is further supported with the presence of petechiae. Meningococcal meningitis is more common in children, but can occur in any age group.

15 Answer b

The antibiotic of choice for patients with meningococcal meningitis is penicillin.

16 Answer b

Rocky Mountain spotted fever should be considered in the differential diagnosis of meningococcal meningitis. Rocky

Mountain spotted fever is an acute febrile illness, which may present with complaints of headache, macular or petechial rash, lethargy, and stiff neck.

17   Answer b
The finding of a systolic ejection murmur in this patient may be an age-related finding secondary to calcification and sclerosis of the aortic valve, and is considered an innocent systolic murmur of the elderly. Endocarditis may produce a murmur, but it would be a regurgitant lesion. The location of the murmur does not support a diagnosis of mitral or aortic regurgitation.

18   Answer a
S4, which is an atrial gallop, is present in conditions in which the left ventricle hypertrophies, for example, hypertension, aortic stenosis, and ischemic heart disease.

19   Answer a
Meningitis or meningeal irritation is associated with a positive Kernig's sign, positive Brudzinski sign, and nuchal rigidity. A positive Romberg sign is not associated with meningitis, but is rather a test of cerebellar function.

20   Answer d
Contacts of persons with meningococcal meningitis should take rifampin 600 mg twice daily for 2 days.

21   Answer c
The most likely cause of this patient's change in mental status is a stroke. Medications, particular narcotics, and electrolyte imbalances may contribute to the patient's confusion, but not the reported motor deficits. The patient's blood pressure is elevated, but does not represent a hypertensive crisis.

22   Answer b
The risk factor for stroke in this patient is hypertension.

23   Answer a
The initial plan of care for this patient should include obtaining a neurology consultation. There is no indication for lumbar puncture, or emergency magnetic resonance imaging (MRI). The patient's blood pressure is elevated, but does not warrant the intervention of nitroprusside (Nipride). Lowering of the blood pressure too rapidly may lead to cerebral hypoperfusion and worsening of the stroke.

24   Answer b
If the patient has a right middle cerebral infarct, he may develop left homonymous hemianopia.

25   Answer a
Left homonymous hemianopia indicates damage to the optic nerve, which is the second cranial nerve.

26   Answer a
The patient seems to have an evolving stroke, and aspiration precautions should be initiated and intubation for airway protection considered.

27   Answer b
The patient described should have a head computed tomography (CT) scan once he can be transported.

28   Answer d
The Glasgow Coma Scale measures eye opening and motor and verbal responses.

29   Answer b
Acquired immunodeficiency syndrome (AIDS) dementia complex is associated with a CD4 count less than 200.

30   Answer d
AIDS dementia complex is a neuropsychiatric complication of human immunodeficiency virus (HIV) infection. It is associated with cognitive deficits such as confusion, memory loss, impaired concentration, depression, agitation, and motor symptoms such as weakness, unsteady gait, and ataxia. Paralysis is not associated with AIDS dementia complex.

31   Answer c
The most common fungal infection of the central nervous system in patients who are positive for human immunodeficiency virus is cryptococcus.

32   Answer d
Factors that may predispose a patient to delirium include advancing age, head injury, and a history of substance abuse.

33   Answer c
Renal failure may produce changes in mental status, including coma. Other causes of coma may be trauma, metabolic factors, infection, psychiatric factors, stroke, alcohol and substance abuse, and lack of oxygen. Coma is a depressed mental state.

34   Answer c
Diagnostic tests that should be obtained on the patient described include serum electrolytes and glucose levels. A head computed tomography (CT) scan should be done only if there is suspicion for a structural lesion or evidence of head trauma. If there is a suspicion of a central nervous system infection, a lumbar puncture should be done. There is no indication for an electroencephalogram.

35   Answer b
The treatment for suspected ingestion of Percocet is naloxone (Narcan).

36   Answer b
Treatment of hypoglycemia should include the administration of 1 ampule of D5W.

37   Answer a
The patient with signs of increased intracranial pressure (ICP) should receive mannitol, and be intubated and hyperventilated to decrease arterial PCO_2 to levels of 25–28.

Bibliography

Ancoli-Israel, S: Sleep problems in older adults: Putting myths to bed. Geriatr 52:20–30, 1997.

Dunphy, L: Management Guidelines for Adult Nurse Practitioners. FA Davis, Philadelphia, 1999.

Goroll, A, et al: Primary Care Medicine Office Evaluation and Management of the Adult Patient, 4th ed. Lippincott Williams & Wilkins, Philadelphia, 2000.

Fauci, AS, et al: Harrison's Principles of Internal Medicine, 14th ed. McGraw-Hill Book Company, New York, 1998.

Mayo-Smith, MF: Pharmacological management of alcohol withdrawal. JAMA 278:144–151, 1997.

17

Shock

1 *Shock is defined as:*

a systolic blood pressure more than 90 mm Hg.
b diastolic blood pressure more than 50 mm Hg.
c a state in which oxygen delivery is inadequate for metabolic needs.
d cardiac output more than 1.8 L/min.

2 *The Frank-Starling law reflects:*

a left ventricular ejection.
b physiologic changes in the heart during systole.
c normal changes that occur in shock states.
d the preload dependence of cardiac contractility.

3 *The primary mechanism in cardiogenic shock is:*

a volume contraction.
b pump failure.
c volume loss.
d increased venous capacitance.

4 *A 50-year-old woman who has had stem-cell transplantation and chemotherapy for breast carcinoma has a fever of 103°F, a pulse of 130, a respiratory rate of 24, and blood pressure of 80/50 mm Hg. Which classification of shock is she exhibiting?*

a Obstructive shock
b Cardiogenic shock
c Hypovolemic shock
d Distributive shock

Questions 5–7 refer to the following scenario:

A 25-year-old man is seen in the emergency department after a stab wound to the chest wall. In the emergency department, he is awake but lethargic. Vital signs are a pulse of 52, a respiratory rate of 32, and blood pressure of 70/50 mm Hg. Physical exam reveals muffled heart tones and elevated neck veins.

5 *What is the most likely diagnosis?*

a Cardiac tamponade
b Hemithorax
c Tension pneumothorax
d Cardiac contusion

6 *Which type of shock is this patient exhibiting?*

a Obstructive shock
b Cardiogenic shock
c Hypovolemic shock
d Distributive shock

7 *Beck's triad, which is associated with cardiac tamponade, consists of distended neck veins, along with the following symptoms:*

a tachycardia and a bounding pulse.
b bradycardia and S_3 heart sounds.
c oliguria and distant heart tones.
d hypotension and distant heart tones.

8 *Causes of distributive shock include all of the following EXCEPT:*

a sepsis.
b drug overdose.
c blood loss.
d autonomic blockade.

Questions 9–13 apply to the following scenario:

A 50-year-old woman with a history of three episodes of deep-vein thrombosis (DVT) in the past year is seen in the emergency department with complaints of progressive shortness of breath for the past 4 hours. Vital signs are a pulse of 120, a respiratory rate of 28, and blood pressure of 80/50 mm Hg. She has no other past medical history except the DVT and no allergies. Medications include aspirin and a daily multivitamin. Arterial blood gas (ABG) results reveal severe hypoxemia. A pulmonary artery catheter is inserted and reveals a pulmonary artery pressure of 50/30, a right atrial pressure of 26, a cardiac index of 1.8 L/min per mm², and mixed venous saturation of 40%.

9 Based on the above data, the nurse practitioner suspects:

a obstructive shock.
b neurogenic shock.
c septic shock.
d cardiogenic shock.

10 What is the most likely cause of this patient's shock?

a Cardiac tamponade
b Myocardial infarction (MI)
c Pulmonary embolus
d Sepsis

11 Treatment options for this patient include:

a thrombolytics, volume replacement, oxygen therapy, and vasopressors.
b volume replacement and oxygen therapy.
c vasopressors.
d oxygen therapy and intra-aortic balloon pump (IABP) counterpulsation.

12 Which valvular lesion would you expect to find in the patient with acute pulmonary embolus?

a Mitral stenosis
b Tricuspid regurgitation
c Aortic regurgitation
d Mitral regurgitation

13 Which inotropic option would be the best option for the patient described in the scenario above?

a Epinephrine
b Norepinephrine (Levophed)
c Dopamine (Intropin)
d Dobutamine (Dobutrex)

14 Symptoms related to decreased organ perfusion include:

a decreased urine output.
b mental status changes.
c clammy extremities.
d all of the above.

15 Hemodynamic features of cardiogenic shock include:

a hypotension.
b decreased pulmonary capillary wedge pressure (PCWP).

c decreased systemic vascular resistance.
d increased cardiac output.

16 A 70-year-old man with a blood pressure reading of 70/50 mm Hg, a cardiac output of 10 L/min, and a systemic vascular resistance (SVR) of 400 dyne-s/cm⁵ is exhibiting:

a Cardiogenic shock
b Hypovolemic shock
c Distributive shock
d Obstructive shock

Questions 17–20 refer to the following scenario:

A 55-year-old man is seen in the emergency department with complaints of midsternal chest discomfort associated with shortness of breath for the past hour. He took 650 mg of aspirin without relief of pain. An electrocardiogram (ECG) in the emergency department reveals an acute MI. Vital signs are a heart rate of 110 and blood pressure of 80/50 mm Hg. He is placed on intravenous nitroglycerin and heparin and has relief of pain. Over the next hour, the patient becomes progressively hypotensive with a blood pressure of 60/40 mm Hg. A pulmonary artery catheter is inserted and reveals a cardiac index of 1.2 L/min per mm², a PCWP of 35%, mixed venous saturation of 35%, and systemic vascular resistance of 2400 dyne-s/cm⁵.

17 What is the most appropriate initial response for this patient?

a Stop the nitroglycerin and start epinephrine.
b Start thrombolytic therapy.
c Administer 2 L of D5W.
d Administer morphine sulfate.

18 The patient described is exhibiting:

a distributive shock.
b neurogenic shock.
c obstructive shock.
d cardiogenic shock.

19 The priority for the care of the patient described is to:

a restore coronary blood flow.
b provide volume resuscitation.
c identify the septic focus.
d replace electrolytes.

20 Initial management of a patient with a suspected right ventricular MI should include:

a administration of vasopressors.
b volume resuscitation.
c administration of antibiotics.
d insertion of a ventricular assist device.

21 *A patient with an acute cervical spinal cord injury will exhibit:*

a cardiogenic shock.
b hypovolemic shock.
c distributive shock.
d obstructive shock.

22 *Causes of cardiogenic shock in trauma patients may include all of the following* **EXCEPT:**

a pericardial tamponade.
b cardiac contusion.
c pulmonary embolus.
d tension pneumothorax.

23 *The normal central venous pressure (CVP) is:*

a 5–12 mm Hg.
b 10–20 mm Hg.
c 20–30 mm Hg.
d 2.0 mm Hg.

24 *The patient with septic shock will have:*

a an increased SVR.
b a decreased SVR.
c a decreased cardiac output.
d bradycardia.

25 *Hemodynamic findings associated with hypovolemic shock include:*

a tachycardia and hypotension.
b bradycardia and increased cardiac index.
c tachycardia and elevated PCWP.
d elevated central venous pressure and hypotension.

26 *All of the following vasoactive substances are released in sepsis* **EXCEPT:**

a endotoxins.
b endorphins.
c histamines.
d bradykinins.

27 *A patient in cardiogenic shock who has an elevated left ventricular end diastolic pressure (LVEDP) is best treated with:*

a dopamine.
b epinephrine.
c dobutamine and IABC.
d dopamine and diuretics.

Questions 28–29 refer to the following scenario:

A 24-year-old man is brought to the emergency department after a gunshot wound to the chest and abdomen. His systolic blood pressure is 40 mm Hg.

28 *Which of the following should be started?*

a Normal saline infused at a wide-open rate and type O– blood
b Mannitol
c 4 L of D5W
d 4 L of lactated Ringer's injection

29 *Which type of shock is this patient exhibiting?*

a Distributive shock
b Cardiogenic shock
c Obstructive shock
d Hypovolemic shock

30 *Initial treatment of anaphylaxis should include the administration of:*

a steroids.
b epinephrine.
c dopamine.
d dobutamine.

31 *A 25-year-old man is seen in the emergency department with an anaphylactic reaction to penicillin. He suddenly develops upper airway obstruction and stridor. What is the most appropriate treatment?*

a Administration of epinephrine and emergency intubation or cricothyrotomy
b Administration of steroids and epinephrine
c Administration of dopamine and fluids
d Administration of epinephrine only

32 *The most likely acid-base disturbance in the end stages of shock is:*

a metabolic alkalosis.
b metabolic acidosis.
c respiratory acidosis.
d respiratory alkalosis.

33 *A 45-year-old man is brought to the emergency department after a gunshot wound to his left chest. He is cyanotic with agonal breathing. He has absent breath sounds on the left side, and lung sounds are dull on percussion. Vital signs are a pulse of 100 and blood pressure of 60/40 mm Hg. What is the most likely diagnosis?*

a Tension pneumothorax
b Cardiac tamponade
c Hemothorax
d Diaphragmatic laceration

34 *Hemodynamic indications for use of ventricular assist devices include all of the following* **EXCEPT:**

a cardiac index less than 2.0 L/min per m^2.
b atrial pressure more than 20 mm Hg.
c SVR less than 1200 dyne-s/cm^5.
d urine output less than 20 cc/h.

35 *The most significant physiologic manifestation of massive hemothorax is:*

a hypovolemia.
b cardiac tamponade.
c tension pneumothorax.
d reduction of left ventricular ejection fraction.

36 *The impedance to ventricular ejection is referred to as:*

a preload.
b afterload.
c oxygen consumption.
d contractility.

37 *Which of the following would increase CVP readings?*

a Vasodilator drugs
b Diuretics
c Positive-pressure ventilation
d Transducer positioned too high

Answers

1 Answer c
Shock is defined as a state in which oxygen delivery is inadequate for metabolic needs.

2 Answer d
The Frank-Starling law reflects the preload dependence of cardiac contractility.

3 Answer b
The primary mechanism in cardiogenic shock is pump failure, which may be caused by MI, arrhythmias, and/or heart failure.

4 Answer d
The patient described is exhibiting signs of sepsis, which is a form of distributive shock.

5 Answer a
The most likely diagnosis for the patient described is cardiac tamponade. The patient has muffled heart tones and elevated neck veins along with bradycardia and hypotension.

6 Answer a
The type of shock the patient described is exhibiting is obstructive shock, in which there is impedance of the blood to the heart, secondary to blood accumulation in the pericardium. This will result in circulatory collapse.

7 Answer d
Beck's triad, which is associated with cardiac tamponade, consists of (1) distended neck veins, (2) hypotension, and (3) distant, or muffled, heart tones.

8 Answer c
Causes of distributive shock include sepsis, drug overdose,

and autonomic blockade. Distributive shock is not caused by blood loss, which is a form of hypovolemic shock.

9 Answer a
This patient described is exhibiting obstructive shock. This form of shock is caused by an extracardiac obstruction of blood flow.

10 Answer c
The most likely cause of this patient's shock is pulmonary embolus. Based on the patient's history of DVT and acute shortness of breath with hypoxemia, pulmonary embolus is the most likely cause.

11 Answer a
Treatment options for this patient include thrombolytics, volume replacement, oxygen therapy, and vasopressors.

12 Answer b
The patient with acute pulmonary embolus may have tricuspid regurgitation secondary to right ventricular dilatation.

13 Answer d
The best inotropic option for the patient described is dobutamine.

14 Answer d
Symptoms related to decreased organ perfusion include decreased urine output, mental status changes, and clammy extremities.

15 Answer a
Hemodynamic features of cardiogenic shock include hypotension. Other features of cardiogenic shock include elevated PCWP, decreased cardiac output and cardiac index, and elevated SVR. The SVR is usually markedly elevated. The elevation is a reflex attempt to maintain perfusion pressure.

16 Answer c
The patient described who has hypotension and an elevated cardiac output with decreased SVR is exhibiting distributive shock.

17 Answer a
The most appropriate initial response for the patient described is to stop the nitroglycerin and start epinephrine therapy.

18 Answer d
The patient described is exhibiting cardiogenic shock, secondary to MI.

19 Answer a
The priority for the care of the patient described is to restore coronary blood flow, which may be achieved by coronary angioplasty or emergency coronary artery bypass surgery.

20 Answer b
Initial management of a patient with a suspected right ventricular MI should include volume resuscitation.

21 Answer c
A patient with an acute cervical spinal cord injury will exhibit distributive shock. In spinal cord injuries, there is loss of sympathetic tone distal to the lesion, resulting in arteriolar and venous dilatation.

22 Answer c
Causes of cardiogenic shock in the trauma patient may in-

clude pericardial tamponade, cardiac contusion, and tension pneumothorax. Pulmonary embolus will result in obstructive shock.

23 Answer a

The normal central venous pressure is 5–12 mm Hg.

24 Answer b

The patient with septic shock will have a decreased SVR.

25 Answer a

Hemodynamic findings associated with hypovolemic shock include tachycardia and hypotension.

26 Answer b

Sepsis causes the release of endotoxin, histamine, and bradykinin; it does not cause the release of endorphins.

27 Answer c

A patient in cardiogenic shock who has an elevated LVEDP is best treated with dobutamine, diuretics, and IABC.

28 Answer a

Normal saline infused at a wide-open rate and type O– blood should be given to the patient described.

29 Answer d

The patient described is exhibiting hypovolemic shock.

30 Answer b

Initial treatment of anaphylaxis should include the administration of epinephrine.

31 Answer a

The treatment for anaphylaxis associated with upper airway obstruction and stridor includes the administration of epinephrine and emergency intubation and/or cricothyrotomy.

32 Answer a

The most likely acid-base disturbance in the end stages of shock is metabolic acidosis.

33 Answer c

Based on the nature of the injury, and the hemodynamic compromise, the most likely diagnosis for the patient described is hemothorax. Tension pneumothorax would exhibit tracheal displacement away from the affected side, and hyper-resonant percussion. Cardiac tamponade and diaphragmatic laceration may account for the hemodynamic compromise, but probably would not account for the pulmonary compromise exhibited by this patient.

34 Answer c

Hemodynamic indications for use of ventricular assist devices include cardiac index less than 2.0 L/min per m², atrial pressure more than 20 mm Hg, urine output less than 20 cc/h, and a SVR of more than 2000 dyne-s/cm⁵.

35 Answer a

The most significant physiologic manifestation of massive hemothorax is loss of circulating blood volume and hypovolemia.

36 Answer b

The impedance to ventricular ejection is referred to as afterload.

37 Answer c

Positive pressure ventilation would increase CVP readings.

Bibliography

Fauci, AS, et al: Harrison's Principles of Internal Medicine, 14th ed. McGraw-Hill Book Company, New York, 1998.
Kline, JA: Emergency Medicine: Concepts and Clinical Practice, 4th ed. Mosby, St. Louis, 1998.

18
Nutritional Imbalances

1 *The recommended daily allowance (RDA) of protein per day for the adult is:*

a 0.75 gm/kg.
b 10 gm/kg.
c 5 gm/kg.
d 2.5 gm/kg.

2 *Which of the following proteins is synthesized by the liver and requires vitamin K to become an active protein?*

a Factor VIII
b Factor X
c Factor XIII
d Factor V

3 *A 70-year-old man is 2 weeks post stroke and has suffered pharyngeal paralysis. He is unable to eat food without aspiration. What is the most appropriate method to provide nutrition to this patient?*

a Total parenteral nutrition (TPN)
b Surgical gastrostomy
c Nasogastric tube
d Peripheral parenteral nutrition (PPN)

4 *A 40-year-old woman with a gunshot wound to the abdomen had a resection of half of her colon. It has been 4 months since the trauma, and she is unable to maintain weight on oral feedings. What is the appropriate method to provide nutrition to this patient?*

a Nocturnal feedings via a nasoduodenal tube
b PPN
c Surgical gastrostomy tube placement
d TPN

5 *Zinc deficiency is characterized by:*

a anemia and neutropenia.
b perioral rash, hair loss, and poor wound healing.
c hair loss and blurred vision.
d nausea and vomiting.

6 *Symptoms of protein malnutrition may include:*

a weakness and edema.
b fever and chills.
c skin rashes and hair loss.
d muscle wasting and hair loss.

Questions 7 and 8 refer to the following scenario:

An 80-year-old man is admitted to your nurse practitioner service with a diagnosis of pneumonia. His past medical history includes type 2 diabetes, hypothyroidism, and anemia. His current medications include glyburide (DiaBeta), levothyroxine (Synthroid), and multivitamins. His daughter states that she is concerned about her father's forgetfulness because he has had periods of disorientation over the past 3 months.

7 *What is the most likely vitamin deficiency in this patient?*

a Vitamin C
b Vitamin B_{12}
c Vitamin E
d Vitamin D

8 *Which of the following anemias is associated with this patient's vitamin deficiency?*

a Sickle cell anemia
b Iron-deficiency anemia
c Thalassemia minor
d Pernicious anemia

9 *The most common causes of iron deficiency in the elderly include:*

a gastric carcinoma.
b inadequate iron intake.
c renal failure.
d bone marrow suppression.

10 *Which of the following vitamin deficiencies may impair iron absorption?*

a Vitamin D
b Vitamin C
c Vitamin A
d Vitamin E

11 *Which of the following diets has been associated with lowering the risk of colorectal cancer?*

a High-fat diet
b High-carbohydrate diet
c High-protein diet
d High-fiber diet

Questions 12–15 refer to the following scenario:

A 65-year-old man is admitted to your service with a diagnosis of acute pancreatitis. His past medical history includes hypertension, alcohol use, and gastritis. He states he went to a birthday party 5 days ago and drank for a 24-hour period. His current medications include enalapril (Vasotec), famotidine (Pepcid), and metoprolol (Lopressor).

12 *What is the best way to initially provide nutrition to this patient?*

a Oral feedings
b Nasogastric tube placement
c TPN
d PPN

13 *Which of the following enzyme levels should be periodically checked in patients with acute pancreatitis?*

a Lipase and amylase
b Creatine kinase (CK)
c Lactate dehydrogenase (LDH)
d C-reactive protein

14 *What in the patient's history is identified as a risk factor for pancreatitis?*

a Age
b Hypertension
c Use of enalapril
d Alcohol intake

15 *Which of the following electrolyte abnormalities is commonly observed in patients with acute pancreatitis?*

a Hyponatremia
b Hyperglycemia
c Hypocalcemia
d Hypermagnesemia

16 *Which of the following diets should be implemented in patients with pancreatitis?*

a Low-fat diet

b High-fat diet
c Low-carbohydrate diet
d High-protein diet

17 *All of the statements concerning a high fiber diet are true* **EXCEPT:**

a fiber increases the intestinal transit time.
b high-fiber diets may be associated with increased flatulence and diarrhea.
c high-fiber diets improve bowel function.
d high-fiber diets may be associated with increased absorption of glucose and cholesterol.

Questions 18 and 19 refer to the following scenario:

A 25-year-old woman is diagnosed with celiac disease. She has no other health problems.

18 *The recommended diet for a patient with celiac disease is a:*

a high-fat diet.
b high-fiber diet.
c gluten-free diet.
d high-protein diet.

19 *Which of the following foods should be avoided in a patient with celiac disease?*

a Wheat bread
b Rice
c Potatoes
d Soybeans

20 *Vitamin A deficiency is associated with:*

a a sore throat.
b recurrent urinary tract infections (UTIs).
c night blindness.
d iron-deficiency anemia.

21 *Contraindications to enteral feedings include:*

a paralytic ileus.
b ischemic bowel.
c severe diarrhea.
d all of the above.

Questions 22–27 refer to the following scenario:

A 65-year-old man with diabetes is admitted to the intensive care unit with pneumonia and congestive heart failure (CHF). His condition deteriorates to respiratory failure, and he is placed on a ventilator. After 2 weeks, he remains dependent on the ventilator and has a tracheotomy performed.

22 *Which of the following assessments would be important in determining the route of nutrition for this patient?*

a Mental status
b Presence of bowel sounds
c Previous gallbladder surgery
d Ability to open the mouth

23 *The route of nutritional support for this patient should be:*

a oral.
b enteral feeding via gastrostomy.
c TPN.
d none of the above.

24 *Benefits of enteral feeding for this patient include:*

a fewer fluid and electrolyte disturbances.
b worsened glucose control.
c decreased protein synthesis.
d decreased nitrogen balance.

25 *Three days after initiating enteral feedings, the patient develops a high gastric residual. What are its possible causes?*

a High osmolarity formulas
b Low-fat feedings
c Isotonic formulas
d Bolus feedings

26 *Which of the following medications may be used to stimulate gastric emptying?*

a Cimetidine (Tagamet)
b Metoclopramide (Reglan)
c Famotidine
d Ranitidine (Zantac)

27 *What in the patient's history makes him likely to have problems with gastric emptying?*

a Ventilator dependence
b CHF
c Age
d Diabetes mellitus

Questions 28–30 refer to the following scenario:

A 70-year-old man had cardiac surgery 3 days ago and is complaining of an inability to eat because of nausea and loss of appetite. The patient has no prior history of gastric problems. His current medications include aspirin, ferrous sulfate, metoprolol, acetaminophen with codeine (Tylenol #3), and docusate sodium (Colace).

28 *Potential causes of this patient's gastrointestinal symptoms include:*

a medications.
b a gastric ulcer.
c right coronary artery ischemia.
d all of the above.

29 *Which of the following laboratory tests would be the most helpful in evaluating this patient's nutritional status?*

a Hemoglobin
b Prealbumin, albumin, and calcium levels
c Calcium and phosphorous levels
d Total protein level

30 *Steps helpful in the management of this patient include:*

a obtaining daily calorie counts.
b ordering nutritional supplements.
c holding the patient's medications (aspirin, ferrous sulfate, and acetaminophen with codeine).
d all of the above.

31 *Causes of malabsorption include:*

a pancreatic insufficiency.
b peptic ulcer disease.
c duodenal ulcer.
d cholelithiasis.

32 *An 80-year-old man who has been dependent on a ventilator for 2 weeks is extubated. What should be done to evaluate if the patient can safely eat?*

a Start him on a liquid diet.
b Check the patient's gag reflex; if absent, start the patient on regular food.
c Obtain a swallowing evaluation.
d All of the above.

33 *A 45-year-old woman with human immunodeficiency virus (HIV) infection is intubated and has been on a ventilator for 2 weeks because of acute respiratory distress syndrome (ARDS). She is malnourished. Which of the following nutritional factors may affect respiratory muscles?*

a Hypocalcemia
b Hypermagnesemia
c Hyperphosphatemia
d Hyperkalemia

34 *All of the statements concerning malnutrition and the pulmonary system are true* **EXCEPT:**

a patients with chronic respiratory problems are prone to the development of malnutrition.
b malnutrition may lead to impairment of respiratory muscle function.
c malnutrition is associated with increased production of surfactant.
d malnutrition may lead to difficulty in weaning intubated patients.

35 *Which of the following diets are recommended for the prevention of coronary artery disease?*

a   A low-fat diet
b   A calorie-restricted diet.
c   A high-carbohydrate diet.
d   A diet that emphasizes fruits, vegetables, and low amounts of unsaturated fat.

36 *Which of the following diets should be prescribed for a patient with Crohn's disease and an intestinal fistula?*

a   High-protein and high-fat diet
b   Low-residue diet
c   Regular diet
d   Gluten-free diet

37 *Which of the following vitamins should not be given to patients with end-stage renal failure who are on dialysis?*

a   Vitamin B
b   Vitamin C
c   Vitamin E
d   Vitamin A

Answers

1   Answer a
The RDA of protein for the adult is 0.75 gm/kg.

2   Answer b
Factor X is synthesized by the liver and requires vitamin K to become an active protein.

3   Answer b
The most appropriate way to provide nutrition to the patient described is by surgical gastrostomy.

4   Answer d
The appropriate method to provide nutrition to the patient described who has had a partial colon resection and is unable to sustain weight with oral feedings should include TPN. Attempts at continuing to nourish via the gastrointestinal tract will not produce significant changes in weight. There is probably a malabsorption phenomenon caused by the colon resection.

5   Answer b
Zinc deficiency is characterized by perioral rash, hair loss, and poor wound healing. Anemia and neutropenia characterize copper deficiency. Hair loss, dermatitis, paraesthesia, and blurred vision characterize linoleic acid deficiency.

6   Answer a
Symptoms of protein malnutrition may include weakness and edema. Other symptoms include lassitude, muscle wasting, skin rashes, and poor healing.

7   Answer b
The most likely vitamin deficiency in the patient described is vitamin B_{12} deficiency. Vitamin B_{12} deficiency in the elderly is

usually associated with impairment of cognitive function, dementia, and complaints of fatigue.

8   Answer d
Pernicious anemia is associated with vitamin B_{12} deficiency.

9   Answer b
The most common causes of iron deficiency in the elderly population include inadequate iron intake, acute blood loss, and chronic disease states.

10   Answer b
Vitamin C deficiency may impair iron absorption.

11   Answer d
A high-fiber diet has been associated with lowering the risk of colorectal cancer.

12   Answer c
The best way to initially provide nutrition to the patient described is by TPN. Oral or gastric feedings may increase the activation and secretion of pancreatic enzymes and stimulate the cycle of pancreatic autodigestion, inflammation, and necrosis. Treatment is aimed at pancreatic rest, which can be achieved by placing the patient on a nothing by mouth (NPO) diet.

13   Answer a
Serum lipase and amylase levels should be periodically checked in patients with acute pancreatitis.

14   Answer d
Alcohol ingestion is identified as a risk factor for acute and chronic pancreatitis. Other risk factors include hypercalcemia, gallstones, and hypertriglyceridemia. Medications associated with pancreatitis include thiazide diuretics, estrogens, azathioprine, and steroids.

15   Answer b
Patients with acute pancreatitis will commonly have hyperglycemia.

16   Answer a
The patient with pancreatitis should be on a low-fat diet to lessen pancreatic stimulation.

17   Answer d
A high-fiber diet is not associated with increased absorption of glucose and cholesterol but rather with decreased absorption.

18   Answer c
The recommended diet for a patient with celiac disease is a gluten- and gliadin-free diet.

19   Answer a
The patient with celiac disease should not eat wheat bread.

20   Answer c
Vitamin A deficiency is associated with night blindness. Vitamin A is important in the function of rhodopsin, a vision pigment important for vision in dim light. Vitamin A deficiency results in a squamous metaplasia of the respiratory and urinary tracts, resulting in recurrent respiratory infections and an increased frequency of urinary stones.

21   Answer d
Contraindications to enteral feedings occur when the gas-

trointestinal tract is nonfunctional, for instance, in such conditions as paralytic ileus, ischemic bowel, and severe diarrhea.

22 Answer b

The presence of bowel sounds would be important in determining the route of nutrition for the patient described. If the stomach is working, it is the preferred route of nutritional support.

23 Answer b

The route of nutritional support for the patient described should be enteral feeding via gastrostomy because of the risk of aspiration.

24 Answer a

Benefits of enteral feeding for the patient described include fewer fluid and electrolyte disturbances.

25 Answer a

Possible causes of a high gastric residual after the initiation of enteral feedings may be related to high-osmolarity and high-fat formulas.

26 Answer b

Metoclopramide, which is a prokinetic drug, may be used to stimulate gastric emptying. Cimetidine, famotidine, and ranitidine are all histamine blockers.

27 Answer d

A history of diabetes may produce gastric paresis and delayed gastric emptying.

28 Answer d

Potential causes of the patient's gastrointestinal symptoms include medications, a gastric ulcer, and right coronary artery ischemia.

29 Answer b

The most helpful tests in evaluating nutritional status are prealbumin, albumin, and calcium levels.

30 Answer d

Steps helpful in the management of the patient described include obtaining daily calorie counts, ordering nutritional supplements, and discontinuing medications (aspirin, ferrous sulfate, and acetaminophen with codeine) to see if symptoms improve.

31 Answer a

Causes of malabsorption include factors that affect the intraluminal and mucosal phases of digestion, such as pancreatic insufficiency, surgical defects, inflammatory bowel disease, and malignancy.

32 Answer c

A swallowing evaluation should be done to evaluate whether or not an elderly patient who has been intubated for 2 weeks can safely eat.

33 Answer a

Hypocalcemia, which may occur as a result of malnutrition, may affect respiratory muscles.

34 Answer c

Malnutrition is associated with a decreased (not increased) production of surfactant, which may lead to decreased lung compliance and thus increase the work of breathing.

35 Answer d

The diet that is recommended for the prevention of coronary heart disease is a diet that emphasizes fruits, vegetables, and low levels of unsaturated fat.

36 Answer b

The recommended diet for a patient with Crohn's disease and an intestinal fistula is a low-residue diet.

37 Answer d

Patients with end-stage renal failure who are on dialysis should not receive vitamin A, which is a fat-soluble vitamin.

Bibliography

Goroll, A, et al: Primary Care Medicine Office Evaluation and Management of the Adult Patient, 4th ed. Lippincott Williams & Wilkins, Philadelphia, 2000.

Grimble, RF: Effect of antioxidative vitamins on immune function with clinical applications. Int J Vitam Nutr Res 67(5):312–320.

Latifi, R, and Dudrick, SJ: Current Surgical Nutrition, RG Landes, Austin, Texas, 1996.

Mahan, LK, and Escott-Stump, S: Krause's Food, Nutrition, and Diet Therapy, 10th ed. Harcourt, Philadelphia, 2000.

US Department of Health and Human Services Public Health Services: Healthy People 2000: National Health Promotion and Disease Prevention Objectives, Pub. No. 91–50212. US Government Printing Office, Washington, DC, 1990.

19

Fluid, Electrolyte, and Acid-Base Imbalances

Questions 1–5 refer to the following scenario:

An 85-year-old woman is admitted to the intensive care unit from a nursing home with a 4-day history of confusion and change in mental status. The patient is afebrile with a pulse of 120, respiratory rate of 20, and blood pressure of 90/60 mm Hg. Laboratory data reveals the following levels: sodium of 158, blood urea nitrogen (BUN) of 30, potassium of 4.0, creatinine of 2.4, urine sodium of 15, and a urine osmolarity of 500.

1 What is the most likely cause of this patient's change in mental status?

a Hypernatremia
b Elevated CK level
c Dementia
d Elevated BUN level

2 The most likely cause of this patient's problem is:

a Diabetes insipidus.
b a decrease in renal perfusion.
c limited access to water.
d heat stroke.

3 Clinical manifestations of hypernatremia include:

a seizure.
b coma.
c vomiting.
d all of the above.

4 How rapidly should you correct hypernatremia in this patient?

a Within 12 hours
b Within 6 hours
c Between 48 and 72 hours
d Within 18 hours

5 Which of the following intravenous fluids should be used to correct hypernatremia?

a Normal saline (NS) solution
b Albumin
c Dextrose in water (D5W) solution
d Lactated ringer's injection

6 Which of the following intravenous fluids most closely resembles the plasma composition?

a NS solution
b D5W solution
c Lactated ringer's solution
d 5% dextrose in normal saline solution (D5NS)

7 A 55-year-old woman is seen in the emergency department with complaints of fatigue and dizziness. Her blood pressure is 100/60 mm Hg and her pulse is 64. Laboratory data reveal a sodium level of 116, potassium level of 4.1, serum osmolarity of 280, and urine osmolarity of 500. What is the most likely cause of the hyponatremia?

a Metabolic acidosis
b Syndrome of inappropriate antidiuretic hormone (SIADH)
c Central polydipsia
d Diabetic insipidus

8 Which of the following acute *acid-base imbalances* causes increased urinary potassium excretion?

a Metabolic alkalosis
b Metabolic acidosis
c Respiratory acidosis
d Respiratory alkalosis

9 Treatment of hypervolemic hypernatremia includes:

a using diuretics.
b administering vasopressin (Pitressin).
c restricting water intake.
d encouraging fluid intake.

10 *All of the statements concerning diabetes insipidus are true* **EXCEPT:**

a diabetes insipidus results from a deficiency in the secretion of antidiuretic hormone (ADH).
b nephrogenic diabetes insipidus may result from defects in the hypothalamic secretion of ADH.
c patients may present with polyuria and polydipsia.
d patients may present with hypernatremia.

11 *All of the statements concerning metabolic alkalosis are true* **EXCEPT:**

a compensation is mostly done by the kidneys.
b it often results from prolonged nasogastric suctioning.
c it results from the loss of bicarbonate.
d it may occur with renal tubular damage.

12 *A 50-year-old woman had gastric resection surgery 2 weeks ago and is readmitted to your unit with a 5-day history of persistent vomiting. Which of the following acid-base abnormalities would you expect to find?*

a Hyperkalemic, hypochloremic metabolic acidosis
b Hypokalemic, hypochloremic metabolic alkalosis
c Hypokalemic, hyperchloremic metabolic alkalosis
d Hyperkalemic, hyperchloremic metabolic alkalosis

13 *Which of the following statements concerning potassium is* **TRUE?**

a More than 90% of potassium in the body is located in the extracellular fluid compartment.
b In patients with normal renal function, the majority of ingested potassium is excreted in the urine.
c Symptoms of hyperkalemia are primarily neuromuscular.
d Normal dietary intake of potassium is 200–250 mEq/L daily.

14 *Treatment of hyperkalemia may include the use of:*

a NS solution.
b sodium polystyrene sulfonate (Kayexalate).
c insulin.
d magnesium.

15 *Calcium gluconate is administered in patients with hyperkalemia to:*

a stimulate the uptake of dextrose.
b raise the serum pH.
c counteract the myocardial effects of hyperkalemia.
d shift potassium into the cells.

16 *A 55-year-old coal miner with chronic lung disease is admitted to the unit with a bacterial pneumonia. His initial laboratory data reveals a sodium level* of 135, potassium level of 5.0, chloride level of 95, bicarbonate level of 24, CK level of 1.0, glucose level of 80, arterial pH of 7.15, and partial pressure of carbon dioxide (P_{CO_2}) of 60. Which of the following acid-base disturbances is this patient exhibiting?

a Respiratory alkalosis
b Respiratory acidosis
c Metabolic acidosis with a high anion gap and chronic respiratory acidosis
d Respiratory alkalosis and metabolic acidosis

17 *Manifestations of nephrotic syndrome may include all of the following* **EXCEPT:**

a hyperlipidemia.
b hyperalbuminemia.
c generalized edema.
d hypoalbuminemia.

18 *A 45-year-old woman who has had streptococcal pharyngitis is being evaluated for complaints of generalized body edema. She is found to have hyponatremia. What is the most likely diagnosis?*

a Nephrotic syndrome
b Acute renal failure
c SIADH
d Congestive heart failure (CHF)

19 *The normal anion gap is:*

a 1–4 mEq/L.
b 10–20 mEq/L.
c 5–10 mEq/L.
d 8–16 mEq/L.

20 *Causes of proximal renal tubular acidosis include all of the following* **EXCEPT:**

a nephrotic syndrome.
b amyloidosis.
c vitamin D deficiency.
d lithium (Eskalith) ingestion.

21 *Which of the following symptoms may be seen in a patient with hypomagnesemia?*

a Muscle weakness and paralysis
b Nystagmus and paralysis
c Seizures and cardiac arrhythmias
d Excessive thirst and confusion

22 *Patients with acute respiratory distress syndrome (ARDS) typically exhibit:*

a hypercapnia.
b hypoxemia.
c hypocapnia with hypoxemia.
d hypocarbia.

23 *A 75-year-old man who has had femoral artery bypass surgery develops acute tubular necrosis (ATN). Which of the following is NOT consistent with early ATN?*

a Oliguria
b Urine osmolarity less than 200 mOsm/L
c Creatinine clearance of 100 mL/min
d Urinary sodium greater than 5 mEq/L

24 *Which of the following findings would you expect to find in a patient with respiratory acidosis?*

a Elevated lactic acid level
b Elevated bicarbonate level
c Elevated Pco_2 level
d Low Po_2 level

25 *A 25-year-old woman with panic disorder is seen in the emergency department with complaints of chest pain and shortness of breath. As the nurse practitioner, you suspect anxiety but order electrolytes and an arterial blood gas measurement. Which of the following findings would you expect to see on the arterial blood gas results?*

a Increased bicarbonate
b Decreased Pco_2 level
c Decreased pH
d Decreased Po_2 level

26 *A 70-year-old patient is admitted to the hospital with decompensated heart failure. Which of the following laboratory data is consistent with a prerenal state?*

a Sodium level of 140, potassium level of 4.0, BUN of 100, and creatinine clearance of 5.8
b Sodium level of 140, potassium level of 3.8, BUN of 100, creatinine clearance of 2.0
c Sodium level of 132, potassium level of 4.0, BUN of 50, creatinine clearance of 3.1
d Sodium level of 130, potassium level of 4.0, BUN of 30, creatinine clearance of 2.5

27 *Which of the following medications can produce nephrogenic diabetes insipidus?*

a Furosemide (Lasix)
b Lithium (Eskalith)
c Enalapril (Vasotec)
d Amlodipine (Norvasc)

28 *Which of the following conditions is associated with an increased total body sodium level?*

a Nephrotic syndrome
b SIADH
c Diabetes insipidus
d CHF

29 *An increase in the serum anion gap means that there is an increase in:*

a potassium concentration.
b BUN.
c chloride concentration.
d the concentration of unmeasured anions.

30 *The most common cause of metabolic acidosis with a normal anion gap is:*

a renal tubular acidosis.
b lactic acidosis.
c acute renal failure.
d aspirin overdose.

31 *Which of the following conditions produces a metabolic acidosis with an increased anion gap?*

a Hyperparathyroidism
b Hypoaldosteronism
c Diabetic ketoacidosis
d Small-bowel fistula

Questions 32–35 refer to the following scenario:

A 30-year-old woman is admitted to the hospital with complaints of severe abdominal pain and vomiting for the past 5 days. She has not been able to retain any food or fluids for the past 5 days. She has no previous health history. Her last menopausal period was 4 days prior to admission. She does not take medications, and her vital signs are a temperature of 100°F, a pulse of 120, a respiratory rate of 20, and blood pressure of 100/60 mm Hg. Laboratory data reveal a sodium level of 138, potassium level of 3.0, chloride level of 87, bicarbonate level of 34, BUN of 40, and a creatinine clearance of 1.6. An arterial blood gas reading without oxygen revealed a pH of 7.5, a Pco_2 of 45, and a Po_2 of 80.

32 *What is the acid-base disturbance in this patient?*

a Metabolic acidosis
b Metabolic alkalosis
c Respiratory alkalosis
d Respiratory alkalosis and metabolic acidosis

33 *The causes of this patient's acid-base disturbance is:*

a fever.
b tachycardia.
c inadequate oral intake and vomiting.
d abdominal pain.

34 *Causes of sodium chloride–resistant metabolic alkalosis include all of the following EXCEPT:*

a Cushing's syndrome.
b excessive licorice intake.
c antacid use.
d profound potassium depletion.

35 *The most common finding in a patient with sodium chloride–responsive metabolic alkalosis is:*

a fever.
b intravascular volume depletion.
c hypokalemia.
d hyponatremia.

36 *The most common cause of hyponatremia in hospitalized patients is:*

a diuretic use.
b vomiting and diarrhea.
c respiratory failure.
d SIADH.

37 *Pulmonary disorders associated with SIADH include all of the following* **EXCEPT:**

a tuberculosis.
b pulmonary abscess.
c pneumonia.
d pulmonary embolus.

Answers

1 Answer a
The most likely cause of the patient's described change in mental status is hypernatremia. The BUN and creatinine clearance are only mildly elevated.

2 Answer c
The most likely cause of the patient's described problem of hypernatremia is dehydration and limited fluid intake.

3 Answer d
Clinical manifestations of hypernatremia include seizure, coma, and vomiting.

4 Answer c
The correction of hypernatremia in the patient described should proceed over a 48–72 hour period. Rapid correction in less than 24 hours may lead to cerebral edema.

5 Answer c
The fluid that should be used to correct the hypernatremia is D5W solution. NS has 154 mEq/L of sodium, and Ringer's lactate injection has 130 mEq/L of sodium.

6 Answer c
Lactated Ringer's injection is very similar to and most closely resembles plasma composition.

7 Answer b
The most likely cause of the hyponatremia is SIADH.

8 Answer a
Acute metabolic alkalosis causes increased urinary potassium excretion.

9 Answer c
The treatment of hypervolemic hypernatremia includes correcting the underlying disorder and restricting water intake.

10 Answer b
Nephrogenic diabetes insipidus is usually the result of renal tubular resistance to the effects of circulating ADH, not from defects in hypothalamic secretion of ADH. Diabetes insipidus results from a deficiency in the secretion of ADH, and patients may present with polyuria, polydipsia, or hypernatremia.

11 Answer c
Metabolic alkalosis is the result of a gain of bicarbonate rather than a loss of bicarbonate. Compensation is mostly done by the kidneys, it often results from prolonged nasogastric suctioning, and it may occur with renal tubular damage.

12 Answer b
The patient with persistent vomiting would be expected to have hypokalemic, hypochloremic metabolic alkalosis. The patient with persistent emesis compensates for the high loss of chloride from the stomach by losing bicarbonate in the urine.

13 Answer b
Patients with normal renal function excrete the ingested potassium via the urine. More than 90% of potassium in the body is located in the intracellular, not the extracellular, fluid compartment. Symptoms of hyperkalemia are primarily cardiac and gastrointestinal, not neuromuscular. The normal dietary intake of potassium is 50–100 mEq/L daily, not 200–250 mEq/L.

14 Answer b
Treatment of hyperkalemia may include the use of cation-exchange resins such as sodium polystyrene sulfonate (Kayexalate). Other treatments may include a solution of calcium gluconate, dextrose, and insulin, and sodium lactate.

15 Answer c
Calcium gluconate is administered to patients with hyperkalemia to counteract the myocardial effects of hyperkalemia.

16 Answer c
This patient is exhibiting metabolic acidosis with a high anion gap and chronic respiratory acidosis.

17 Answer b
Manifestations of nephrotic syndrome may include hyperlipidemia, generalized edema, and hypoalbuminemia, but not hyperalbuminemia.

18 Answer a
The most likely diagnosis in a patient with generalized edema with hyponatremia after a streptococcal infection is nephrotic syndrome.

19 Answer d
The normal anion gap is 8–16 mEq/L.

20 Answer d
Causes of proximal renal tubular acidosis include nephrotic syndrome, amyloidosis, and vitamin D deficiency. Lithium ingestion produces a distal renal tubular acidosis.

21 Answer c
The patient with hypomagnesemia may exhibit seizures and

cardiac arrhythmias, as well as confusion, irritability, vertigo, muscle tremors, nystagmus, hypotension, and tachycardia.

22 Answer c
Patients with ARDS typically exhibit hypocarbia with hypoxemia.

23 Answer c
A creatinine clearance of 100 mL/min is normal and is not consistent with ATN. A urine osmolarity less than 350 mOsm/L represents the inability of the renal tubule to reabsorb sodium and concentrate urine.

24 Answer c
A patient with respiratory acidosis will have an elevated P_{CO_2}.

25 Answer b
The findings you would expect to see on the arterial blood gas results of the patient described is a decreased P_{CO_2}.

26 Answer b
The laboratory data that is most consistent with a prerenal state is a serum sodium level of 140, potassium level of 3.8, BUN of 100, and creatinine clearance of 2.0.

27 Answer b
Lithium has been found to cause renal tubular toxicity and nephrogenic diabetes insipidus.

28 Answer d
CHF is associated with an increased total body sodium level.

29 Answer d
A serum anion gap means that there is a serum increase in the concentration of unmeasured anions.

30 Answer a
The most common cause of metabolic acidosis with a normal anion gap is renal tubular acidosis. Lactic acidosis, acute renal failure, and aspirin overdose produce metabolic acidosis with an increased anion gap.

31 Answer c
Diabetic ketoacidosis will produce a metabolic acidosis with an increased anion gap.

32 Answer b
This patient described has metabolic alkalosis. The serum bicarbonate level is elevated to 34, and the P_{CO_2} is also elevated, both of which support metabolic alkalosis.

33 Answer c
The cause of this patient's acid-base disturbance is inadequate oral intake and vomiting of 5 days duration.

34 Answer c
Causes of sodium chloride–resistant metabolic alkalosis include Cushing's syndrome, excessive licorice intake, and profound potassium depletion. Antacids are not a cause.

35 Answer b
The most common finding in a patient with sodium chloride-responsive metabolic alkalosis is the presence of intravascular volume depletion.

36 Answer d
The most common cause of hyponatremia in hospitalized patients is SIADH.

37 Answer d
Pulmonary disorders associated with SIADH include pneumonia, pulmonary abscess, tuberculosis, aspergillosis, positive-pressure breathing, and respiratory failure. Pulmonary embolus is not associated with SIADH.

Bibliography

Goroll, A, et al: Primary Care Medicine Office Evaluation and Management of the Adult Patient, ed 4. Lippincott Williams & Wilkins, Philadelphia, 2000.

Narins, RG, Jones, ER, Stom, MC, et al: Diagnostic Strategies in Disorders of Fluid, Electrolyte and Acid-Base Homeostasis. Am J Med 77:496–519, 1982.

Orth DN: Current Therapy in Endocrinology and Metabolism, 6th ed. Mosby, St. Louis, 1997.

20

Poisoning and Drug Toxicities

Questions 1–9 refer to the following scenario:

A 60-year-old woman is brought to the emergency room by her daughter with a suspected salicylate overdose. She is awake, but anxious. Her vital signs are a temperature of 100°F, pulse of 100, respiratory rate of 32, and blood pressure of 100/60 mm Hg.

1   Which of the following products contains salicylate?

a   Green tea
b   Calcium carbonate (Maalox)
c   Bismuth subsalicylate (Pepto-Bismol)
d   Simethicone (Mylanta)

2   Which of the following central nervous system (CNS) symptoms may occur as a result of salicylate toxicity?

a   Delirium and tinnitus
b   Seizures
c   Coma
d   All of the above

3   What is the most common acid-base disturbance found in the early presentation of salicylate toxicity?

a   Metabolic acidosis
b   Respiratory alkalosis
c   Respiratory acidosis
d   Metabolic alkalosis

4   Which of the following laboratory abnormalities may occur in salicylate overdose?

a   Leukopenia
b   Thrombocytosis
c   Thrombocytopenia
d   A decrease in the production of factor V

5   The initial treatment for acute ingested salicylate overdose is:

a   an infusion of normal saline with sodium bicarbonate.
b   administration of activated charcoal, either orally or via gastric lavage, and administration of a cathartic.
c   administration of naloxone (Narcan).
d   ultrafiltration.

6   Indications for hemodialysis in patients with acute salicylate overdose include:

a   the presence of tinnitus.
b   a salicylate level greater than 50 mg/dL 6 hours after ingestion.
c   refractory metabolic acidosis with a pH less than 7.0.
d   the presence of metabolic alkalosis.

7   Treatment for topical salicylate toxicity is:

a   administering activated charcoal.
b   washing the skin with tap water.
c   washing the skin with antibiotic ointment.
d   administering oral sorbitol.

8   All of the statements concerning salicylate toxicity are true EXCEPT:

a   acute salicylate toxicity may cause rhabdomyolysis.
b   salicylate toxicity may cause fever.
c   chronic salicylate toxicity may be manifested as a change in mental status.
d   the serum salicylate level reflects tissue distribution of the drug.

9   Which of the following acid-base imbalances is seen in chronic salicylate toxicity?

a   Metabolic acidosis
b   Metabolic alkalosis
c   Anion gap metabolic acidosis
d   Respiratory alkalosis

10 A 24-year-old college student is seen in the emergency room with suspected carbon monoxide poisoning. What is the antidote for carbon monoxide poisoning?

a Activated charcoal
b N-acetylcysteine (Mucomyst)
c Sodium bicarbonate
d Oxygen

11 All of the statements concerning early acetaminophen toxicity are true **EXCEPT:**

a patients with acetaminophen toxicity may present with seizures and change in mental status.
b it is the drug most commonly involved in acute analgesic ingestions.
c hepatotoxicity is the major feature of acetaminophen toxicity.
d toxicity in children is rare.

12 Which of the following medications may accelerate acetaminophen toxicity?

a Ranitidine (Zantac)
b Phenytoin (Dilantin)
c Cimetidine (Tagamet)
d Aspirin

13 The specific antidote for acetaminophen overdose is:

a activated charcoal.
b magnesium sulfate.
c naloxone (Narcan)
d N-acetylcysteine (Mucomyst).

14 Common side effects associated with N-acetylcysteine administration include:

a seizures and coma.
b nausea, vomiting, and bronchospasm.
c tinnitus.
d hearing loss.

15 The primary symptoms associated with ibuprofen (Motrin) toxicity are:

a nausea, vomiting, and headaches.
b nausea, vomiting, hematemesis, and acute renal failure.
c seizures and fever.
d tinnitus and hearing loss.

16 Toxicities associated with aminoglycosides include:

a hepatic failure.
b nephrotoxicity and ototoxicity.
c coma.
d depression.

17 Which of the following factors are associated with an increased incidence of digoxin (Lanoxin) toxicity?

a Advanced age and renal insufficiency
b Congestive heart failure (CHF)
c Renal calculi and use of amiodarone (Cordarone)
d Advanced age and history of hepatitis

18 Which of the following patients should **NOT** be given activated charcoal as a poisoning antidote?

a A 50-year-old woman who ingested a bottle of bleach
b A 65-year-old woman with an aspirin overdose
c A 30-year-old man with who overdosed on acetaminophen 2 hours ago
d A 40-year-old woman with aspirin overdose.

19 All of the statements concerning drug overdose are true **EXCEPT:**

a blood toxicology screens may be helpful.
b drug toxicity may cause cardiac arrhythmias.
c an overdose of amitriptyline (Elavil) may cause heart block.
d 20% of poisons have antidotes.

20 All of the following medications may interact with alcohol **EXCEPT:**

a Warfarin (Coumadin)
b Digoxin (Lanoxin)
c Metronidazole (Flagyl)
d Glyburide (DiaBeta)

Questions 21–25 refer to the following scenario:

A 30-year-old man is seen in the emergency room with complaints of chest pain. While obtaining his history, you find out that he used cocaine up until 2 years ago but denies using it since that time. The patient's electrocardiogram (ECG) is normal.

21 What is the most likely cause of this patient's chest pain?

a Myocardial infarction (MI)
b Coronary artery vasoconstriction
c Pulmonary embolus
d Pleural effusion

22 The coronary artery most commonly involved in patients with a history of cocaine use and MI is the:

a right coronary artery.
b posterior descending coronary artery.
c left main coronary artery.
d left anterior descending coronary artery.

23 Which of the following medications is contraindicated in the treatment of cocaine-related chest pain?

a Nitroglycerin
b Heparin
c Diltiazem (Cardizem)
d Metoprolol (Lopressor)

24 *Symptoms commonly associated with cocaine abuse include:*

a hallucinations.
b panic attacks.
c severe depression.
d dementia.

25 *The medication approved for treatment of cocaine addiction is:*

a amitriptyline (Elavil).
b nothing. There are no approved medications for the treatment of cocaine addiction.
c fluoxetine (Prozac).
d bromocriptine (Parlodel).

Questions 26–31 refer to the following scenario:

A 25-year-old man, who is agitated and hallucinating, is brought by the police to the emergency room. He is suspected of using drugs. He is found on physical exam to have bidirectional nystagmus.

26 *Which of the following drugs will produce the findings in the patient described?*

a Alcohol
b Cocaine
c lysergic acid diethylamide (LSD)
d 1-phenylcyclohexyl piperidine (PCP)

27 *Management of a patient with PCP intoxication includes:*

a placing the patient in a quiet environment.
b administering haloperidol (Haldol) for treatment of hallucinations.
c providing supportive care.
d all of the above.

28 *The antidote for PCP is:*

a naloxone (Narcan).
b haloperidol (Haldol).
c nothing; there is no antidote.
d activated charcoal.

29 *Which of the following are commonly associated with PCP intoxication?*

a Hypertension, hallucinations, and muscle rigidity
b Hallucination and renal failure
c MI
d Hematemesis and hallucinations.

30 *Hypertensive crisis in a patient with PCP intoxication should be treated with:*

a diuretics.
b intravenous fluids.
c nitroprusside (Nipride).
d haloperidol (Haldol)

31 *A positive urine test for PCP usually indicates drug use within the past:*

a 24 hours.
b 24–48 hours.
c month.
d week.

32 *Which of the following medications are used in opiate withdrawal treatment?*

a lorazepam (Ativan) and haloperidol.
b clonidine (Catapres) and methadone (Dolophine).
c methadone and lorazepam.
d lorazepam and alprazolam (Xanax).

33 *Common manifestations in patients with mild withdrawal from opiates include:*

a tachycardia and hypertension.
b irritability and vomiting.
c yawning and dilated pupils.
d insomnia and dilated pupils.

34 *Symptoms associated with mushroom poisoning include:*

a seizures.
b ataxia.
c diarrhea.
d all of the above.

35 *Which of the following pulmonary complications have been observed in patients after an overdose of opioids?*

a Pneumothorax
b Pleural effusion
c Pulmonary edema
d Pleurisy

Questions 36–37 refer to the following scenario:

A 70-year-old man is brought to the emergency room after being bitten by a black widow spider (Latrodectus envenomation).

36 *Typical manifestations of a black widow spider bite include:*

a muscle cramps and spasm.
b scarlatiniform rash.
c a bull's eye lesion.
d fever.

37 *All of the statements concerning black widow spider bites are true* **EXCEPT:**

a the initial bite is usually painless.

b the mortality associated with black widow spider bites may exceed 40%.

c muscle relaxants may be helpful in treating muscle cramps and spasm.

d diffuse abdominal spasm may mimic an acute abdomen.

Answers

1   Answer c

Pepto-Bismol contains 130 mg per tablespoon of salicylate.

2   Answer d

Central nervous system symptoms that may occur as a result of salicylate toxicity include delirium, tinnitus, seizures, irritability, confusion, and coma.

3   Answer b

The most common acid-base disturbance found in the early presentation of salicylate toxicity is respiratory alkalosis, which is due to stimulation of the respiratory center.

4   Answer c

Thrombocytopenia may occur in salicylate overdose. It is also associated with a decrease in the function of the platelets.

5   Answer b

The initial treatment for acute ingested salicylate overdose is the administration of activated charcoal, either orally or via gastric lavage, and the administration of a cathartic (either sorbitol or magnesium sulfate.) The dosage of activated charcoal is l gm/kg of body weight.

6   Answer c

Indications for hemodialysis in patients with acute salicylate overdose include persistent refractory acidosis, renal failure, cardiac arrhythmia, CHF, cardiac arrest, seizures, coma, presence of cerebral edema, and a salicylate level greater than 130 mg/dL 6 hours after the ingestion.

7   Answer b

The treatment for topical salicylate toxicity is vigorous washing of the skin with tap water.

8   Answer d

The serum salicylate level does not reflect the tissue distribution of the drug in acute salicylate toxicity. The salicylate level should be evaluated along with a concurrent elevated blood pH, because an acidotic pH is associated with toxicity regardless of the salicylate level. Acute salicylate toxicity may cause rhabdomyolysis; salicylate toxicity may cause fever; and chronic salicylate toxicity may be manifested as a change in mental status.

9   Answer c

The acid-base imbalance seen in chronic salicylate toxicity is anion gap metabolic acidosis.

10   Answer d

The antidote for carbon monoxide poisoning is the administration of oxygen. Oxygen hastens the breakdown of carboxyhemoglobin and increases the availability of oxygen at the tissue level.

11   Answer a

Acetaminophen toxicity mostly affects the liver; neurologic symptoms such as seizures and change in mental status are rarely observed early in the diagnosis. Hepatic dysfunction may lead to encephalopathy, but this occurs usually 3 to 5 days after ingestion of the acetaminophen. Acetaminophen is the drug most commonly involved in acute analgesic ingestions; hepatotoxicity is the major feature of acetaminophen toxicity; and toxicity in children is rare.

12   Answer b

Phenytoin may accelerate acetaminophen toxicity by inducing the P-450 enzymes, which allow for an increased risk of toxicity.

13   Answer d

The specific antidote for acetaminophen overdose is N-acetylcysteine (Mucomyst). Activated charcoal and magnesium can be administered orally or by lavage, but they are not specific for acetaminophen overdose. Naloxone (Narcan) is used for opioid overdose.

14   Answer b

Common side effects associated with N-acetylcysteine (Mucomyst) administration include nausea, vomiting, and bronchospasm.

15   Answer b

The primary symptoms associated with ibuprofen (Motrin) toxicity are nausea, vomiting, hematemesis, and acute renal failure.

16   Answer b

Toxicities associated with aminoglycosides include nephrotoxicity and ototoxicity.

17   Answer a

The factors that are associated with an increased incidence of digoxin (Lanoxin) toxicity are advanced age, renal insufficiency, and use of medications such as amiodarone (Cordarone), quinidine, and verapamil (Calan).

18   Answer a

The 50-year-old woman who ingested a bottle of bleach should not be given activated charcoal because you would not induce vomiting in a patient who has consumed a corrosive substance.

19   Answer d

Only 5% (not 20%) of poisons have antidotes. Blood toxicology screens may be helpful; drug toxicity may cause cardiac arrhythmias; and an overdose of amitriptyline may cause heart block.

20   Answer b

Warfarin (Coumadin), metronidazole (Flagyl), and glyburide (DiaBeta) may all interact with alcohol; digoxin (Lanoxin) does not. Warfarin prolongs the prothrombin time and may affect the liver enzymes. Metronidazole inhibits the metabolic oxidation of alcohol and may produce an Antabuse effect. Glyburide, which is a sulfonylurea, is altered by the use of alcohol and may lead to hypoglycemia.

21   Answer b

The most likely cause of the chest pain in the patient described is coronary artery vasoconstriction caused by his past history of cocaine use. His electrocardiogram (ECG) is normal, so an MI is unlikely.

22   Answer d

The left anterior descending coronary artery is the coronary artery most commonly involved in patients with a history of cocaine use and MI.

23   Answer d

The beta blocker metoprolol is contraindicated in the treatment of cocaine-related chest pain. Beta blockers may induce coronary vasoconstriction.

24   Answer c

Symptoms commonly associated with cocaine abuse include severe depression. Hallucinations and panic attacks may be seen with LSD, whereas dementia may occur as a result of alcohol ingestion.

25   Answer b

There are no approved medications for the treatment of cocaine addiction. Some research studies have suggested that the use of tricyclic antidepressants, selective serotonin reuptake inhibitors (SSRIs), and medications such as bromocriptine may be effective in reducing the craving of cocaine.

26   Answer d

1-phenylcyclohexyl piperidine (PCP) is the only drug that will produce the finding of bidirectional nystagmus. PCP has anticholinergic, adrenergic, and dopaminergic properties.

27   Answer d

Management of the patient with PCP intoxication includes the use of benzodiazepines and haloperidol (Haldol), as well as the provision of supportive care and placement of the patient in a quiet environment.

28   Answer c

There is no antidote for PCP or any of the other hallucinogenic drugs.

29   Answer a

Hypertension, hallucinations, muscle rigidity, bidirectional nystagmus, hyperthermia, tachycardia, and marked agitation are commonly associated with PCP intoxication.

30   Answer c

Hypertensive crisis in a patient with PCP intoxication should be treated with nitroprusside (Nipride).

31   Answer d

A positive urine test for PCP usually indicates drug use within the past week.

32   Answer b

Clonidine (Catapres) and methadone (Dolophine) are used in opiate withdrawal treatment.

33   Answer c

Common manifestations in patients with mild withdrawal from opiates include yawning and dilated pupils.

34   Answer d

Symptoms associated with mushroom poisoning include diarrhea, nausea, vomiting, ataxia, seizures, and hallucinations. Mushrooms that contain muscimol or psilocybin are responsible for central nervous system symptoms. Mushrooms that contain cyclopeptides cause gastrointestinal symptoms.

35   Answer c

Pulmonary edema may occur as a result of an overdose of opioids such as codeine, methadone, and propoxyphene.

36   Answer a

Typical manifestations of a black widow spider bite include muscle cramps and spasm. A bull's eye lesion, fever, and scarlatiniform rash are seen in brown recluse spider bites.

37   Answer b

The mortality associated with black widow spider bites is low; it does not exceed 40%. The initial bite is usually painless; muscle relaxants may be helpful in treating muscle cramps and spasm; and diffuse abdominal spasm may mimic an acute abdomen.

Bibliography

Bryson, PD: Comprehensive Review in Toxicology for Emergency Clinicians, 3rd ed. Taylor and Francis, Bristol, Penna., 1997.

Ellenhorn, MJ: Ellenhorn's Medical Toxicology: Diagnosis and Treatment of Human Poisoning, 2nd ed. Williams & Wilkins, Baltimore, 1997.

Rosen, P, and Barkin, RM: Emergency Medicine: Concepts and Current Practice, 4th ed. Mosby, St. Louis, 1998.

21

Wound Management

1 *A 40-year-old man is scheduled for an elective hernia repair. Prophylactic antibiotics should be administered:*

a   3 hours before the incision.
b   1 hour after the incision.
c   immediately after the surgical incision.
d   immediately before the surgical incision.

2 *Postoperative wound infections usually develop:*

a   1 to 2 days after surgery.
b   5 to 7 days after surgery.
c   21 days after surgery.
d   28 days after surgery.

3 *All of the following are risk factors for wound dehiscence* **EXCEPT:**

a   diabetes.
b   obesity.
c   malnutrition.
d   hypertension.

4 *The most important factor in wound dehiscence is:*

a   adequacy of closure.
b   infection.
c   obesity.
d   diabetes mellitus.

5 *The most common pathogen in surgical site infection is:*

a   *Streptococcus.*
b   *Enterococcus.*
c   *Staphylococcus.*
d   *Klebsiella.*

6 *A 50-year-old diabetic woman had an abdominal hysterectomy 6 days ago. Wound dehiscence is most likely to occur:*

a   3 to 5 days after surgery.
b   1 to 2 days after surgery.
c   less than 24 hours after surgery.
d   5 to 10 days after surgery.

7 *All of the following are phases of surgical wound healing* **EXCEPT:**

a   inflammation.
b   miosis.
c   epithelialization.
d   collagen synthesis.

8 *In normal healing situations, the maturation phase of healing starts:*

a   24 hours after surgery.
b   3 weeks after surgery.
c   2 to 4 days after surgery.
d   1 week after surgery.

9 *Angiogenesis occurs during which phase of healing?*

a   Proliferative phase
b   Maturation phase
c   Inflammation phase
d   None of the above

10 *A 25-year-old woman, who had a cholecystectomy 1 week ago, inquires about measures to accelerate the healing of her abdominal wound. Which of the following measures will accelerate healing?*

a   Increased doses of vitamin D
b   Increased doses of vitamin A
c   Increased doses of zinc
d   Increased local oxygen tension

11 *A 40-year-old woman who had an abdominal hysterectomy 3 months ago is unhappy with the appearance of her incision. When is it advisable for her to have a revision of the incision?*

a   In 6 months
b   In 2 years
c   In 12 to 18 months
d   In 4 months

12   *A 20-year-old college student is seen in the emergency department after suffering a burn with destruction of varying depths of dermis and blister formation. This type of burn is a:*

a   first-degree burn.
b   second-degree burn.
c   third-degree burn.
d   none of the above.

13   *The most common cause of third-degree burns is:*

a   a scalding injury.
b   an electrical injury.
c   a sunburn.
d   hot oil.

14   *A first-degree burn usually presents as:*

a   painless.
b   mottled.
c   erythematous with no blisters.
d   blistered.

15   *Initial treatment of first-degree burns should include:*

a   debridement and administration of systemic steroids.
b   application of cool saline and administration of analgesia.
c   administration of topical steroids and analgesia.
d   administration of topical antibiotics and immobilization.

16   *A 67-year-old man with an abdominal abscess has had the area surgically debrided. The surgeon decides to have the wound healed by secondary closure, which allows:*

a   for closure of the wound in 3 to 5 days.
b   for closure of the wound margins with staples.
c   the wound to heal by granulation without mechanical manipulation of the wound edges.
d   for closure of the wound margins with continuous suture.

17   *The disadvantages of tissue adhesives for wound closure include:*

a   discomfort to the patient.
b   increased potential for infection.
c   increased costs.
d   dehiscence over high-tension areas.

Questions 18–22 refer to the following scenario:

A 50-year-old man is brought to the emergency department with a circumferential, full-thickness burn to the left lower leg that occurred 4 hours ago. The patient is complaining of pain, weakness, and numbness in the leg. On physical exam, you note that the leg is cool to the touch with absent posterior tibial and pedal pulses.

18   *What is the most likely cause of the patient's symptoms.*

a   Left leg deep-vein thrombosis
b   Compartment syndrome
c   Tibial fracture
d   Fat embolism

19   *Initial management of the patient includes:*

a   an urgent surgical consultation.
b   debridement of the burn area.
c   heparin administration.
d   topical steroid application.

20   *Which of the following laboratory tests may indicate muscle damage in this patient?*

a   Amylase level
b   Urine myoglobin level
c   Serum calcium level
d   Serum creatinine level

21   *The initial fluid management of this patient should include:*

a   total parenteral nutrition (TPN).
b   lactated Ringer's solution.
c   dextrose in water (D5W).
d   albumin.

22   *Hemodynamic parameters associated with the burn injury of this patient may include all of the following EXCEPT:*

a   tachycardia.
b   hypotension.
c   elevated pulmonary capillary wedge pressure (PCWP).
d   decreased right atrial pressure.

23   *All of the statements concerning cat bites are true EXCEPT:*

a   they are usually painful and edematous.
b   they may lead to abscess formation.
c   only immunocompromised persons should be given antibiotics.
d   they are two times more likely to produce infection than dog bites.

24   *The most common pathogen involved in cat bites is:*

a *Pasturella multocida.*
b *Bartonella henselae.*
c *Staphylococcus aureus.*
d Cytomegalovirus (CMV).

25 *The most common cause of foot ulcers in patients with diabetes is:*

a an elevated serum glucose.
b ischemia.
c neuropathy.
d osteomyelitis.

26 *All of the statements concerning foot ulcers in patients with diabetes are true* **EXCEPT:**

a most neuropathic ulcers develop on the soles of the feet.
b neuropathic ulcers have marked keratosis.
c a bone scan is diagnostic in finding deep infections.
d infected ulcers require prompt intervention.

27 *A 90-year-old bedridden nursing home patient with a sacral pressure ulcer is at risk for:*

a acute arterial occlusion.
b sepsis.
c urinary tract infection.
d fat embolism.

28 *The most common symptoms of arterial ulcers are:*

a fever and chills.
b lower extremity edema and pain.
c edema and fever.
d rest pain and claudication.

29 *The most common sites of arterial ulcers include the:*

a sacrum.
b wrist and elbow.
c lateral ankle, toes, and feet.
d hip.

30 *All of the statements concerning venous stasis ulcers are true* **EXCEPT:**

a they are commonly associated with lower extremity edema.
b they are common in bedridden patients.
c they usually involve the saphenous vein system.
d they are associated with hyperpigmentation of the surrounding skin.

31 *Which of the following patients is at greatest risk for developing a pressure ulcer?*

a A 45-year-old man after total knee replacement
b An 85-year-old woman after total hip replacement complicated by a middle cerebral artery stroke
c A 90-year-old ambulatory man with hypertension and diabetes
d A 60-year-old woman 1 day after cholecystectomy

32 *Which of the following types of wound infections may benefit from hyperbaric oxygen therapy?*

a Osteomyelitis
b Diabetic foot ulcers
c Compromised skin grafts
d All of the above

33 *Data points that are important in assessing a wound include:*

a the appearance of the tissue surrounding the wound.
b the anatomic location.
c the size and depth of the wound.
d all of the above.

34 *The treatment of simple wound infections should include all of the following* **EXCEPT:**

a debridement.
b hyperbaric oxygen.
c antibiotics.
d irrigation.

35 *Which of the following patients is at risk for developing cellulitis?*

a A 45-year-old healthy woman
b A 70-year-old man with end-stage renal disease and diabetes
c A 20-year-old healthy man
d A 50-year-old man with hypertension

36 *The most common pathogens in patients with cellulitis are:*

a *Pseudomonas aeruginosa* and *Haemophilus influenzae.*
b Group A streptococci and *S. aureus.*
c Group A streptococci and *P. aeruginosa.*
d *S. aureus* and *Enterococcus.*

37 *A 60-year-old woman is diagnosed with* Hidradenitis suppurativa. *Which of the statements concerning* Hidradenitis *is true?*

a It is caused by a cat scratch.
b It is complicated by streptococcal infections.
c It is treated with hyperbaric oxygen therapy.
d It is caused by the plugging of the apocrine glands in the axilla and groin.

Answers

1 Answer d

Prophylactic antibiotics should be administered immediately before the surgical incision.

2 Answer b

Postoperative wound infections usually develop 5 to 7 days after surgery.

3 Answer d

Risk factors for wound dehiscence include diabetes, obesity, malnutrition, advanced age, use of immunosuppressant agents or corticosteroids, hepatic or renal failure, and radiation. Hypertension is not a risk factor for wound dehiscence.

4 Answer a

The most important factor in wound dehiscence is adequacy of surgical closure.

5 Answer c

The most common pathogen in surgical site infections is *Staphylococcus.*

6 Answer d

Wound dehiscence is most likely to occur 5 to 10 days after surgery, when wound strength is at a minimum.

7 Answer b

The phases of surgical wound healing include inflammation, epithelialization, collagen synthesis, and contraction. Miosis is not a phase of surgical wound healing.

8 Answer b

In normal healing situations, the maturation phase of healing starts 3 weeks after surgery.

9 Answer a

Angiogenesis occurs during the proliferative phase of healing. The first step of angiogenesis is stimulation of endothelial cell proliferation. The angiogenic factors most important to wound healing originate from leukocytes.

10 Answer d

Increased local oxygen tension may help stimulate healing and increase wound strength. Vitamin A and zinc are important in wound healing, but increasing doses do not accelerate healing.

11 Answer c

Revisions of incisional scars should not be undertaken for at least 12 to 18 months to allow natural improvement to take place. Changes in the pliability, pigmentation, and configuration of the incision are termed *scar maturation.*

12 Answer b

A burn with destruction of varying depths of dermis and blister formation is a second-degree burn.

13 Answer b

The common cause of third-degree burns is an electrical injury.

14 Answer c

First-degree burns usually present as erythematous with no blisters and blanching with pressure. Second-degree burns usually present as painful, mottled, and blistered.

15 Answer b

The initial treatment of first-degree burns is generally supportive and includes applications of cool water or saline, and administration of adequate analgesia. In the case of sunburn, antihistamines may be helpful in decreasing edema. Steroid use is controversial in the treatment of first-degree burns.

16 Answer c

Secondary closure is the healing by secondary intention, which allows a wound to heal by granulation without mechanical manipulation (*approximation*) of the wound margins.

17 Answer d

The disadvantages of tissue adhesives for wound closure include the propensity for dehiscence over high-tension areas such as over joint spaces. The advantages of tissue adhesives include patient comfort, the ease of application, decreased incidence of infection, no need for professional removal as in the case of sutures and staples, and low cost.

18 Answer b

The most likely cause of the patient's symptoms is compartment syndrome. Circumferential burns of the extremities can cause neurovascular compromise to the burn site, edema, tissue ischemia, and compartment syndrome.

19 Answer a

Initial management of the patient should include an urgent surgical consultation, in an attempt to salvage the limb.

20 Answer b

A urine myoglobin test may indicate muscle damage in this patient.

21 Answer b

The initial fluid management of this patient should include a balanced salt solution such as lactated Ringer's or normal saline.

22 Answer c

The patient with a circumferential burn may have fluid leaks from the intravascular to the extravascular spaces, and third spacing of fluid. This may lead to hypovolemia, which may be manifested by tachycardia, hypotension, and decreased filling pressures. You would expect to find a lowered PCWP, rather than an elevated one.

23 Answer c

All persons who have a cat bite, not only immunocompromised persons, should be treated with antibiotics. Cat bites are thought to contribute to infection secondary to the sharpness of their teeth and the ability to penetrate tissue and the potential mixed flora infection. Cat bites are usually painful and edematous; they may lead to abscess formation; and they are two times more likely to produce infection than dog bites.

24 Answer a

The most common pathogen involved in cat bites is *P. multocida.* Other pathogens involved in cat bites include *S. aureus,* streptococci, and rarely *B. henselae,* which is associated with cat scratch disease.

25 Answer c

The most common cause of foot ulcers in patients with diabetes is neuropathy.

26 Answer c

The evaluation of deep infections of foot ulcers in patients with diabetes is best done with the use of computed tomography (CT) scanning and magnetic resonance imaging (MRI). Bone scan combined with radiologic labeled white blood cells can produce a higher yield for detecting infection. Most neuropathic ulcers develop on the soles of the feet; neuropathic ulcers have marked keratosis; and infected ulcers require prompt intervention.

27 Answer b

A bedridden patient with a sacral pressure ulcer is at risk for propagation of the wound and sepsis.

28 Answer d

The most common symptoms of arterial ulcers are rest pain and claudication.

29 Answer c

The most common sites of arterial ulcers include the lateral ankle, heels and soles of the feet, the fifth metatarsal, and the head of the first metatarsal.

30 Answer b

Bedridden patients are at risk for pressure ulcers, not venous stasis ulcers. Venous stasis ulcers are common in patients with underlying venous insufficiency, and are manifested by lower extremity edema, stasis dermatitis, and hyperpigmentation. Venous stasis ulcers usually involve the saphenous vein system.

31 Answer b

The patient at greatest risk for developing a pressure is the elderly patient with a new stroke and recent total hip replacement.

32 Answer d

Osteomyelitis, diabetic foot ulcers, compromised skin grafts, necrotizing fasciitis, and clostridial myonecrosis may all benefit from the use of hyperbaric oxygen therapy.

33 Answer d

Data points important in assessing a wound include the appearance of the surrounding tissue, anatomic location, and size and depth of the wound.

34 Answer b

The treatment of simple wound infections should include debridement, irrigation, antibiotics, and the removal of foreign objects. In some cases, antibiotics may not be indicated. Hyperbaric oxygen therapy is often used as an adjunct to complex wound care.

35 Answer b

Patients with chronic diseases or those who are immunocompromised are at risk for developing cellulitis.

36 Answer b

The most common pathogens in patients with cellulitis are group A *Streptococci* and *S. aureus.*

37 Answer d

Hidradenitis suppurativa is caused by the plugging of the apocrine glands in the axilla and the groin. The patient may develop abscesses and draining sinuses. Hidradenitis is commonly secondarily infected with *S. aureus.*

Bibliography

Goroll, A, et al: Primary Care Medicine Office Evaluation and Management of the Adult Patient, 4th ed. Lippincott Williams & Wilkins, Philadelphia, 2000.
Herndon, DN: Total Burn Care. WB Saunders, Philadelphia, 1996.
Lee, JT: Operative complications and quality improvement. Am J Surg 171:545, 1996.
Nichols, RL: Surgical antibiotic prophylaxis. Med Clin North Am 79(3):50, 1995.
Wittman, DH, and Schein, M: Let us shorten antibiotic prophylaxis and therapy in surgery. Am Surg 172(6A):25S–32S, 1996.

22

Comorbidities

1 *A 50-year-old man with known hypertension develops congestive heart failure (CHF). His current medications include 25 mg of metoprolol (Lopressor) twice daily and one tablet of hydrochlorothiazide daily. Which of the following medications should be added to his regimen?*

a   Increase metoprolol to 50 mg twice daily
b   Enalapril (Vasotec)
c   Amlodipine (Norvasc)
d   Diltiazem (Cardizem)

2 *A 65-year-old man with diabetes and a history of chronic cholelithiasis presents with complaints of dull, aching pain in the midepigastrum, weight loss, and jaundice for the past 2 weeks. On physical exam, the gallbladder is palpable. What is the most likely diagnosis?*

a   Gastric ulcer
b   Pancreatic head tumor
c   Hepatic cirrhosis
d   Gallbladder carcinoma

3 *A 30-year-old woman with no known health history presents with complaints of chest pain and shortness of breath. Physical exam reveals reduction of vocal and tactile fremitus and decreased breath sounds on the right side. The most likely diagnosis is:*

a   asthmatic bronchitis.
b   pulmonary embolism.
c   pneumonia.
d   spontaneous pneumothorax.

4 *A 50-year-old man with history of coronary artery disease and hyperlipidemia is started on lovastatin (Mevacor). Side effects commonly associated with this drug include:*

a   lower extremity edema.
b   myalgias.

c   hypertension.
d   tachycardia.

5 *A 30-year-old woman with a history of migraine headaches and new onset of hypertension should be treated with:*

a   enalapril (Vasotec).
b   amitriptyline (Elavil).
c   aspirin.
d   metoprolol.

6 *Exophthalmos may be associated with all of the following conditions* **EXCEPT:**

a   hyperthyroidism.
b   hypothyroidism.
c   rectus muscle paralysis.
d   fibroma.

7 *A 35-year-old man has sickle cell anemia. Which of the following is usually associated with sickle cell anemia in the adult?*

a   Normal reticulocyte count
b   Lower gastrointestinal bleeding
c   Splenomegaly
d   Elevated reticulocyte count

8 *Lung cancer is most commonly associated with:*

a   cigarette smoking.
b   asbestos exposure.
c   acrylic exposure.
d   vitamin E deficiency.

9 *A 40-year-old woman with asthma develops a new onset of hypertension. Which of the following should be avoided in this patient?*

a   Metoprolol (Lopressor)
b   Enalapril (Vasotec)

c Diltiazem (Cardizem)
d Furosemide (Lasix)

10 *A 55-year-old man with hypertension and type 2 diabetes mellitus is seen in the emergency department with complaints of midsternal chest pain. Laboratory tests reveal a serum potassium level of 2.8. Which of the following electrocardiogram (ECG) findings would you expect?*

a Peaked T waves
b U waves
c New Q waves
d Flat T waves

11 *Which of the following medications should be avoided in a patient with gouty arthritis and hypertension?*

a Angiotensin-converting enzyme (ACE) inhibitors
b Beta blockers
c Alpha blockers
d Diuretics

12 *Mesothelioma is associated with exposure to:*

a cigarette smoke.
b asbestos.
c tuberculosis.
d radon.

13 *A 65-year-old man with end-stage renal failure is on hemodialysis. Which of the following diets should be recommended?*

a Low sodium
b High protein
c Low potassium
d Restricted calories

14 *The ocular findings in patients with diabetes mellitus may include all of the following EXCEPT:*

a cotton-wool spots.
b retinal detachment.
c blue scleras.
d cataracts.

15 *A 28-year-old man who presents with a new onset of diabetes, bilateral cataracts, and premature aging most likely has:*

a Turner's syndrome.
b Werner's syndrome.
c Ménière's disease.
d Kleinfelter's syndrome.

16 *A 55-year-old man complains of impotence, pain in both legs with walking, and coolness of the legs. Physical exam reveals absent femoral pulses. What is the most likely diagnosis?*

a Hypertension
b Leriche's syndrome
c Raynaud's disease
d Buerger's disease

17 *Tourette's syndrome is commonly associated with all of the following EXCEPT:*

a mental retardation.
b attention deficit disorder.
c obsessive-compulsive tendencies.
d learning disabilities.

18 *A 65-year-old woman with small-cell lung cancer is seen in the emergency department with confusion, ataxia, nystagmus, peripheral sensory loss, and generalized weakness. The most likely diagnosis is:*

a multiple sclerosis.
b myasthenia gravis.
c paraneoplastic syndromes.
d hypercalcemia.

19 *An 80-year-old woman is hospitalized for pneumonia and treated with an intravenous antibiotic. On the second day of her hospitalization, the patient develops diarrhea and tests positive for Clostridium difficile. What is the best treatment option?*

a Gentamicin (Garamycin)
b Clindamycin (Cleocin)
c Doxycycline (Vibramycin)
d Vancomycin (Vancocin)

20 *A 30-year-old woman is seen in your practice with weight gain, amenorrhea, abdominal striae, and hypertension. Which of the following tests should be ordered?*

a Prolactin level
b Overnight dexamethasone suppression test
c Random cortisol level
d Adrenocorticotropic hormone (ACTH) level

21 *A 40-year-old woman presents with amenorrhea for the past 4 months, along with weight gain, cold intolerance, decreased energy level, and thinning hair. Which of the following tests should be ordered?*

a Thyroid stimulating hormone (TSH) level
b Estrogen level
c Cortisol level
d Rapid plasma reagin (RPR)

22 *Which of the following medications used to treat tuberculosis induces the microsomal cytochrome P-450 enzymes in the liver?*

a Isoniazid (INH)
b Rifampin (Rifadin)
c Vitamin B_6
d Ethambutol (Myambutol)

23 *A 25-year-old woman with myasthenia gravis has autoimmune hemolytic anemia. A routine chest x-ray reveals an anterior mediastinal mass. The most likely diagnosis is:*

a thymoma.
b Hodgkin's disease.
c teratoma.
d sarcoma.

24 *The most common lung cancer associated with hypercalcemia is:*

a small-cell carcinoma.
b epidermoid carcinoma.
c adenocarcinoma.
d squamous cell carcinoma.

25 *A 30-year-old man develops an anaphylactic reaction to penicillin. He is given epinephrine intravenously. Epinephrine works by all of the following mechanisms* **EXCEPT:**

a inhibiting mediator release from mast cells and basophils.
b increasing blood pressure.
c relaxing bronchial smooth muscle.
d decreasing heart rate.

26 *The most common cause of aortic dissection in women under the age of 40 is:*

a Marfan's syndrome.
b pregnancy.
c hypertension.
d Reiter's syndrome.

27 *The most common valvular heart disease in the adult population in the United States is:*

a mitral regurgitation.
b pulmonic stenosis.
c mitral stenosis.
d aortic stenosis.

28 *The medical management of mitral regurgitation and left ventricular dysfunction includes:*

a ACE inhibitors and diuretics.
b calcium channel blockers and beta blockers.
c diuretics and beta blockers.
d alpha blockers and diuretics.

Questions 29–32 relate to the following scenario:

A 60-year-old woman with a history of hypertension and diabetes states she has had epigastric abdominal pain that is unrelieved for the past 6 days by antacids. The pain awakens her at night, and today she experienced an episode of hematemesis, associated with lightheadedness. She smokes a pack of cigarettes per day, drinks three to four beers per day, and takes aspirin once a day. Physical exam reveals a blood pressure of 110/60 mm Hg lying and 90/60 mm Hg standing; abdominal exam reveals epigastric tenderness without a palpable mass; and rectal exam reveals brown stool, which is positive for occult blood.

29 *What in the patient's history is a risk factor for development of peptic ulcer disease?*

a History of diabetes
b History of hypertension
c Cigarette and alcohol use
d Age and sex

30 *Which of the following medications are used in the treatment of peptic ulcer disease?*

a Histamine-2 (H_2)-receptor antagonists
b Proton pump inhibitors
c Antacids
d All of the above

31 *The treatment of choice for patients with Zollinger-Ellison syndrome is:*

a omeprazole (Prilosec).
b cimetadine (Tagamet).
c ranitidine (Zantac).
d trimethoprim sulfamethoxazole (Bactrim DS).

32 *Treatment for* **Helicobacter pylori** *infection consists of:*

a antibiotics only.
b an H_2-receptor antagonist only.
c an H_2-receptor antagonist, proton pump inhibitor, antibiotics, and bismuth compound.
d an H_2-receptor antagonist and antibiotics.

33 *The most common source of pulmonary emboli is:*

a the deep venous system of the legs.
b a central venous catheter.
c the pelvic veins.
d the upper arms.

34 *Signs and symptoms commonly associated with sarcoidosis include all of the following* **EXCEPT:**

a bilateral hilar adenopathy.
b fatigue.
c splenomegaly.
d congestive heart failure.

35 *Treatment of fibromyalgia includes all of the following* **EXCEPT:**

a plasmapheresis.
b nonsteroidal anti-inflammatory drugs (NSAIDs).
c tricyclic antidepressants (TCAs).
d aerobic exercise.

36 *The most common cause of cirrhosis is:*

a hepatitis B.
b hepatitis C.
c Epstein-Barr virus.
d alcoholic hepatitis.

37 *A 60-year-old woman has angina pectoris and hypertension. Her current medications include 325 mg of aspirin 325 daily and 60 mg of isosorbide (Imdur) daily. Her blood pressure is 180/120 mm Hg, and her heart rate is 90. Which of the following medications should be added to her regimen for better blood pressure control?*

a Enalapril (Vasotec)
b Metoprolol (Lopressor)
c Terazosin (Hytrin)
d Amlodipine (Norvasc)

Answers

1 Answer b

A patient with hypertension and the onset of CHF should be treated with enalapril. ACE inhibitors are the standard of care in patients with CHF. Increasing the metoprolol and adding diltiazem and amlodipine may lead to worsening of heart failure.

2 Answer b

The most likely diagnosis for the patient described is pancreatic head tumor. Pancreatic head tumor is frequently found in diabetic men over 60 years of age, and associated with dull pain, weight loss, progressive jaundice, and a palpable gallbladder and liver.

3 Answer d

The most likely diagnosis in a patient with decreased breath sounds and fremitus with onset of acute chest pain and shortness of breath is spontaneous pneumothorax.

4 Answer b

Common side effects associated with lovastatin (Mevacor) include myalgias, elevated liver function tests, gastrointestinal upset, and rashes.

5 Answer d

The medications for treatment of hypertension and migraine headache would include the use of a beta blocker such as metoprolol.

6 Answer b

Exophthalmos is not associated with hypothyroidism. The most common cause of exophthalmos is Graves' disease (hyperthyroidism). Other causes include fibroma, rectus muscle paralysis, myopia, leukemia, and trauma.

7 Answer d

The adult with sickle cell anemia will have a chronically elevated reticulocyte count and a chronic hemolytic anemia. The spleen actually atrophies secondary to chronic infections.

8 Answer a

Lung cancer is commonly associated with cigarette smoking, which is thought to contribute to 90% of all lung cancers. Other exposures that may contribute to lung cancer include nickel, zinc, radon, uranium, asbestosis, iron oxide, and beryllium.

9 Answer a

Metoprolol (Lopressor), which is a beta blocker, should be avoided to prevent bronchospasm in a patient with asthma who also has hypertension.

10 Answer b

Generally, the ECG in a patient with hypokalemia will reveal U waves.

11 Answer d

Diuretics, which may increase uric acid levels, should be avoided in a patient with gouty arthritis and hypertension.

12 Answer b

Mesothelioma, which is a tumor of the pleural surface of the lung, is associated with asbestos exposure.

13 Answer c

The recommended diet in patients with renal failure is a low-potassium diet.

14 Answer c

Ocular findings in patients with diabetes mellitus do not include blue sclerae. Blue sclerae are commonly associated with osteogenia imperfecta. Ocular findings in patients with diabetes may include cotton-wool spots, iris changes, retinal detachment, retinal hemorrhage, and cataracts.

15 Answer b

The most likely diagnosis of the patient with early onset diabetes mellitus, bilateral cataracts, and premature aging is Werner's syndrome. Werner's syndrome is a rare condition with an onset between ages 20 and 30.

16 Answer b

The most likely diagnosis for the patient described is Leriche's syndrome, which is characterized by claudication and impotence. Leriche's syndrome is an aortoiliac occlusive disease usually secondary to atherosclerosis. The physical exam usually demonstrates absence of femoral, popliteal, and pedal pulses.

17 Answer a

Tourette's syndrome is commonly associated with attention deficit disorder, obsessive-compulsive tendencies, and learning disabilities. It is not associated with mental retardation.

18 Answer c

The most likely diagnosis for the patient described is paraneoplastic syndrome.

19 Answer d

The best treatment option for *C. difficile* is the use of oral vancomycin. Other treatment options may include the use of metronidazole (Flagyl).

20 Answer b

The next test in the evaluation of the patient with amenorrhea, weight gain, abdominal striae, and hypertension is an overnight dexamethasone suppression test. This patient most likely has Cushing's syndrome. A random cortisol level and ACTH level is not sufficient to screen for Cushing's syndrome.

21   Answer a

A TSH level should be ordered for the patient described. This patient most likely has hypothyroidism as evidenced by the weight gain, cold intolerance, fatigue, and thinning hair.

22   Answer b

Rifampin, a medication used to treat tuberculosis, induces the P-450 system, which causes an increase in the elimination of medications such as oral contraceptives, anticoagulants, cyclosporine, and ketoconazole.

23   Answer a

The most likely diagnosis for the patient described is thymoma, which is commonly associated with myasthenia gravis.

24   Answer b

The most common lung cancer associated with hypercalcemia is epidermoid carcinoma. It is associated with hypercalcemia due to the metastatic destruction of the bone and ectopic formation of parathyroid hormone.

25   Answer d

Epinephrine works in an anaphylactic reaction by inhibiting mediator release from mast cells, relaxing bronchial smooth muscles, and bolstering blood pressure.

26   Answer b

The most common cause of aortic dissection in women under the age of 40 is pregnancy. The most common cause of aortic dissection in the general population is hypertension, whereas in men under age 40, the most common cause is Marfan's syndrome.

27   Answer d

The most common valvular heart disease in the adult population is aortic stenosis.

28   Answer a

The medical management of mitral regurgitation and left ventricular dysfunction includes afterload reduction, which may be accomplished with ACE inhibitors and diuretics.

29   Answer c

Risk factors for the development of peptic ulcer disease in the patient described include cigarette and alcohol use.

30   Answer d

Treatment of peptic ulcer disease includes the use of H_2-receptor antagonists, proton pump inhibitors, and antacids.

31   Answer a

The treatment of choice for patients with Zollinger-Ellison syndrome is omeprazole (Prilosec), a proton pump inhibitor.

32   Answer c

Treatment of *H. pylori* infection consists of an H_2-receptor antagonist, proton pump inhibitor, antibiotics, and bismuth compound.

33   Answer a

The most common source of pulmonary emboli is the deep venous system of the legs, accounting for approximately 90% of pulmonary emboli.

34   Answer d

Sarcoidosis is commonly associated with bilateral hilar adenopathy (seen on chest x-ray), fatigue, splenomegaly, pigmented papulonodular skin rash, anemia, and elevation in liver function tests. It is not associated with congestive heart failure.

35   Answer a

Treatment of fibromyalgia includes the use of nonsteroidal anti-inflammatory drugs (NSAIDs) and tricyclic antidepressants (TCAs), as well as aerobic exercise. Plasmapheresis is not a treatment modality.

36   Answer d

The most common cause of cirrhosis is alcoholic hepatitis.

37   Answer b

Metoprolol (Lopressor), a beta blocker, should be added to the regimen of the patient described. This medication would be an additive to the angina regimen and would help control the patient's blood pressure.

Bibliography

Centers for Disease Control and Prevention: Guidelines for Prevention of Nosocomial Pneumonia. MMWR 46 (No. RR-01), 1997.

Goroll, A, et al: Primary Care Medicine Office Evaluation and Management of the Adult Patient, 4th ed. Lippincott Williams & Wilkins, Philadelphia, 2000.

Fauci, AS, et al: Harrison's Principles of Internal Medicine, 14th ed. McGraw-Hill, New York, 1998.

Marco, CA, et al: Fever in geriatric emergency patients: Clinical features associated with serious illness. Ann Emerg Med 26:18–24, 1995.

23

Immobility

1 *The most frequently reported complication after total knee replacement surgery is:*

a deep-vein thrombosis (DVT).
b sepsis.
c related to the extensor mechanism.
d fat embolism.

Questions 2–7 refer to the following scenario:

A 90-year-old woman is admitted to your nurse practitioner service from the nursing home. She has a non-healing sacral pressure ulcer, confusion, and a fever of 103°F. The confusion started in the past 24 hours along with the rising temperature. On physical exam, her vital signs are blood pressure of 100/60, and a pulse of 88. The ulcer measures 8 × 8 cm and is oozing purulent material.

2 *The most common site of pressure ulcers is the:*

a sacrum.
b medial malleolus.
c scalp.
d elbow.

3 *Which of the following statements concerning pressure ulcers in the elderly is true?*

a *Streptococcus* is the most common organism associated with septic pressure ulcers.
b Antibiotics should not be used in the treatment of pressure ulcers.
c Good nutrition in the elderly will help prevent pressure ulcers.
d Hypothyroidism predisposes the elderly to pressure ulcers.

4 *Which of the following organisms is commonly associated with septic pressure ulcers?*

a *Bacteroides fragilis*
b *Klebsiella*

c *Streptococcus*
d *Enterococcus*

5 *Which of the following treatments should be initially implemented in this patient?*

a Surgical consultation for debridement and institution of systemic antibiotics
b Hydrotherapy
c Rotational mattress and hydrotherapy
d Debridement only

6 *Complications of pressure ulcers include:*

a septicemia.
b cellulitis.
c osteomyelitis.
d all of the above.

7 *Pressure ulcers occurring in patients in a nursing home may be prevented by:*

a using alcohol rubs to the skin twice daily.
b rotating bedridden patients every 1 to 2 hours.
c checking all pressure points in bedridden patients at least once weekly.
d providing a high-carbohydrate, high-fat diet.

8 *Constipation in the elderly is often associated with:*

a immobility.
b increased fluid intake.
c anxiety.
d a high-protein diet.

9 *Treatments used for patients with ankylosing spondylosis include:*

a gold salts.
b intra-articular corticosteroids.
c systemic steroids.
d nonsteroidal anti-inflammatory drugs (NSAIDs).

10 *Virchow's classic triad for the development of deep-vein thrombosis (DVT) includes:*

a venous stasis, tachycardia, and obesity.
b vascular damage, malignancy, and venous stasis.
c prolonged immobility, venous stasis, and vascular damage.
d venous stasis, vascular damage, and hypercoagulability.

11 *Risk factors associated with an increased risk of development of deep-vein thrombosis (DVT) include:*

a prolonged immobility and surgery in the pelvis or lower extremities.
b obesity and diabetes.
c immobility and arthritis.
d previous history of DVT and renal failure.

12 *An 80-year-old woman had elective total right hip replacement surgery 2 days ago. She complains of pain in the left leg with swelling and a positive Homans' sign. You suspect deep-vein thrombosis (DVT). Which of the statements concerning the development of DVT in patients after hip surgery is correct?*

a DVT occurs in approximately 50% of elective orthopedic procedures.
b Fifty percent of DVT develops in the first 24 hours.
c DVT accounts for approximately 50% of the mortality after total hip surgery.
d All of the above.

13 *A positive Homans' sign is:*

a diagnostic of deep-vein thrombosis (DVT).
b calf pain associated with dorsiflexion of the ankle.
c diagnosed with venous duplex scanning.
d commonly found in patients with peripheral vascular disease.

14 *The most serious complication of deep-vein thrombosis (DVT) is:*

a cerebral embolism.
b myocardial infarction (MI).
c peripheral embolism.
d pulmonary embolism.

15 *Which of the following prophylactic measures should be implemented to prevent deep-vein thrombosis (DVT) in a 70-year-old patient after abdominal surgery?*

a Intravenous heparin 2 hours postoperatively
b Preoperative aspirin use
c Early ambulation
d Compression wrapping of the lower extremities

16 *Which of the following patients should not require deep-vein thrombosis (DVT) prophylaxis?*

a A 70-year-old woman after total knee replacement surgery
b A 35-year-old healthy woman after cholecystectomy
c A 65-year-old man after abdominal aneurysm surgery
d An 80-year-old healthy woman after total hip replacement surgery

17 *A 40-year-old woman is admitted to the hospital after an automobile accident in which she suffered a pelvic fracture. Two days after hospitalization, you are asked to evaluate her because of her complaints of shortness of breath, a temperature of 101.5°F, and confusion. Physical exam reveals a negative Homans' sign and crackles at the bases of both lungs. Chest x-ray reveals diffuse alveolar filling pattern throughout the lung fields. The arterial blood gas reveals hypoxia. What is the most likely diagnosis?*

a Pulmonary embolus
b Fat emboli
c Postoperative atelectasis
d Aspiration pneumonia

18 *Which of the following factors may contribute to postoperative atelectasis?*

a History of smoking and postoperative immobility
b Age greater than 40 years and asthma
c Cardiomyopathy and asthma
d Smoking and history of previous transient ischemic attack (TIA)

19 *A 45-year-old woman has suffered a second-degree burn to her right arm. What is the best way to limit edema in the arm?*

a Compression dressings
b Topical antibiotics
c Elevation and early mobilization
d Casting

20 *A 60-year-old woman has rheumatoid arthritis with boutonnière deformity. Boutonnière deformity is characterized by all of the following EXCEPT:*

a flexion of the proximal interphalangeal (PIP) joints.
b hyperextension of the PIP joints.
c hyperextension of the distal interphalangeal (DIP) joints.
d hyperextension of the metacarpophalangeal (MCP) joints.

21 *A 25-year-old man has cerebral palsy. What is the most common contracture in patients with cerebral palsy?*

a Adduction of the shoulder
b Abduction of the wrist

c Abduction of the hip
d Adduction and flexion of the hip

22 *Which of the following may suggest spinal stenosis?*

a Pain upon awakening in the morning
b Back pain that worsens with standing
c Pain in both arms associated with activity
d Numbness in the legs while sitting

23 *A 35-year-old nurse has a herniated disc at C5 with acute cervical nerve root compression. Which of the following treatments should be implemented?*

a Active resistance exercises
b Cervical collar
c Bed rest and cervical traction
d Systemic steroids to prevent progressive neurologic deficits

24 *Dupuytren's contractures are:*

a the result of repetitive motion of the wrist.
b ischemic injuries.
c deformities associated with humeral fractures.
d treated with physical therapy and steroid injections.

25 *A 50-year-old woman has a history of phospholipid antibody syndrome and is scheduled to undergo abdominal hysterectomy. This patient is at risk for:*

a atelectasis.
b deep-vein thrombosis.
c surgical wound infection.
d surgical wound dehiscence.

26 *Which of the following tests, if positive, indicates hip disease?*

a Phalen's test
b Tinel's sign
c Trendelenburg test
d Kernig's sign

27 *Which of the following should be considered in the differential diagnosis of a patient who presents with low-back pain?*

a MI
b Cholelithiasis
c Osteomyelitis
d Peptic ulcer disease

28 *The most common cause of avascular necrosis of the femoral head is:*

a trauma.
b alcohol abuse.
c steroid use.
d rheumatoid arthritis.

29 *A 50-year-old woman is scheduled for cholecystectomy under general anesthesia. She has a history of rheumatoid arthritis and is on chronic steroid therapy. Which of the following studies should be done preoperatively?*

a Chest x-ray
b Cervical spine x-rays
c Echocardiogram
d Stress thallium test

30 *An 80-year-old nursing home patient had total knee replacement surgery 2 days ago and suffers a stroke with hemiplegia. Which of the following measures will help prevent pressure ulcers?*

a Using a donut cushion
b Eating a high-carbohydrate diet
c Massaging the skin with alcohol
d Turning and repositioning the patient every 2 hours

31 *The most common malignant lesion of the bones is:*

a Ewing's sarcoma.
b metastatic carcinoma.
c multiple myeloma.
d osteosarcoma.

32 *Which of the following statements concerning osteoporosis are true?*

a It affects nearly 25 million Americans.
b It may result in increased bone fragility.
c It may result in fractures.
d All of the above.

33 *Which of the following laboratory tests is a marker of bone osteoblast function?*

a Calcium level
b Alkaline phosphatase level
c Phosphorus level
d Magnesium level

34 *Treatment of carpal tunnel syndrome includes:*

a use of splints.
b use of nonsteroidal anti-inflammatory drugs (NSAIDs).
c surgery.
d all of the above.

35 *Trigger finger deformities are:*

a characterized by stiffness and discoloration in the hand after trauma.
b caused by repetitive use of the hand.
c associated with rheumatoid arthritis.
d frequently treated by splinting.

36 *Which of the following tests are the gold standard for the diagnosis of deep-vein thrombosis (DVT)?*

a Physical examination
b Venogram
c Duplex ultrasound
d D-dimer measurements

37 *Which of the following patients should be considered for an inferior vena caval (IVC) filter placement?*

a A 55-year-old woman after abdominal hysterectomy with a left lower extremity DVT.
b A 45-year-old woman after appendectomy with hyperphospholipid syndrome.
c A 65-year-old man after coronary bypass surgery with gastrointestinal bleeding and documented pulmonary embolus.
d An 80-year-old woman 2 days after total knee replacement who has deep-vein thrombosis (DVT).

Answers

1 Answer c

The most frequently reported complication after total knee replacement is related to the extensor mechanism with a range of 1.5 to 12% in some centers.

2 Answer a

The most common site of pressure ulcers is the sacrum. Other common sites include the greater trochanter, lateral malleolus, and calcaneus.

3 Answer c

Pressure ulcers in the elderly can be prevented with good nutrition consisting of a high-protein, high-vitamin diet. An adequate diet prevents anemia and hypoalbuminemia, which are both risk factors for the development of pressure ulcers.

4 Answer a

The organism most commonly associated with septic pressure ulcers is *B. fragilis.* Other common organisms include *Proteus mirabilis, Staphylococcus aureus,* and *Pseudomonas.*

5 Answer a

The treatment of the patient described should include a surgical consultation for debridement of the pressure ulcer and institution of systemic antibiotics. The use of a rotational mattress and hydrotherapy may be helpful in the healing of the ulcer, but the immediate need is to control the sepsis associated with this ulcer.

6 Answer d

Complications of pressure ulcers include septicemia, cellulitis, and osteomyelitis.

7 Answer b

Prevention of pressure ulcers in patients in a nursing home may be achieved by rotating bedridden patients every 1 to 2 hours. Other preventive measures include checking all pressure points at least twice daily, avoiding alcohol rubs, using

hydrotherapy and exercises, and providing a high-protein, high-vitamin diet.

8 Answer a

Constipation in the elderly is often associated with immobility. Other factors include decreased fluid intake, depression, laxative abuse, and poor nutrition.

9 Answer d

Nonsteroidal anti-inflammatory drugs (NSAIDs) and physical therapy are used in the management of ankylosing spondylosis.

10 Answer d

Virchow's classic triad for the pathogenesis of deep-vein thrombosis (DVT) includes venous stasis, vascular damage, and hypercoagulability.

11 Answer a

Prolonged immobility and surgery in the pelvis or lower extremities are risk factors associated with the development of deep-vein thrombosis (DVT). Other risk factors include previous history of DVT or pulmonary embolus, pregnancy, congestive heart failure, obesity, malignancy, varicose veins, hypercoagulable states, and use of oral contraceptives.

12 Answer d

Deep-vein thrombosis (DVT) after hip surgery can occur in 50 to 70% of patients, with most DVTs occurring in the first 24 hours and with associated mortality of 50%.

13 Answer b

A positive Homans' sign is calf pain associated with dorsiflexion of the ankle, but the presence is not diagnostic of deep-vein thrombosis (DVT).

14 Answer d

The most serious complication of deep-vein thrombosis (DVT) is the development of pulmonary embolism.

15 Answer c

Measures that should be implemented to prevent deep-vein thrombosis (DVT) include early ambulation, as well as elastic or pneumatic stockings and range-of-motion exercises.

16 Answer b

A 35-year-old healthy woman should not require deep-vein thrombosis (DVT) prophylaxis after cholecystectomy. Generally, patients younger than 40 years of age undergoing uncomplicated abdominal procedures do not require DVT prophylaxis.

17 Answer b

The most likely diagnosis for the patient described is fat emboli. Fat emboli usually develop 24 to 48 hours after the injury and may be accompanied by fever, alterations in mental status, hypoxia, hypocapnia, and alveolar filling pattern throughout the lung fields.

18 Answer a

Factors that may contribute to postoperative atelectasis include a history of smoking and postoperative immobility. Other factors include obstructive and restrictive lung disease, thoracotomy incision, upper abdominal surgery, obesity, and age older than 70 years.

19 Answer c

The best way to limit edema in the extremity is elevation and early mobilization. Compression dressings and casting are contraindicated because of the potential for compromised circulation.

20 Answer b

Boutonnière deformity is a progressive condition seen in patients with rheumatoid arthritis. It is characterized by flexion of the interphalangeal (PIP) joints, hyperextension of the distal interphalangeal (DIP) joints, and hyperextension of the metacarpophalangeal (MCP) joints.

21 Answer d

The most common contracture in patients with cerebral palsy is adduction and flexion of the hip.

22 Answer b

Spinal stenosis is a degenerative disease of the spine and is associated with back pain and paraesthesias that worsen with standing but are not present when sitting.

23 Answer c

The treatment of a herniated disc with acute nerve root compression should include bed rest and cervical traction. Other treatment modalities include intrathecal steroids and surgical intervention.

24 Answer d

Dupuytren's contracture is a contracture of the palmar fascia and is associated with tuberculosis, alcoholism, and epilepsy. Treatment of this disorder includes physical therapy, steroid injections, and palmar fasciectomy.

25 Answer b

The patient with phospholipid antibody syndrome who is immobile after abdominal surgery is at risk for the development of deep-vein thrombosis (DVT).

26 Answer c

Trendelenburg test is done to assess for hip disease. To perform the test, ask the patient to stand on one foot. When the patient does so, the contralateral hip should normally pull upward. If the hip the patient is standing on pulls downward, this is a positive test and indicates hip disease.

27 Answer c

The differential diagnosis of a patient with low-back pain should include osteomyelitis, pyelonephritis, malignancy, aortic aneurysm, and unstable spinal fractures.

28 Answer a

The most common cause of avascular necrosis of the femoral head is trauma. Other causes include alcohol use, steroid use, radiation, and sickle cell disease.

29 Answer b

Cervical spine x-rays should be performed preoperatively in patients with rheumatoid arthritis to assess for the stability of the cervical spine prior to neck extension for intubation.

30 Answer d

Turning and repositioning of the patient every 2 hours may be beneficial in preventing pressure ulcers. Donut cushions should be avoided because they lead to ischemia. A well-rounded diet should be encouraged to provide adequate nutrition. Massaging the skin with alcohol may lead to drying and subsequent skin breakdown.

31 Answer b

The most common malignant lesion of the bones is metastatic carcinoma.

32 Answer d

Osteoporosis is a metabolic skeletal disorder characterized by increased bone fragility and the potential for fractures. It affects nearly 25 million Americans.

33 Answer b

Alkaline phosphatase is a marker of bone osteoblast formation and helps to identify patients with high-turnover osteoporosis.

34 Answer d

Treatment of carpal tunnel syndrome includes the use of splints, NSAIDs, and surgery.

35 Answer b

Trigger finger deformities are caused by repetitive use of the hand. They involve a tendon nodule at the opening of the flexor sheath at the level of the distal palmar crease. Treatment may include surgical release or injections into the sheath.

36 Answer b

The gold standard for the diagnosis of deep-vein thrombosis (DVT) is a venogram. Whereas other methods such as duplex ultrasound and impedance plethysmography may detect 90% of acute proximal DVT, venogram remains the gold standard. The diagnostic accuracy of D-dimer measurements has not been confirmed.

37 Answer c

The patient who should be considered for an IVC filter is the patient with gastrointestinal bleeding in which heparin would be contraindicated, and who already has evidence of pulmonary embolus.

Bibliography

Canale, ST: Campbell's Operative Orthopedics, 9th ed. Mosby, St. Louis, 1998.

Goroll, A, et al: Primary Care Medicine Office Evaluation and Management of the Adult Patient, 4th ed. Lippincott Williams & Wilkins, Philadelphia, 2000.

Simon, RR, and Koenigsknect, SJ: Emergency Orthopedics: The Extremities, 3rd ed. Appleton & Lange, Norwalk, Conn., 1995.

Sumner, DS: Diagnosis of deep venous thrombosis. In Rutherford, RB (ed): Vascular Surgery, 5th ed. WB Saunders, Philadelphia, 2000.

24

Infections

Questions 1–3 refer to the following scenario:

A 25-year-old bisexual man presents with complaints of fever, chills, bloody diarrhea, midsternal burning, decreased appetite, and difficulty swallowing. ELISA and Western Blot assays are positive for human immunodeficiency virus (HIV) infection.

1 Which of the following CD4 counts would define this patient as a patient with acquired immunodeficiency syndrome (AIDS)?

a 600
b 180
c 250
d 300

2 The most likely cause of this patient's diarrhea is:

a *Cryptosporidium parvum.*
b *Clostridium difficile.*
c *Shigella.*
d *Giardia lamblia.*

3 The most common cause of dysphagia in a patient with human immunodeficiency virus (HIV) infection is:

a Kaposi's sarcoma.
b hairy leukoplakia.
c herpes virus.
d candidal esophagitis.

4 A 20-year-old male college student has the following serologies: Monospot positive, positive anti–viral capsid antigen (anti–VCA), and negative anti–Epstein-Barr nuclear antigen. Which of the following statements is true concerning this patient?

a He has hepatitis.
b He previously had cytomegalovirus (CMV) infection.
c He previously had Epstein-Barr virus infection.
d He has Epstein-Barr virus infection.

5 A 25-year-old woman is diagnosed with pyelonephritis. What is the most likely responsible organism?

a *Streptococcus.*
b *Staphylococcus.*
c *Escherichia coli.*
d *Klebsiella.*

6 A 20-year-old woman consumed unpasteurized milk. Which of the following pathogens is found in unpasteurized milk?

a *Bartonella henselae.*
b *Brucella abortus.*
c *Staphylococcus aureus.*
d *Mycoplasma.*

7 A 25-year-old woman complains of a curdlike vaginal discharge. The most likely cause is:

a *Trichomonas vaginalis.*
b Human papilloma virus (HPV).
c *Candida albicans.*
d Syphilis.

8 A 30-year-old man complains of burning on urination. Physical exam reveals a chancre on the penis. The most likely etiology of the chancre is:

a *Treponema pallidum.*
b *Neisseria Neisseria.*
c Human papilloma virus (HPV).
d Herpes zoster.

9 A 55-year-old man is admitted to your nurse practitioner service with complaints of fever, chills, and a productive cough with "currant jelly" sputum. A chest x-ray reveals a left lower lobe (LLL) pneumonia. Which of the following pathogens is most likely responsible?

a *Staphylococcus aureus.*
b *Klebsiella pneumoniae.*

c *Mycoplasma pneumoniae.*
d Acid-fast bacilli.

10 *An 18-year-old woman with pelvic inflammatory disease (PID) is admitted with fever, abdominal pain, and vomiting. The pathogen commonly associated with PID is:*

a *Candida albicans.*
b *Neisseria gonorrhoeae.*
c *Chlamydia trachomatis.*
d *Escherichia coli.*

11 *A 45-year-old woman is admitted to your nurse practitioner service with complaints of abdominal pain and fever. The patient's laboratory tests reveal the following: negative hepatitis B surface antigen (HBsAg), positive anti-HBs, negative anti-hepatitis B core antigen (anti-HBc IgM), and positive anti-HBc (IgG). According to these results, the patient has a(n):*

a acute hepatitis B infection.
b acute hepatitis C infection.
c chronic hepatitis B infection.
d previous hepatitis B infection.

12 *A 28-year-old woman with acquired immunodeficiency syndrome (AIDS) has been diagnosed with retinitis. What is the most common cause of retinitis in a patient with AIDS?*

a Herpes simplex virus (HSV)
b Epstein-Barr virus (EBV)
c Cytomegalovirus (CMV)
d *Staphylococcus*

13 *A 30-year-old woman presents with complaints of fever, weight loss, night sweats, and enlarged nodes in the neck. Examination of the patient reveals white plaque on the tongue and palate. What test(s) should be performed to confirm your suspected diagnosis?*

a Purified protein derivative (PPD)
b Hepatitis serologies
c Enzyme-linked immunosorbent assay (ELISA) test for HIV
d Monospot

14 *Which of the following organisms is endemic to the soil in the Ohio valley?*

a *Aspergillus*
b *Histoplasma capsulatum*
c *Candida albicans*
d *Mycoplasma*

Questions 15–16 refer to the following scenario:

A 40-year-old previously healthy woman is seen in the clinic with complaints of fever, fatigue, cough, and generalized myalgias that have occurred for the past 2

weeks. A chest x-ray reveals diffuse interstitial pneumonia in the right lower lobe of the lung, and the complete blood count (CBC) is normal.

15 *What is the most likely diagnosis of this patient?*

a Pneumococcal pneumonia
b *Legionella pneumophila*
c *Mycoplasma pneumoniae*
d Herpes pneumonia

16 *The antibiotic choice for this patient is:*

a erythromycin (E-Mycin).
b ampicillin (Omnipen).
c penicillin.
d trimethoprim sulfamethoxazole (Bactrim DS).

17 *Helicobacter pylori has been implicated in:*

a bacterial vaginosis.
b hepatitis C infection.
c gastric ulcers.
d cervical dysplasia.

18 *Clinical manifestations of mediastinal chest infections after coronary bypass surgery include:*

a fever only.
b sternal pain, fever, and drainage.
c bradycardia.
d sharp pleuritic pain.

19 *A 65-year-old man is being evaluated for prostatitis. All of the following clinical manifestations may be seen EXCEPT:*

a urinary urgency.
b abdominal bruit.
c dysuria.
d perianal pain.

20 *Use of a Wood's lamp would be important in the diagnosis of:*

a tinea infections.
b herpes simplex virus (HSV) infection.
c rabies.
d cytomegalovirus (CMV) infection.

21 *A positive Tzanck test is seen in:*

a cytomegalovirus (CMV) infection.
b hepatitis B infection.
c herpes zoster infection.
d Epstein-Barr virus (EBV) infection.

22 *A positive Kernig's sign is seen in patients with:*

a meningitis.
b an *Escherichia coli* infection.

c   peritonitis.
d   acute cholecystitis.

23   *Acute rheumatic fever is a late sequela of which of the following infections?*

a   *Streptococcus* infection.
b   methicillin-resistant *Staphylococcus aureus* (MRSA) infection.
c   *Staphylococcus epidermidis* infection.
d   *Enterococcus* infection.

24   *A 65-year-old man is admitted to the intensive care unit with bilateral pneumonia. You suspect Legionnaire's disease in the differential diagnosis and want to provide antibiotic coverage for this possibility. All of the following antibiotics would be appropriate* **EXCEPT:**

a   erythromycin (E-Mycin).
b   levofloxacin (Levaquin).
c   ciprofloxacin (Cipro).
d   trimethoprim sulfamethoxazole (Bactrim DS).

25   *The preferred initial treatment of* Clostridium difficile *infection is:*

a   levofloxacin (Levaquin).
b   metronidazole (Flagyl).
c   trimethoprim sulfamethoxazole (Bactrim DS).
d   amoxicillin (Amoxil).

26   *All of the following antibiotics are excreted by the kidneys* **EXCEPT:**

a   imipenem (Primaxin).
b   ciprofloxacin (Cipro).
c   trimethoprim sulfamethoxazole (Bactrim DS).
d   rifampin (Rifadin).

27   *An antibiotic you would like to prescribe to a pregnant patient has a Food and Drug Administration (FDA) X rating. This rating means that:*

a   controlled studies show no risk to the fetus.
b   data show that there is risk to the fetus, but the potential benefits outweigh the risk.
c   the drug is contraindicated in pregnancy.
d   there is no evidence of risk to humans.

28   *Which of the following medications is most commonly used to treat invasive fungal infections?*

a   Fluconazole (Diflucan).
b   Amphotericin B (Amphocin).
c   Gentamicin (Garamycin).
d   Ampicillin (Omnipen).

29   *Which of the following side effects are associated with amphotericin B?*

a   Hypokalemia and nephrotoxicity
b   Fever and hyperkalemia
c   Hypermagnesemia and hyperkalemia
d   Hyponatremia and hyperkalemia

30   *The primary mode of transmission of* Giardia lamblia *is:*

a   water.
b   oral-fecal.
c   blood.
d   sexual contact.

31   *Reiter's syndrome is associated with urethritis, uveitis, conjunctivitis, and:*

a   diabetes mellitus.
b   peptic ulcer disease.
c   arthritis.
d   mitral stenosis.

32   *The most common cause of food poisoning is:*

a   *Staphylococcus aureus.*
b   *Streptococcus.*
c   *Clostridium difficile.*
d   nontyphoidal salmonellosis.

33   *The most common site of embolization in patients with infective endocarditis is the:*

a   retinal artery.
b   kidney.
c   spleen.
d   brain.

34   *All of the statements concerning ventilator-associated pneumonia are true* **EXCEPT:**

a   mortality is high in patients with gram-negative pneumonias.
b   postoperative atelectasis may contribute to the development of ventilator-associated pneumonia.
c   aspiration is the most common mechanism for development of pneumonia.
d   use of famotidine (Pepcid) for gastrointestinal prophylaxis may decrease the incidence of ventilator-associated pneumonia.

35   *All of the following statements concerning scabies are true* **EXCEPT:**

a   it is caused by infestation with the itch mite.
b   it causes intense pruritus.
c   the rash most commonly occurs on the face.
d   the treatment of choice is permethrin (Elimite).

36   *All of the following are major Jones criteria for the diagnosis of rheumatic fever* **EXCEPT:**

a   polyarthritis.

b fever.
c carditis.
d erythema marginatum.

37 *Negri bodies are seen on autopsy in persons with:*

a meningitis.
b rabies.
c tuberculosis.
d herpes encephalitis.

Answers

1   Answer b
A CD4 count less than 200 would define the patient with HIV infection as having AIDS.

2   Answer a
The most likely cause of the patient's diarrhea is *Cryptosporidium parvum.*

3   Answer d
The most common cause of dysphagia in a patient with HIV infection is candidal esophagitis.

4   Answer d
The patient described has a current Epstein-Barr virus infection as demonstrated by the serologies (Monospot positive, anti-VCA positive, and anti-EBNA negative).

5   Answer c
The most likely organism responsible for pyelonephritis is *Escherichia coli.*

6   Answer b
Brucella abortus is found in unpasteurized dairy products.

7   Answer c
The patient with a curdlike vaginal discharge most likely has a *Candida* vaginal infection.

8   Answer a
The most likely etiology of a chancre on the penis is *Treponema pallidum.*

9   Answer b
The most likely pathogen causing the pneumonia in the patient described is *Klebsiella pneumoniae.* Currant jelly sputum is characteristic of *K. pneumoniae.*

10   Answer c
Pelvic inflammatory disease (PID) is commonly caused by *Chlamydia trachomatis.*

11   Answer d
The laboratory tests of the patient described indicate that the patient has had a previous hepatitis B infection.

12   Answer c
The most common cause of retinitis in patients with AIDS is cytomegalovirus.

13   Answer c
The test that should be performed on the patient described is the ELISA test for HIV. If the test is positive, then a western blot assay should be performed. The symptoms of the patient described may be seen with tuberculosis, but the *Candida* infection in the mouth makes HIV infection the most likely diagnosis.

14   Answer b
Histoplasma capsulatum is endemic in the Ohio valley.

15   Answer c
The most likely diagnosis of the patient described is *Mycoplasma pneumoniae,* commonly termed "walking pneumonia," which can commonly persist up to 2 weeks if not treated.

16   Answer a
The antibiotic of choice for a patient with *Mycoplasma pneumoniae* is erythromycin. The organism lacks a cell wall and is resistant to the penicillins.

17   Answer c
Helicobacter pylori has been implicated in gastric ulcers.

18   Answer b
Clinical manifestations of mediastinal chest infections after coronary bypass surgery include sternal pain, fever, and drainage.

19   Answer b
Prostatitis may be associated with urinary urgency, dysuria, and perianal pain; an abdominal bruit is not associated with prostatitis.

20   Answer a
A Wood's ray would be important in the diagnosis of tinea infections.

21   Answer c
A positive Tzanck test is seen in a herpes zoster infection. The test would demonstrate multinucleated giant cells.

22   Answer a
A positive Kernig's sign is seen in patients with meningitis.

23   Answer a
Acute rheumatic fever is a late sequela of group A streptococcus infection.

24   Answer d
The appropriate coverage of *Legionella pneumophila* includes the macrolides such as erythromycin, quinolones such as ciprofloxacin and levofloxacin, and tetracyclines in combination with rifampin.

25   Answer b
The preferred initial treatment of *Clostridium difficile* infection is metronidazole (Flagyl).

26   Answer d
Rifampin (Rifadin) is excreted by the liver. Imipenem (Primaxin), ciprofloxacin (Cipro), and trimethoprim sulfamethoxazole (Bactrim DS) are all excreted by the kidneys.

27   Answer c
An FDA X rating for an antibiotic means that the drug is con-

traindicated in pregnancy because the risk to the fetus outweighs any possible benefit to the mother.

28 Answer b

The medication most commonly used to treat invasive fungal infections is amphotericin B (Amphocin).

29 Answer a

Side effects associated with amphotericin B infusion include fever, chills, hypokalemia, and nephrotoxicity.

30 Answer a

The primary mode of transmission of *Giardia lamblia* is water.

31 Answer c

Reiter's syndrome is associated with urethritis, uveitis, conjunctivitis, and arthritis. Reiter's syndrome is usually preceded by a sexually transmitted disease or bacterial gastroenteritis.

32 Answer d

The most common cause of food poisoning is nontyphoidal salmonellosis.

33 Answer c

The most common site of embolization in patients with infective endocarditis is the spleen.

34 Answer d

Sucralfate (Carafate) use, not famotidine (Pepcid) use, for gastrointestinal prophylaxis may decrease the incidence of ventilator-associated pneumonia. Mortality is high in patients with gram-negative pneumonias; postoperative atelectasis may contribute to the development of ventilator-associated pneumonia; and aspiration is the most common mechanism for development of pneumonia.

35 Answer c

Scabies can occur on any portion of the body, but it is most commonly seen in the finger webs, wrists, waist, axillae, buttocks, and umbilical area—not in the face. Scabies is caused by infestation with the itch mite. It causes intense pruritus, and the treatment of choice is permethrin (Elimite).

36 Answer b

Major Jones criteria for the diagnosis of rheumatic fever include polyarthritis, carditis, and erythema marginatum. Fever is not part of the major Jones criteria for the diagnosis of rheumatic fever.

37 Answer b

Negri bodies are seen on autopsy in the brain of persons with rabies.

Bibliography

Bennett, JV, and Brachman, PS: Hospital Infections, 4th ed. Lippincott Williams & Wilkins, Philadelphia, 1998.

Edmond, MB, et al: Vancomycin-resistant *Staphylococcus aureus:* Perspectives on measures needed for control. Ann Intern Med 124: 329–334, 1996.

Fekety, R: Guidelines for the diagnosis and management of *Clostridium difficile*–associated diarrhea and colitis. Am J Gastroenterol 92:739–750, 1997.

Gold, HS, and Moellering, RC: Antimicrobial drug resistance. N Engl J Med 335:1445–1453, 1996.

Goroll, A, et al: Primary Care Medicine Office Evaluation and Management of the Adult Patient, 4th ed. Lippincott Williams & Wilkins, Philadelphia, 2000.

Hirschmann, JV: Fever of unknown origin in adults. Clin Infect Dis 24:291–302, 1997.

Mandell, GI, et al: Principles and Practice of Infectious Disease, 5th ed. Churchill Livingstone, New York, 2000.

Pinner, RW, et al: Trends in infectious diseases mortality in the United States. JAMA 275:189–193, 1996.

Quagliarello, VJ, and Scheld, WM: Treatment of bacterial meningitis. N Engl J Med 336:708–716, 1997.

Raviglione, MC, et al: A global epidemiology of tuberculosis. JAMA 273:220–226, 1995.

Royce, RA, et al: Current concepts: Sexual transmission of HIV. N Engl J Med 336:1072–1078, 1997.

25

Dermatologic Problems

1 *A 60-year-old woman has had dry skin on the soles of her feet for the past 5 years. She presents now during the summer months with complaints of an itchy scaly rash around her ankles. She used steroid cream for the past 5 days without any change. She states she had this rash last year during the summer and fall, and that it disappeared in the winter. What is the most likely diagnosis?*

a Psoriasis
b *Candida albicans*
c Tinea pedis
d Lichen planus

2 *Vitiligo is commonly associated with:*

a diabetes mellitus.
b hypothyroidism.
c hypertension.
d renal failure.

3 *Tinea versicolor is caused by:*

a cytomegalovirus (CMV).
b *Streptococcus.*
c *Candida albicans.*
d *Pityrosporum orbiculare.*

4 *Stevens-Johnson syndrome is commonly caused by:*

a sulfa drugs.
b penicillin.
c vancomycin (Vancocin).
d aspirin.

5 *A 30-year-old woman presents with complaints of fatigue and a macular eruption on her face that appears in a butterfly pattern. What is the most likely diagnosis?*

a Scleroderma
b Psoriasis
c Systemic lupus erythematosus (SLE)
d Impetigo

6 *A 25-year-old woman presents with complaints of scattered vesicular lesions around the mouth and nose for the past week. Her physical exam reveals yellow, honey-colored crusts around the mouth with erosions in some of the lesions. Culture reveals Staphylococcus aureus. What is the most likely diagnosis?*

a Herpes simplex
b Herpes zoster
c Impetigo
d Rosacea

7 *A vesicle filled with purulent material is referred to as a:*

a papule.
b wheal.
c plaque.
d pustule.

8 *A nonpalpable lesion less than 1 cm in size is referred to as a:*

a papule.
b macule.
c patch.
d bullae.

9 *A 50-year-old man has pneumonia and disseminated intravascular coagulation (DIC). Which of the following dermatologic manifestations would you expect to see?*

a Petechiae and purpura
b Spider angiomas
c A maculopapular rash
d Fissures

10 *A 50-year-old deer hunter is diagnosed with Lyme disease. The rash of Lyme disease is:*

a difficult to treat.
b painful.

c an annular erythematous patch.
d associated with tissue necrosis.

11 *A purplish red tumor that may occur in patients with acquired immunodeficiency syndrome (AIDS) is:*

a seborrheic dermatosis.
b Kaposi's sarcoma.
c pityriasis rosea.
d varicella.

12 *All of the following statements concerning pityriasis rosea are true* **EXCEPT:**

a it is a maculopapular red eruption.
b it most often occurs on the trunk.
c it is most likely caused by a virus.
d it may mimic a *Candida albicans* infection.

13 *Erysipelas is caused by:*

a *Staphylococcus aureus.*
b group A *Streptococcus.*
c *Pseudomonas.*
d herpes simplex.

14 *The most common bullous disease is:*

a pemphigus vulgaris.
b dermatitis herpetiformis.
c erythema multiforme.
d Stevens-Johnson syndrome.

15 *The treatment of chickenpox in the adult should include:*

a ganciclovir (Cytovene).
b acyclovir (Zovirax).
c aspirin therapy.
d penicillin.

16 *Which of the following may be used to treat postherpetic neuralgia?*

a Steroids
b Acyclovir
c Amitriptyline (Elavil)
d All of the above

17 *The clinical presentation of shingles is characterized by all of the following* **EXCEPT:**

a a unilateral vesicular eruption.
b pain during the eruption only.
c vesicular eruption in a dermatomal distribution.
d potential involvement of the cranial nerves.

18 *A 40-year-old woman complains of recurrent pruritic vesicles on the elbows and knees. What is the most likely diagnosis?*

a Steven-Johnson syndrome
b Herpes zoster
c Dermatitis herpetiformis
d Psoriasis

19 *A 50-year-old man is found on a snow bank and is brought to the emergency department. He has frostbite and clear blisters on his arm. The blisters are debrided. Which of the following medications should be applied to the blistered areas?*

a Dapsone
b Dermaide
c Erythromycin (E-Mycin)
d Isotretinoin (Accutane)

20 *The most common bite wounds seen in urban emergency departments are:*

a human bites.
b dog bites.
c cat bites.
d spider bites.

21 *The most common organism cultured from human bite wounds is:*

a *Streptococcus.*
b *Enterococcus.*
c *Staphylococcus.*
d *Proteus.*

22 *The topical treatment of acne vulgaris is best achieved with:*

a erythromycin (E-Mycin).
b gentamicin (Garamycin).
c polymycin.
d vancomycin (Vancocin).

23 *The antibiotic of choice for the systemic treatment of acne vulgaris is:*

a erythromycin (E-Mycin).
b clindamycin (Cleocin).
c ciprofloxacin (Cipro).
d cephalexin (Keflex).

24 *Complications of dermabrasion therapy used in treating acne include:*

a infection.
b hyperpigmentation.
c hypertrophic scarring.
d all of the above.

25 *The treatment of choice for recalcitrant nodulocystic acne is:*

a erythromycin (E-Mycin).
b tetracycline (Achromycin).

c isotretinoin (Accutane).
d chloramphenicol (Chloromycetin).

26 *Which of the following laboratory tests should be monitored in patients taking isotretinoin?*

a Serum triglyceride and liver enzyme levels
b Complete blood count
c Renal function tests
d Platelet count

27 *Treatment of acne includes:*

a gentle facial washing.
b using water-based cosmetics.
c eating a well-balanced diet.
d all of the above.

28 *A 50-year-old woman complains of a pruritic skin rash after exposure to cold water that lasts for 2 to 3 hours. What is the most likely diagnosis?*

a Cold-induced urticaria
b Contact dermatitis
c Psoriasis
d Raynaud's syndrome

29 *Lyme disease is caused by:*

a *Rickettsia rickettsii.*
b *Staphylococcus aureus.*
c *Borrelia burgdorferi.*
d Epstein-Barr virus (EBV).

30 *Common warts are caused by:*

a Epstein-Barr virus (EBV).
b cytomegalovirus (CMV).
c human papilloma virus (HPV).
d tinea pedis.

31 *Common warts are usually found on the:*

a dorsal surface of the hands and fingers.
b buttocks.
c anterior chest.
d feet.

32 *Which of the following persons are at risk for melanoma?*

a Persons with blond hair
b Fair skinned, blue-eyed, and freckled persons
c Persons with a previous history of squamous cell carcinoma
d African-Americans

33 *All of the statements concerning basal cell carcinoma are true EXCEPT:*

a it is the most common cutaneous malignancy.
b it is associated with chronic sun exposure.
c it is most commonly found on the abdomen and trunk.
d it may be difficult to differentiate from malignant melanoma.

34 *Diagnosis of malignant melanoma is made by:*

a a Wood's ray test.
b potassium hydroxide preparation.
c excisional biopsy.
d cryotherapy.

35 *Which of the following suggests a diagnosis of malignant melanoma?*

a Lesion with border irregularity
b Lesion diameter less than 0.2 cm
c Lesion on the face
d Light color lesion

36 *Which of the following diseases are associated with pitting of the nailbeds?*

a Diabetes mellitus
b Psoriasis
c Hyperthyroidism
d Hypertension

Answers

1 Answer c
The most likely diagnosis for the patient described is tinea pedis.

2 Answer b
Vitiligo is commonly associated with metabolic disorders such as hypothyroidism, adrenocortical insufficiency, scleroderma, and alopecia areata. The lesions of vitiligo are white, contain no pigment, and are seen in the periorbital area, hands, axillas, perineum, and neck.

3 Answer d
Tinea versicolor is caused by *Pityrosporum orbiculare.*

4 Answer a
Stevens-Johnson syndrome is commonly caused by sulfa drugs. It is usually associated with a fever and ulcerations in the mucous membranes of the lips, eyes, buccal cavity, and genitalia.

5 Answer c
The most likely diagnosis for the patient described is systemic lupus erythematosus (SLE).

6 Answer c
The most likely diagnosis for the patient described is impetigo. Impetigo can be caused by *Staphylococcus* and *Streptococcus*

organisms. It is most common in children, but can also occur in adults.

7   Answer d

A vesicle filled with purulent material is referred to as a pustule.

8   Answer b

A nonpalpable lesion less than 1 cm in size is referred to as a macule.

9   Answer a

Dermatologic manifestations of disseminated intravascular coagulation (DIC) include petechiae and purpura.

10   Answer c

The rash of Lyme disease is an annular erythematous patch. The rash is usually easily treated with doxycycline (Vibramycin), is painless, and is not associated with tissue necrosis.

11   Answer b

Kaposi's sarcoma is a purplish tumor that may occur anywhere on the body in patients with AIDS.

12   Answer d

Pityriasis rosea is a maculopapular red, scaling eruption that is commonly found on the trunk and is caused by a virus. The rash may mimic syphilis but not a *Candida albicans* infection.

13   Answer b

Erysipelas is caused by group A *Streptococcus* and is commonly associated with an upper respiratory infection. Treatment may include penicillin or a cephalosporin.

14   Answer c

The most common bullous disease is erythema multiforme.

15   Answer b

Treatment of chickenpox in the adult should include the use of acyclovir (Zovirax).

16   Answer d

Postherpetic neuralgia may be treated with the use of steroids, acyclovir, and amitriptyline.

17   Answer b

The clinical presentation of shingles is not characterized by pain during the eruption only. The pain of shingles may last months after the resolution of the vesicular eruption. Shingles are a unilateral vesicular eruption that occurs in a dermatomal distribution and has potential involvement of the cranial nerves.

18   Answer c

The most likely diagnosis for the patient described is dermatitis herpetiformis, which usually involves the elbows, interscapular area, lower back, and knees.

19   Answer b

Dermaide, which is topical aloe vera, should be applied to the blisters. Dermaide acts as a thromboxane inhibitor, which may help to minimize arachidonic acid breakdown and subsequent skin loss.

20   Answer a

The most common bite wounds seen in the urban emergency department are human bites.

21   Answer a

The most common organism cultured from human bite wounds is *Streptococcus*.

22   Answer a

The topical treatment of acne vulgaris is best achieved with erythromycin. Other medications that may be used include topical tetracycline and clindamycin.

23   Answer a

The antibiotic of choice for the systemic treatment of acne vulgaris is erythromycin. Tetracycline may also be used.

24   Answer d

Complications of dermabrasion include infection, hyperpigmentation, hypopigmentation, and hypertrophic scarring.

25   Answer c

The treatment of choice for recalcitrant nodulocystic acne is isotretinoin (Accutane).

26   Answer a

Serum triglycerides and liver enzymes should be monitored in patients taking isotretinoin (Accutane).

27   Answer d

Treatment of acne includes using water-based cosmetics, gentle facial washing, and eating a well-balanced diet.

28   Answer a

The most likely diagnosis for the patient described is cold-induced urticaria (CIU). The cause of CIU is unknown, but it occurs in the rewarming phase of cold exposure.

29   Answer c

Lyme disease is caused by *Borrelia burgdorferi*.

30   Answer c

Common warts are caused by human papilloma virus (HPV).

31   Answer a

Common warts are usually found on the dorsal surface of the hands and fingers.

32   Answer b

Melanoma is more likely to develop in people who are fair skinned, blue-eyed, red-haired, and freckled. Persons with atypical moles or large congenital nevus, who have a family history of melanoma, or who are immunocompromised are at risk for the development of melanoma.

33   Answer c

Basal cell carcinoma is the most common cutaneous malignancy, associated with chronic sun exposure. It is commonly found on the head and neck, not the abdomen or trunk. It is heavily pigmented and difficult at times to differentiate from malignant melanoma.

34   Answer c

Diagnosis of malignant melanoma is made by excisional biopsy.

35   Answer a

A diagnosis of malignant melanoma is suggested by lesion asymmetry, border irregularity, dark color, and a diameter of more than 0.6 cm.

36   Answer b

Psoriasis is associated with pitting of the nailbeds.

Bibliography

Freedberg, IM: Fitzpatrick's Dermatology in General Medicine, 5th ed. McGraw-Hill, New York, 1999.

Goroll, A, et al: Primary Care Medicine Office Evaluation and Management of the Adult Patient, 4th ed. Lippincott Williams & Wilkins, Philadelphia, 2000.

Lesher, JL: Recent developments in antifungal therapy. Derm Clin 14:163–169, 1996.

Sontheimer, RD, and Provost, TT: Cutaneous Manifestations of Rheumatic Disease. Williams & Wilkins, Baltimore, 1996.

26

Palliative Care

1 *Palliative care is defined as:*

a a referral service for patients with a terminal illness.
b advanced cancer care.
c the active total care of patients; control of pain; and minimization of emotional, social, and spiritual problems at a time when disease is not responsive to active treatment.
d the use of church groups in caring for patients.

2 *The goals of palliative care include:*

a providing relief from pain and other distressing symptoms.
b maintaining quality of life.
c integrating psychosocial and spiritual aspects of patient care.
d all of the above.

3 *The most common cause of malignant pleural effusion is:*

a lung cancer.
b metastatic breast cancer.
c abdominal cancer.
d hepatic carcinoma.

4 *A 45-year-old woman with metastatic ovarian carcinoma has ascites. Pharmacologic management of the ascites includes:*

a digoxin (Lanoxin).
b furosemide (Lasix) and spironolactone (Aldactone).
c enalapril (Vasotec).
d mannitol (Osmitrol).

5 *Which of the following are classifications of pain in the patient with cancer?*

a Visceral pain
b Somatic pain
c Psychogenic pain
d All of the above

6 *The pain of bone metastasis is referred to as:*

a visceral pain.
b somatic pain.
c neuropathic pain.
d central pain.

7 *A 70-year-old man with a history of prostate cancer treated with radiation now presents with metastasis to the bone and signs of impending spinal cord compression. Which of the following treatments should be instituted?*

a Epidural analgesia
b Intravenous corticosteroids
c Chemotherapy
d Lumbar traction

8 *The most commonly used steroid in treatment of spinal cord compression is:*

a prednisone.
b methylprednisolone succinate (Solumedrol).
c hydrocortisone succinate (Solu-Cortef).
d dexamethasone (Decadron).

9 *The most common tumors associated with superior vena cava syndrome are:*

a breast and ovarian carcinoma.
b lung and bone carcinoma.
c lung carcinoma and lymphoma.
d lung and abdominal carcinoma.

10 *Common clinical manifestations associated with superior vena cava syndrome include:*

a nausea, vomiting, and chest pain.
b engorgement of the neck veins, swollen face, and shortness of breath.
c palpitations and syncope.
d shortness of breath and hemoptysis.

11 *The advantage(s) of radiation therapy in the treatment of cancer is(are) that it:*

a provides pain relief.
b allows for direct treatment of the tumor.
c is associated with limited toxicity.
d all of the above.

12 *Which of the following instructions should be given to a patient receiving radiation therapy?*

a Take cold showers.
b Massage the treated area three times daily.
c Do not apply creams to the treated skin areas prior to radiation treatment.
d Scrub the treated area with soap and water.

13 *The most common cause of hemoptysis is:*

a lung carcinoma.
b lymphoma.
c tuberculosis.
d histoplasmosis.

14 *A 45-year-old woman has a 1-cm squamous cell tumor resected from her lung. The margins are free of tumor and have no evidence of metastasis. Which of the following adjunctive therapies should be used?*

a Radiation.
b Chemotherapy.
c Radiation and chemotherapy.
d No further treatment is needed.

15 *The treatment for oral candidiasis in a patient on chemotherapy is:*

a acyclovir (Zovirax).
b clotrimazole (Mycelex).
c magnesium hydroxide (Maalox).
d phenazopyridine (Pyridium).

16 *Which of the following therapies may be implemented in palliative care?*

a Guided imagery
b Reflexology
c Visualization
d All of the above

17 *Which of the following statements concerning therapeutic touch is true?*

a Therapeutic touch is massage therapy.
b Therapeutic touch incorporates music.
c Therapeutic touch is based on the belief that energy fields surround us and are constantly changing according to our emotions.
d The therapeutic touch practitioner is usually an internal medicine physician.

18 *A 55-year-old man had a resection of a gastric carcinoma 2 months ago. He complains of dysphagia. Which of the following tests should be done initially to evaluate the dysphagia?*

a Abdominal computed tomography (CT) scan
b Barium swallow
c Colonoscopy
d A trial of a liquid diet

19 *The most common fear(s) of patients at end of life include the fear of:*

a pain.
b suffering.
c isolation.
d all of the above.

20 *One of the major causes of insomnia in palliative care patients is:*

a anxiety.
b headaches.
c chest pains.
d palpitations.

21 *A 35-year-old woman with metastatic breast cancer has requested that you help her to die because of the constant pain she is feeling. What is the most appropriate response?*

a Inform the patient that she is too young to die.
b Inform the patient that euthanasia is illegal, but you will use measures to ensure her comfort.
c Inform the patient that the staff nurse will make her comfortable.
d Ask the patient how she would like to die.

22 *A 65-year-old man with metastatic lung cancer has chronic pain. Which of the following statements concerning morphine in the treatment of cancer pain is true?*

a Morphine produces rapid tolerance.
b There is no maximum morphine dosage.
c Morphine may produce euphoria.
d Morphine should not be used for cancer pain.

23 *The goals of pain management in palliative care include:*

a preventing the pain.
b defining the cause of the pain.
c erasing the memory of the pain.
d all of the above.

24 *Which of the following medications can be used in conjunction with analgesics for the management of cancer pain?*

a Metoprolol (Lopressor)
b Amitriptyline (Elavil)
c Furosemide (Lasix)
d Metoclopramide (Reglan)

25 *Which of the following agents may be used to treat nausea and vomiting in palliative care patients?*

a Metoclopramide (Reglan) and prochlorperazine (Compazine)
b Prochlorperazine and docusate sodium (Colace)
c Psyllium (Metamucil) and metoclopramide
d Famotidine (Pepcid) and prochlorperazine

26 *Treatment of a partial bowel obstruction in a patient with metastatic brain cancer should include:*

a intravenous steroids.
b placement of a gastrotomy tube.
c a colonoscopy.
d decreased fluid intake.

27 *The World Health Organization (WHO) guidelines for evaluating pain include all of the following* **EXCEPT:**

a taking a detailed history of pain.
b considering alternative methods of pain relief.
c questioning the patient's report of pain.
d performing a thorough physical examination.

28 *Side effects associated with morphine use include all of the following* **EXCEPT:**

a constipation.
b urinary retention.
c myoclonic jerks.
d myalgias.

29 *The most common cause of sore mouth in patients in palliative care is from:*

a a monilial infection.
b a nasogastric tube.
c a vitamin A deficiency.
d improperly fitting dentures.

30 *Which of the following nurse practitioner– and physician-related factors may prevent referrals to hospice care?*

a Perceived loss of control
b Lack of knowledge concerning services
c Appearance of giving up on the patient
d All of the above

31 *All of the statements concerning hospice care are true* **EXCEPT:**

a it is provided to terminally ill patients.

b the Medicare guidelines state that life expectancy should be 6 months or less.
c referrals can be initiated only by physicians.
d most patients have a cancer diagnosis.

32 *A 60-year-old woman with metastatic ovarian carcinoma has developed a bowel obstruction. What are the common symptoms of bowel obstruction?*

a Abdominal pain, vomiting, and intestinal colic
b Fever and abdominal pain
c Diarrhea, fever, and abdominal pain
d Hematemesis and abdominal pain

33 *Which of the following patients is an appropriate hospice referral?*

a A 50-year-old woman with congestive heart failure, metastatic breast cancer, and a life expectancy of 3 months
b A 45-year-old man who has human immunodeficiency virus (HIV) infection
c A 55-year-old man following coronary bypass surgery
d An 80-year-old healthy man.

34 *A 40-year-old woman with acquired immunodeficiency syndrome (AIDS) is in a vegetative state on a ventilator in the intensive care unit and is expected to live less than 48 hours. She develops upper gastrointestinal (GI) bleeding and has a hemoglobin of 7.5 g/dL. A family member who has durable power of attorney for health care has signed a do not resuscitate (DNR) form and requests supportive care only. Which of the following treatments should be instituted to treat the GI bleed?*

a Transfuse to a hemoglobin greater than 10.
b Consult gastroenterology and general surgery.
c Recheck the hemoglobin in 2 hours.
d No further treatment should be instituted.

35 *Durable power of attorney refers to a:*

a person's next of kin.
b person who represents the family without any legal authority.
c care provider for patients in hospice care.
d person who makes decisions for the patient when they become incompetent.

36 *Patients in palliative care may fail to thrive. All of the following are characteristics of failure to thrive in palliative care* **EXCEPT:**

a signs of hopelessness.
b inability to concentrate.
c weight gain.
d loss of appetite.

Answers

1 Answer c
Palliative care, as defined by the World Health Organization, is the active total care of patients; control of pain; and minimization of emotional, social, and spiritual problems at a time when disease is not responsive to active treatment.

2 Answer d
The goals of palliative care include providing relief from pain and other distressing symptoms, maintaining quality of life, integrating psychosocial and spiritual aspects of care, and offering support systems to the family.

3 Answer b
The most common cause of malignant pleural effusion is metastatic breast cancer.

4 Answer b
The pharmacologic management of ascites includes the use of furosemide (Lasix) and spironolactone (Aldactone). Other measures may include paracentesis and placement of a permanent drain.

5 Answer d
Classifications of pain in the patient with cancer include visceral, somatic, and psychogenic pain.

6 Answer b
The pain of bone metastasis is referred to as somatic pain.

7 Answer b
For the patient described with impending spinal cord compression, corticosteroids should be instituted because they are thought to decrease edema and irritation around the nerve roots.

8 Answer d
The most commonly used steroid in the treatment of spinal cord compression is dexamethasone (Decadron).

9 Answer c
The most common tumors associated with superior vena cava syndrome are lung carcinoma and lymphomas.

10 Answer b
Common clinical manifestations associated with superior vena cava syndrome include engorgement of the neck veins, a swollen face, and shortness of breath.

11 Answer d
The advantages of radiation therapy in the treatment of cancer are that it provides pain relief, allows for direct treatment of the tumor, and is associated with limited toxicity.

12 Answer c
Instructions that should be given to patients receiving radiation therapy include not applying creams to the treated skin areas prior to radiation treatment. The application of creams may contribute to burns.

13 Answer a
The most common cause of hemoptysis is lung carcinoma.

14 Answer d
The patient with a totally resected lung tumor with no evi-

dence of metastasis would need no adjunctive therapy. The patient should have oncology follow-up and studies per protocol.

15 Answer b
The treatment for oral candidiasis in a patient on chemotherapy is clotrimazole (Mycelex), which is an antifungal agent. Acyclovir (Zovirax) is used to treat herpetic infections. Magnesium hydroxide (Maalox), with a combination of Benylin and Xylocaine liquid may be used in patients with esophagitis. Phenazopyridine (Pyridium) is a urinary tract analgesic.

16 Answer d
Alternative therapies that may be implemented in palliative care include guided imagery, reflexology, visualization, biofeedback, music therapy, and therapeutic touch.

17 Answer c
Therapeutic touch is based on the belief that energy fields surround us and are constantly changing according to our emotions. When we are sick, the energy fields contract and we feel closed in. The therapeutic touch practitioner places his or her hands a few centimeters from the body and passes them over the patient to detect the energy fields. Most therapeutic touch practitioners are nurses.

18 Answer b
A barium swallow should be done to evaluate a patient with dysphagia. Dysphagia may lead to aspiration and pneumonia. Abdominal CT scan would not be the initial test. Colonoscopy is not indicated because this is an upper GI issue. A trial of liquid diet would be inappropriate and may increase the incidence of aspiration.

19 Answer d
The most common fears of patients at the end of life are the fears of pain, suffering, abandonment, isolation, and loss of control.

20 Answer a
One of the major causes of insomnia in patients in palliative care is anxiety. Other causes include depression, pain, dyspnea, and disruption of the sleep-wake cycle.

21 Answer b
Euthanasia is illegal in this country, so this needs to be communicated to the patient in a concise manner. At the same time, you must assure the patient that you will make efforts to relieve her pain and suffering.

22 Answer b
There is no maximum morphine dosage because the dosage needs to be individualized for each patient to achieve pain control. All of the other statements are commonly held myths about morphine usage and are not applicable in palliative care.

23 Answer d
The goals of pain management in palliative care are to define the cause of pain, prevent the pain, erase the memory of pain, and allow the patient to remain cognitively intact.

24 Answer b
Amitriptyline (Elavil), a tricyclic antidepressant, is effective as an adjunct to narcotics for pain control and is referred to as a co-analgesic. Amitriptyline works synergistically with analgesics to decrease the pain threshold. Other groups of med-

ications that work similarly are corticosteroids, antiseizure medications such as carbamazepine (Tegretol) and phenytoin (Dilantin), and benzodiazepines.

25   Answer a

Metoclopramide (Reglan) and prochlorperazine (Compazine) may be used to treat nausea and vomiting in palliative care. These agents work on the chemoreceptor areas in the medulla and have a sedating effect. The metoclopramide works in the stomach to increase gastric peristalsis.

26   Answer d

Treatment of a partial bowel obstruction in a patient with metastatic cancer should include limiting fluid intake to minimize emesis. Intake may have to be intravenous. A partial bowel obstruction may be temporary, so placement of a gastrotomy tube is not indicated. Colonoscopy is also not indicated.

27   Answer c

The World Health Organization guidelines for evaluating pain include taking a detailed history of pain, considering alternative methods of pain relief, believing the patient's report of pain, and performing a thorough physical examination.

28   Answer d

Side effects associated with morphine use include constipation, urinary retention, and myoclonic jerks; they do not include myalgias.

29   Answer a

The most common cause of sore mouth in patients in palliative care is from a monilial infection.

30   Answer d

Nurse practitioner– and physician-related factors that may prevent referrals to hospice care include the perceived loss of control, lack of knowledge concerning services, and the appearance of giving up on (or failure to save) the patient.

31   Answer c

Patients, families, or health-care providers can make referrals to hospice care; however, the physician is needed to certify that the illness has a terminal prognosis.

32   Answer a

The common symptoms of bowel obstruction are abdominal pain, vomiting, and intestinal colic.

33   Answer a

An appropriate hospice referral would be a patient with less than a 6-month life expectancy who has a terminal illness.

34   Answer d

A patient with gastrointestinal bleeding and a limited life expectancy of less than 2 days should not receive transfusions for perceived short-term gains. The efforts seem futile.

35   Answer d

Durable power of attorney is that of a person who makes decisions for the patient when he or she becomes incompetent.

36   Answer c

Failure to thrive in palliative care may be characterized by loss of appetite, weight loss, inability to concentrate, increased tendency for falls, and signs of hopelessness and helplessness.

Bibliography

Angell, M: The Supreme Court and physician-assisted suicide: The ultimate right. N Engl J Med 336:50–53, 1997.
Asch, DA, et al: Decisions to limit or continue life-sustaining treatment by critical care physicians in the United States: Conflicts between physicians' practices and patients' wishes. Am J Respir Crit Care Med 151:288, 1995.
Goroll, A, et al: Primary Care Medicine Office Evaluation and Management of the Adult Patient, 4th ed. Lippincott Williams & Wilkins, Philadelphia, 2000.
Jadad, AR, and Bowman, GP: The WHO analgesic ladder for cancer pain management: Stepping up the quality of its evaluation. JAMA 274:1870–1873, 1995.
Latimer, EJ: Ethical care at the end of life. CMAJ 158:1741, 1998.
Quill, TE, and Brody, H: Physician recommendations and patient autonomy. Finding a balance between physician power and patient choice. Ann Intern Med 125:763, 1996.

27

Management of Rapidly Changing Situations

1 *A 55-year-old man is admitted to the intensive care unit with upper gastrointestinal (GI) bleeding and is receiving a blood transfusion. In the middle of the transfusion, he complains of shortness of breath, and his vital signs reveal a temperature of 103°F, a pulse of 130, a respiratory rate of 28, and blood pressure of 60/40 mm Hg. What is the most appropriate response?*

a Slow the transfusion and give intravenous steroids.
b Stop the transfusion and administer fluids.
c Stop the transfusion and give potassium chloride.
d Continue the transfusion and give intravenous diphenhydramine (Benadryl).

2 *The most specific diagnostic modality for pulmonary embolism is a:*

a physical exam.
b chest x-ray.
c ventilation perfusion scan.
d pulmonary angiogram.

3 *The most common symptom associated with acute mesenteric ischemia is:*

a nausea/vomiting.
b diarrhea.
c severe periumbilical pain.
d fever.

4 *A 65-year-old man has been treated with prednisone for the past 3 years because of systemic lupus erythematosus (SLE). He was involved in a motor vehicle accident and required an emergency splenectomy. Postoperatively, he developed abdominal pain and fever. Laboratory studies reveal a serum sodium level of 124, potassium level of 6.0, and glucose level of 50. Initial management of this patient should include administration of:*

a saline, glucose, and corticosteroids.

b glucose only.
c corticosteroids.
d diuretics.

5 *A 30-year-old woman is seen in your clinic with paroxysmal hypertension and anxiety. Diagnostic workup reveals elevated urinary metanephrines and vanillylmandelic acid (VMA). What is the most likely diagnosis?*

a Hyperaldosteronism
b Pheochromocytoma
c Cushing's syndrome
d Hyperthyroidism

6 *The most common cause of bloody nipple discharge is:*

a breast feeding.
b intraductal papilloma.
c fibrocystic breast disease.
d menopause.

7 *A 50-year-old woman has left upper quadrant (LUQ) abdominal pain. The most likely diagnosis is:*

a appendicitis.
b pancreatitis.
c diverticulitis.
d pelvic inflammatory disease (PID).

8 *A 25-year-old man is seen in the emergency department with a stab wound on the left anterior chest wall. He is unresponsive and his blood pressure is 60 mm Hg systolic. This suggests which type of shock?*

a Septic shock
b Neurogenic shock
c Cardiogenic shock
d Hypovolemic shock

Questions 9–10 refer to the following scenario:

A 75-year-old man had surgery 2 months ago for repair of a descending thoracic aortic aneurysm repair. He is seen in your practice with a 3-day history of bilious vomiting and pain in the right lower quadrant (RLQ). Vital signs reveal a temperature of 102°F, a pulse of 110, a respiratory rate of 24, and blood pressure of 110/76 mm Hg. The patient's past medical history is significant for hypertension and type 2 diabetes. His current medication is 25 mg of atenolol (Tenormin) daily. Physical exam reveals a swollen, erythematous, and tender right groin. The patient also has rebound tenderness and guarding of the right side.

9 What is the most likely diagnosis?

a Appendicitis
b Strangulated inguinal hernia
c Diverticulitis
d Rupture of the aortic aneurysm

10 What is the highest priority for this patient's care?

a Abdominal computed tomography (CT) scan
b Surgical consultation
c Nasogastric tube placement
d Peritoneal lavage

11 *Clinical manifestations of tension pneumothorax may include all of the following* **EXCEPT:**

a anxiety.
b pleuritic chest pain.
c dullness on the affected side.
d hypotension.

12 *Which of the following statements concerning partial pressure of oxygen (Pao$_2$) readings are true?*

a Pao$_2$ increases with age.
b A lower than normal Pao$_2$ indicates hypoxemia.
c The Pao$_2$ reflects alveolar ventilation.
d Tissue oxygenation is reduced when the Pao$_2$ decreases to less than 100 mm Hg.

13 *The most serious complication occurring in patients on peritoneal dialysis is:*

a hypotension.
b abdominal pain.
c hyperkalemia.
d peritonitis.

14 *A 45-year-old man had a parathyroid adenoma removed. Which of the following electrolyte abnormalities would you expect to find postoperatively?*

a Hypocalcemia
b Hypercalcemia

c Hypomagnesemia
d Hyperkalemia

15 *Emergency treatment of hypercalcemia includes all of the following* **EXCEPT:**

a administration of diuretics.
b administration of plicamycin (Mithracin).
c administration of vitamin D.
d infusion of normal saline solution.

16 *A 40-year-old woman presents to the emergency department with complaints of shortness of breath and confusion. Laboratory studies reveal a serum sodium level of 135, potassium level of 4.0, sodium bicarbonate level of 18, and chloride level of 97. The arterial blood gas reveals a pH of 7.3 and Pco$_2$ of 24. The acid-base imbalance shows:*

a combined metabolic acidosis and respiratory alkalosis.
b respiratory alkalosis.
c metabolic acidosis.
d respiratory acidosis.

17 *Adult respiratory distress syndrome (ARDS) is:*

a right ventricular failure with pulmonary hypertension.
b a form of respiratory failure with hypoxia, loss of lung compliance, and pulmonary edema.
c an autosomal recessive disease with obstruction of the lungs and pancreas.
d a reversible airway obstruction.

18 *A 55-year-old man had mitral valve replacement surgery for mitral valve stenosis 8 hours ago. The patient awakens but is unable to move his right leg on command. The most likely reason for the patient's condition is:*

a a stroke.
b because of the effects of analgesia.
c because of the effects of anesthesia.
d none of the above.

Questions 19–22 refer to the following scenario:

A 25-year-old man was admitted to the intensive care unit after a motor vehicle accident from which he suffered a flail chest, cardiac contusion, and a broken right wrist. Over a 4-hour period he becomes progressively hypoxic and requires intubation. The ventilator settings are fraction concentration of inspired oxygen (Fio$_2$), 100%; tidal volume, 750; assist control, 10; and positive end expiratory pressure (PEEP), 10 cm H$_2$O. A pulmonary artery catheter has been placed and reveals a pulmonary artery pressure (PAP) of 40/20, pulmonary capillary wedge pressure (PCWP) of 20, and cardiac index of 2.3. Vital signs reveal a temperature of 100.5°F, pulse of 120, and blood pressure of 80/60 mm Hg.

19 *What is the most likely cause of this patient's deteriorating pulmonary status?*

a Pneumothorax
b Sepsis
c ARDS
d Atelectasis

20 *Which of the following measures should be initiated to treat the patient's hypotension?*

a Start a nitroglycerine drip.
b Give a liter fluid challenge with saline.
c Decrease the PEEP.
d Start a dopamine infusion.

21 *Which of the following chest x-ray findings would you expect in this patient?*

a Bilateral pleural effusions
b Patchy, diffuse bilateral fluffy infiltrates
c Left lower collapse
d Empyema

22 *An 80-year-old man is admitted to the hospital with pneumococcal pneumonia. On hospital day 4, the patient develops severe diarrhea, and the stool culture is positive for* Clostridium difficile *toxin. What is the best treatment for this condition?*

a Oral vancomycin (Vancocin)
b Intravenous vancomycin
c Doxycycline (Vibramycin)
d Trimethoprim sulfamethoxazole (Bactrim-DS)

Questions 23–26 refer to the following scenario:

A 25-year-old woman with a history of intravenous drug use is seen in the emergency department with complaints of fever, chills, abdominal pain, and swelling in her ankles for the past 7 days. She has no previous medical history and is not taking any current prescription medications. Physical exam reveals a woman in moderate distress with a temperature of 102°F, a pulse of 120, a respiratory rate of 24, and blood pressure of 100/60 mm Hg. The head and neck examination is normal. The lungs are clear. Cardiac exam reveals the apical impulse, and the first and second heart sounds to be normal. There are no third nor fourth heart sounds. The abdominal exam reveals a tender abdomen in the right upper quadrant without rebound, and normoactive bowel sounds. The extremities reveal bilateral pedal edema without clubbing and cyanosis.

23 *What should be your initial approach to this patient?*

a Order an abdominal computed tomography (CT) scan.
b Order blood cultures, a complete blood cell count, electrolyte level, and liver function tests.

c Obtain a surgical consultation.
d Start broad-spectrum antibiotics.

24 *You are called to see this patient 48 hours after admission because of the patient's complaints of shortness of breath and temperature of 103°F. Physical exam reveals decreased breath sounds at the right base and a new holosystolic murmur at the left sternal border that increases with inspiration. You also note petechiae on her anterior chest. What is the most likely diagnosis?*

a Pneumonia
b Pulmonary embolus
c Acute bacterial endocarditis
d Acute pancreatitis

25 *What is the heart valve pathology in this patient?*

a Mitral regurgitation
b Aortic regurgitation
c Mitral stenosis
d Tricuspid regurgitation

26 *The usual management of tricuspid valve endocarditis is:*

a the administration of antibiotics.
b a tricuspid valve replacement.
c a heart transplantation.
d all of the above.

27 *A 50-year-old man who had a renal transplantation 6 weeks ago is receiving intravenous steroids for acute rejection without resolution. Which of the following should be ordered?*

a Azathioprine (Imuran)
b Cyclophosphamide (Cytoxan)
c OKT3.
d Increasing doses of cyclosporine (Neoral)

28 *Septic shock is associated with all of the following* **EXCEPT:**

a an increased cardiac index.
b increased cardiac output.
c hypotension.
d increased systemic vascular resistance (SVR).

29 *A 68-year-old man with a history of chronic obstructive pulmonary disease (COPD) is ventilator dependent and has been in intensive care for the past 4 weeks for treatment of pneumonia. This morning, you note that his hemoglobin is 8 g/mL, whereas 2 days ago it was 11 g/mL. What is the appropriate initial step in the management of this patient?*

a Order a stat surgical consultation.
b Insert a nasogastric tube, and check the patient's stool for blood.

c   Transfuse the patient with 2 units of packed cells.
d   Repeat the hemoglobin.

30   *A 40-year-old woman had a kidney-pancreas transplantation. Which of the following laboratory tests should be followed to track for pancreatic rejection?*

a   Serum creatinine level
b   Serum amylase level
c   Liver function tests
d   Urinary glucose levels

Questions 31–34 refer to the following scenario:

A 30-year-old man with a 6-day history of flulike symptoms and a change in mental status over the last 4 hours is seen at your clinic. Vital signs reveal a temperature of 103.5°F, a pulse of 120, a respiratory rate of 20, and blood pressure of 130/70 mm Hg. The patient has no previous health history and is not taking any medications.

31   *What is the initial plan of care for this patient?*

a   Order blood cultures, administer antibiotics, and perform a lumbar puncture.
b   Order a magnetic resonance imaging (MRI) scan of the head.
c   Order antibiotics only.
d   Observe the patient.

32   *Which of the following tests should be performed before a lumbar puncture?*

a   Electroencephalogram (EEG)
b   magnetic resonance imaging of the head
c   computed tomography of the head
d   All of the above

33   *All of the following signs are associated with meningitis* **EXCEPT:**

a   Kernig's sign.
b   Murphy's sign.
c   Brudzinski sign.
d   Nuchal rigidity.

34   *The most common complication after lumbar puncture is:*

a   headache.
b   paralysis.
c   spinal hematoma.
d   fever.

35   *The leading cause of spinal cord injuries is:*

a   diving accidents.
b   motor vehicle accidents.
c   gun violence.
d   sports injuries.

36   *A 40-year-old man is seen in the emergency department with a complaint of severe low back pain for 4 days, which is worse with sitting and better when lying flat on his back. He also admits to a loss of bowel and bladder function over the past 24 hours. What is the most likely diagnosis?*

a   Urinary tract infection
b   Prostatitis
c   Herniated lumbar disk with cauda equina compression
d   Arthritis

Answers

1   Answer b

The patient described is experiencing a blood transfusion reaction, and the appropriate response is to stop the transfusion and administer fluids. Other measures may include the use of steroids and diphenhydramine (Benadryl), but stopping the infusion is the most appropriate first response. The management of the circulatory and respiratory compromise caused by a blood transfusion is paramount in the management of these patients.

2   Answer d

The most specific diagnostic modality for pulmonary embolism is a pulmonary angiogram. The chest x-ray may show defects suggestive of pulmonary embolism, but it is nonspecific. The physical exam is also nonspecific. In patients with a history suspicious for pulmonary embolus, a ventilation perfusion scan is helpful, because it has a high yield, but it is not the most specific diagnostic modality.

3   Answer c

The most common symptom associated with acute mesenteric ischemia is severe periumbilical pain.

4   Answer a

Initial management of the patient described should include the administration of saline, glucose, and corticosteroids. This patient has acute adrenal insufficiency.

5   Answer b

The most likely diagnosis for the patient described is pheochromocytoma. Complaints of paroxysmal hypertension in persons younger than age 30 years should raise the suspicion of pheochromocytoma. Increased levels of catecholamine-breakdown products (vanillylmandelic acid and metanephrines) in the urine confirm the diagnosis.

6   Answer b

The most common cause of bloody nipple discharge is intraductal papilloma.

7   Answer b

The most likely diagnosis in a patient with left upper quadrant (LUQ) abdominal pain is pancreatitis with another likely diagnosis being a perforated gastric ulcer. Appendicitis and pelvic inflammatory disease usually present with right lower quadrant (RLQ) abdominal pain. Diverticulitis presents with left lower quadrant (LLQ) abdominal pain.

8 Answer d

The history and clinical manifestations of the patient described suggest hypovolemic shock secondary to blood loss from a chest injury.

9 Answer b

The most likely diagnosis for the patient described is a strangulated inguinal hernia. The presence of a hernia in conjunction with fever and rebound tenderness suggests the strangulated hernia. Strangulation occurs when there is a decrease in perfusion of the incarcerated bowel, resulting in necrosis. Appendicitis is a possible etiology, but there would be a tender, erythematous, and swollen area in the right groin. Diverticulitis produces left lower quadrant pain. The patient is too stable for a ruptured aortic aneurysm and would not have the abdominal findings as above.

10 Answer b

The highest priority for this patient's care is immediate surgical consultation and operative intervention to correct the hernia defect, and possibly resection of bowel.

11 Answer c

Clinical manifestations of a tension pneumothorax may include anxiety, pleuritic chest pain, hypotension, dyspnea, elevated jugular venous pressure, absent breath sounds, and hyperresonance (not dullness) on the affected side.

12 Answer b

The statement, "A lower than normal Pao_2 indicates hypoxemia" is true. Pao_2 decreases (not increases) with age because of loss of lung elasticity, and tissue oxygenation is affected when the Pao_2 is less than 60 mm Hg (not less than 100 mm Hg). The partial pressure of carbon dioxide ($Paco_2$), not oxygen, reflects alveolar ventilation.

13 Answer d

The most serious complication occurring in patients on peritoneal dialysis is peritonitis. Other less serious complications may include hypotension, abdominal pain, back pain, and malposition of the catheter.

14 Answer a

You would expect to find hypocalcemia in a patient postoperative from the removal of a parathyroid adenoma.

15 Answer c

Emergency treatment of hypercalcemia may include the administration of diuretics and plicamycin and infusion of normal saline solution. Vitamin D is not a treatment for hypercalcemia, and would increase calcium levels. Hydration with normal saline and diuretics increases the renal excretion of calcium and subsequent decrease in serum levels. Plicamycin (Mithracin) lowers serum calcium levels by inhibiting osteoclastic bone resorption.

16 Answer a

The acid-base imbalance in the patient described is a combined metabolic acidosis and respiratory alkalosis.

17 Answer b

Adult respiratory distress syndrome (ARDS) is a form of respiratory failure with hypoxia, loss of lung compliance, and pulmonary edema. Cor pulmonale is right ventricular failure with pulmonary hypertension. Cystic fibrosis is an autosomal recessive disease with dysfunction of the exocrine glands with obstruction of the lungs and pancreas. Asthma is a reversible airway obstruction.

18 Answer a

The most likely reason for the described patient's condition is the presence of a stroke. Patients with mitral stenosis may have a calcified mitral valve annulus, which may lead to debris going to the brain during surgery. The presence of bilateral findings would raise the suspicion of analgesia and anesthesia effects.

19 Answer c

The most likely cause of this patient's deteriorating pulmonary status is Adult respiratory distress syndrome (ARDS). The requirement for high oxygen levels in a patient with a flail chest injury makes ARDS the most likely diagnosis.

20 Answer d

The measure that should be initiated to treat the patient's hypotension is to start a dopamine infusion to increase blood pressure. Nitroglycerin would serve to further decrease the blood pressure. The administration of further fluid challenges would cause leaking of fluid into the alveoli from the damaged pulmonary capillaries, making the patient's condition worse. Decreasing the PEEP may improve the blood pressure and cardiac index, but may worsen oxygenation.

21 Answer b

The classic chest x-ray finding in patients with adult respiratory distress syndrome (ARDS) is a patchy, diffuse bilateral fluffy infiltrative pattern.

22 Answer a

The best treatment for *Clostridium difficile* infection is oral vancomycin (Vancocin).

23 Answer b

The initial approach to the patient described should be to order blood cultures, a complete blood cell count, electrolyte level, and liver function tests. The patient has right upper quadrant pain but without rebound, so it is prudent to review liver function tests before proceeding to surgical consultation. There is no indication for an abdominal computed tomography scan. Broad-spectrum antibiotics should not be initiated prior to obtaining blood cultures.

24 Answer c

The most likely diagnosis in this patient is acute bacterial endocarditis. The history of drug use, fever, petechiae, and new heart murmur all lead to the diagnosis of endocarditis.

25 Answer d

The heart valve pathology in the patient described is tricuspid regurgitation. The patient has a holosystolic murmur that increases with inspiration accompanied by hepatic congestion and lower extremity edema. Mitral regurgitation would produce a holosystolic murmur without the accompanying right heart symptoms. Aortic regurgitation and mitral stenosis are diastolic murmurs.

26 Answer a

The usual management of tricuspid valve endocarditis is the administration of antibiotics.

27 Answer c

Acute transplant rejection unresponsive to intravenous steroids should be treated with OKT3, which is a monoclonal antibody directed against the CD3 complex. Cyclosporine and azathioprine (Imuran) are effective in the induction and maintenance of patients after transplant but have no role in treating acute rejection. Cyclophosphamide (Cytoxan) may be used for vascular rejection, but it is associated with hemorrhagic cystitis.

28   Answer d

Septic shock is associated with a decrease in systemic vascular resistance (SVR), increased cardiac output, and hypotension.

29   Answer b

The initial step in the management of the patient described is to determine the source of blood by inserting a nasogastric tube as well as to check the patient's stool for occult blood. Acute stress gastritis is common in intensive-care-unit patients. A transfusion may be appropriate, but the initial measure is to attempt to ascertain the source of the blood loss. A surgical consultation is not indicated at this time.

30   Answer a

When a combined kidney-pancreas transplant is performed, the rejection of the renal graft usually precedes the pancreatic rejection; therefore, serum creatinine levels could be followed. Serum amylase levels, liver function tests, and urinary glucose levels are not reflective of pancreatic rejection.

31   Answer a

The initial plan of care for the patient described should include ordering blood cultures, administering antibiotics, and performing a lumbar puncture.

32   Answer c

A computed tomography (CT) of the head should be per-formed before a lumbar puncture is done. The purpose of the CT scan is to rule out subarachnoid hemorrhage.

33   Answer b

Murphy's sign is not associated with meningitis, but rather with acute cholecystitis. Kernig's sign is pain in the hamstrings when the knees are extended with the hips flexed at 90°. Brudzinski's sign is flexion of the hips caused by passive flexion of the neck. Nuchal rigidity is neck stiffness.

34   Answer a

The most common complication after lumbar puncture is headache.

35   Answer b

The leading cause of spinal cord injuries is motor vehicle accidents.

36   Answer c

The most likely diagnosis for the patient described is a herniated lumbar disk with cauda equina compression. The fact that the pain is worse with sitting and improved with lying supine is not particularly helpful in suggesting the cause of the patient's back pain. Pain associated with loss of bladder or bowel control suggests a midline lumbar disk herniation with spinal cord compression.

Bibliography

Goroll, A, et al: Primary Care Medicine Office Evaluation and Management of the Adult Patient, 4th ed. Lippincott Williams & Wilkins, Philadelphia, 2000.

Fauci, AS, et al: Harrison's Principles of Internal Medicine, 14th ed. McGraw-Hill, New York, 1998.

28

Age- and Culture-Related Considerations

1 *Falls among elderly patients are more likely to occur:*

a in public places.
b at home.
c in a hospital.
d in the workplace.

2 *Common ophthalmologic changes in the elderly patient include all of the following EXCEPT:*

a arcus senilis.
b reduced tear formation.
c presbyopia.
d retinal detachment.

3 *An 80-year-old man is having tooth loss. What is the most common cause of tooth loss in the elderly patient?*

a Vitamin D deficiency
b Chronic periodontal disease
c Gastroesophageal reflux disease (GERD)
d Vitamin A deficiency

4 *A 90-year-old woman reported that 1 month ago at a health fair she was told that her cholesterol was elevated. She has no health history and takes only an aspirin and multivitamin daily. What is her appropriate medication regime?*

a 300 mg of gemfibrozil (Lopid) daily
b 20 mg of pravastatin (Pravachol) daily
c No medications
d 2 tablespoons of psyllium (Metamucil) daily

5 *Which of the following hematologic changes would you expect in the elderly patient?*

a Thrombocytopenia
b Anemia
c Leukopenia
d Unchanged hemoglobin concentration

6 *Which of the following diseases are more prevalent in the Hispanic population?*

a Hypertension
b Myocardial infarction
c Cerebrovascular accident
d Diabetes mellitus

7 *Lactose intolerance is more common in:*

a Asians.
b Caucasians.
c African-Americans.
d Hispanics.

8 *Sickle cell anemia is more common in:*

a Caucasians.
b African-Americans.
c Asians.
d persons of Mediterranean descent.

9 *Depression in the elderly patient most commonly presents with:*

a weight loss.
b cognitive impairment.
c nausea and vomiting.
d a shuffling gait.

10 *The first drug of choice for treatment of depression in the elderly patient is:*

a amitriptyline (Elavil).
b desipramine (Norpramin).
c benztropine (Cogentin).
d L-dopa.

11 *A 50-year-old Cambodian woman is seen for a routine physical exam. She is a nonsmoker and does not drink alcohol. You notice that she has cigarette* *burns on her abdomen and areas of circular ecchymo-sis on her posterior chest. How would you proceed?*

a Report the situation to adult protective services.
b Notify the local police.
c Obtain further history.
d Start antibiotics.

12 *The most common health problem in Native-Americans is:*

a coronary artery disease.
b hypertension.
c diabetes.
d alcohol abuse.

13 *Components of a functional assessment in the el-derly patient include:*

a assessment of the ability to perform activities of daily living.
b a baseline electrocardiogram (ECG).
c pulmonary function testing.
d a baseline ophthalmology exam.

14 *An 85-year-old woman living independently at home is brought to the emergency department by her daughter with a complaint of a change in mental sta-tus over the past 6 hours. Which of the following should be considered in the differential diagnosis?*

a Electrolyte imbalances
b Infection
c Intoxication
d All of the above

15 *All of the statements concerning falls in the el-derly patient are true* **EXCEPT:**

a poor lighting and throw rugs may contribute to falls in the home.
b 50% of falls result in hip fractures.
c anxiolytics are associated with falls.
d an abnormal gait may contribute to falls.

16 *A 65-year-old man in your practice wants infor-mation about an advance care directive. You tell him that an advanced directive is a written document:*

a that is also witnessed and that specifies treatment preferences in the event that the person becomes incompetent and unable to make decisions.
b that expresses conditions in which a do not resus-citate (DNR) order should be instituted.
c in which the health-care provider gives direction and authority to caregivers in the event of an emergency.
d that allows one to institute hospice care.

17 *Immunizations in the elderly patient should in-clude:*

a a yearly influenza vaccination.
b a yearly pneumonia vaccination (Pneumovax).
c tetanus boosters every 5 years.
d all of the above.

18 *An 80-year-old woman is brought to the clinic with suspicion of having Alzheimer's disease. Which of the following laboratory tests should be ordered to identify potentially reversible causes of alteration in mental status?*

a Serum calcium level
b Thyroid function tests
c Serum glucose level
d All of the above

19 *A 75-year-old woman is seen by the nurse practi-tioner for a routine physical exam. The family notes that the patient has had memory loss, urinary inconti-nence, and gait disturbances for the past 6 months. What is the most likely diagnosis?*

a Alzheimer's disease
b Normal pressure hydrocephalus
c Myasthenia gravis
d Parkinson's disease

20 *Constipation in the elderly patient may be associ-ated with:*

a laxative abuse.
b depression.
c poor nutritional intake.
d all of the above.

21 *The leading cause of death in African-American men aged 15 to 34 years is:*

a suicide.
b homicide.
c acquired immunodeficiency syndrome (AIDS).
d testicular carcinoma.

22 *In the elderly patient, which of the following medications may cause depression?*

a Enalapril (Vasotec)
b Hydrochlorothiazide (HCTZ)
c Clonidine (Catapres)
d Amitriptyline

23 *The most common skin complaint in the elderly patient is:*

a pruritus.
b oily skin.
c wart formation.
d rashes.

24 *Which of the following is important in the man-agement of the patient with dementia?*

a Maintaining a routine for the patient
b Making the environment safe
c Providing support for the family
d All of the above

25 *The treatment of choice for community-acquired pneumonia in the elderly patient is:*

a penicillin G.
b vancomycin (Vancocin).
c erythromycin (E-Mycin).
d trimethoprim sulfamethoxazole (Bactrim-DS).

26 *Which of the following may predispose the elderly patient to urinary tract infections?*

a Increased prostatic secretion (for men)
b Increased vaginal pH (for women)
c Increased bladder emptying
d Diarrhea

27 *The most common pathogen associated with urinary tract infection in the elderly patient is:*

a *Staphylococcus.*
b *Escherichia coli.*
c *Streptococcus.*
d *Klebsiella.*

28 *An 85-year-old woman is seen in the clinic with a 7-day history of fever to 102°F, chills, confusion, dysuria, decreased appetite, abdominal pain, and diarrhea. Physical exam reveals an ill-appearing woman with a temperature of 103°F, blood pressure of 100/60 mm Hg, and a heart rate of 110 and regular. Lung and heart exam is normal. Abdominal exam reveals mild epigastric tenderness and normal bowel sounds. No costovertebral angle (CVA) tenderness is found. What is the most likely diagnosis?*

a Acute pyelonephritis
b Viral gastroenteritis
c Pneumonia
d Urinary tract infection

29 *An uncomplicated urinary tract infection in the elderly patient may be treated with:*

a no antibiotic.
b a single dose of trimethoprim sulfamethoxazole (Bactrim-DS).
c ampicillin for 14 days.
d penicillin plus an aminoglycoside for 10 days.

30 *All of the following may contribute to urinary incontinence in the elderly patient EXCEPT:*

a increased ability of the kidneys to concentrate urine.
b decreased bladder capacity.
c decreased mobility.
d use of diuretics.

31 *The most common side effect of vasodilators in the elderly patient is:*

a fever.
b orthostatic hypotension.
c hypertension.
d renal failure.

32 *All of the following physiologic changes of aging may affect nutritional status EXCEPT:*

a a decreased number of olfactory nerve endings.
b increased gastric emptying.
c a reduction of albumin synthesis.
d a decrease in the number of taste buds.

33 *The most common nutritional problem(s) in the elderly population is(are):*

a malnutrition and obesity.
b anorexia.
c bulimia.
d all of the above.

34 *Patients over age 80 years undergoing cardiac surgery are at an increased risk for the complication of:*

a mediastinitis.
b myocardial infarction.
c stroke.
d low cardiac output syndrome.

35 *The most common health problem seen in persons from Indochina is:*

a hypertension.
b ascariasis.
c diabetes mellitus.
d hyperthyroidism.

36 *A 75-year-old man is seen for a routine exam, and you note that he is confabulating. Confabulating is associated with:*

a Alzheimer's disease.
b Parkinson's disease.
c delirium.
d Korsakoff's psychosis.

Answers

1 Answer b

Falls among elderly patients are more likely to occur at home.

2 Answer d

Common ophthalmologic changes in the elderly patient include presbyopia, reduced tear formation, arcus senilis, ectropion, and entropion; they do not include retinal detachment.

3   Answer b

The most common cause of tooth loss in the elderly patient is chronic periodontal disease.

4   Answer c

The patient should receive no medications. You should recheck her lipid profile because the screening of cholesterol in the healthy elderly patient is controversial. First-line treatment would include dietary counseling.

5   Answer d

Hematologic changes in the elderly patient include unchanged hemoglobin concentration, platelet count, blood volume, hematocrit, and white blood cell count.

6   Answer d

Of the diseases presented, diabetes mellitus is more prevalent in the Hispanic population.

7   Answer a

Lactose intolerance is more common in Asian patients.

8   Answer b

Sickle cell anemia is more common in African-Americans.

9   Answer a

Depression in the elderly patient most commonly presents with weight loss, and it is less likely to present with symptoms of worthlessness.

10   Answer b

The first drug of choice for treatment of depression in the elderly patient is desipramine. Desipramine has a low side effect profile and a low incidence of postural hypotension, anticholinergic effects, and sedation.

11   Answer c

Cigarette burns are a traditional means of folk healing in some Asian populations. The dermal-abrasive practices are seen as a method to relieve headaches, muscle pains, colds, fever, diarrhea, shortness of breath, and sinusitis. A tradition known as cupping involves placing a heated cup on the skin through which the illness is allowed to leave the body. This results in circular ecchymosis of the skin.

12   Answer d

The most common health problem in Native-Americans is alcohol abuse.

13   Answer a

Functional assessment in the elderly patient includes assessing the person's ability to perform activities of daily living.

14   Answer d

Differential diagnosis of a change in mental status in the elderly patient may include electrolyte imbalances, infection, intoxication, medication-related changes, cerebral hypoperfusion, hypothermia, and hyperthermia. Electrolyte and metabolic abnormalities such as hyponatremia, hypernatremia, hypoglycemia, hyperglycemia, hypoxia, hypercapnia, and hypocalcemia may all present as a change in mental status.

15   Answer b

The number of falls in elderly patients that may lead to fracture is 5%, not 50%.

16   Answer a

An advanced directive is a written and witnessed document that specifies treatment preferences in the event that the person becomes incompetent and is unable to make decisions. There are two forms of advanced directives: a living will and durable power of attorney. A living will is effective when the patient is either terminally ill or incompetent. The durable power of attorney is the appointment of a surrogate decision maker and the expression of treatment preferences. The implementation of advanced directives differs from state to state.

17   Answer a

Immunizations in the elderly patient should include a yearly influenza vaccination, a pneumonia vaccination (which may be repeated every 10 years—however, this is an area of controversy), and a tetanus booster every 10 years.

18   Answer d

The workup for alteration in mental status should include serum electrolytes, calcium and glucose levels, and evaluation of thyroid function tests.

19   Answer b

The most likely diagnosis for the patient described is normal-pressure hydrocephalus. Normal-pressure hydrocephalus is characterized by gait disturbances, dementia, and urinary incontinence without signs of increased intracranial pressure.

20   Answer d

Constipation in the elderly patient may be associated with laxative abuse, decreased mobility, dehydration, depression, and poor nutritional intake.

21   Answer b

The leading cause of death in African-American men aged 15 to 34 years is homicide.

22   Answer c

Clonidine (Catapres), a centrally acting agent used to treat hypertension, may cause depression in the elderly, as well as in other populations. Other common agents associated with depression in the elderly include histamine blockers, estrogens, beta blockers, and calcium channel blockers.

23   Answer a

The most common skin complaint in the elderly is pruritus. The etiology of pruritus may be multifactorial.

24   Answer d

Management of the patient with dementia includes maintaining a routine for the patient, making the environment safe, and providing support for the family.

25   Answer a

The treatment of choice for community-acquired pneumonia in the elderly is penicillin G or ampicillin.

26   Answer b

Increased vaginal pH and decreased vaginal glycogen may predispose elderly women to urinary tract infections. Other factors may include decreased functional ability, decreased bladder emptying, use of indwelling catheters, and decreased prostatic secretions in men.

27   Answer b

The most common pathogen associated with urinary tract infection in the elderly patient is *E. coli.* Other pathogens may include *Klebsiella, Proteus,* and *Pseudomonas.*

28 Answer a

The most likely diagnosis is acute pyelonephritis. Patients with pyelonephritis usually present with fever, chills, flank pain, and dysuria. Elderly patients may present with changes in mental status as the only symptom of pyelonephritis. Elderly patients with pyelonephritis are at risk for septic shock.

29 Answer b

An uncomplicated urinary tract infection in the elderly patient may be treated with a single dose of trimethoprim sulfamethoxazole (Bactrim-DS), the same as in younger individuals.

30 Answer a

Decreased bladder capacity, decreased mobility, and use of diuretics may contribute to urinary incontinence in the elderly patient. The decreased ability of the kidney (not increased ability) to concentrate urine may also contribute to incontinence.

31 Answer b

The most common side effect of vasodilators in the elderly patient is orthostatic hypotension.

32 Answer b

Physiologic changes of aging that may affect nutritional status in the elderly patient include decreased gastric emptying (not increased), a decrease in olfactory nerve endings, a decrease in taste and the number of taste buds (papilla) on the tongue, a decline in oral health, an impairment of thirst response, decreased vitamin D synthesis, and a reduction of albumin synthesis.

33 Answer a

The most common nutritional problems in the elderly population are malnutrition and obesity.

34 Answer c

Patients over the age of 80 undergoing cardiac surgery are at increased risk for stroke.

35 Answer b

From the list provided, the most common health problem seen in persons from Indochina is ascariasis. Intestinal parasites are the most common health problem seen in persons from Indochina and may include *Ascaris, Trichuris, Giardia lamblia,* hookworm, and *Entamoeba.*

36 Answer d

Confabulation is associated with Korsakoff's psychosis. Confabulation is an unconscious filling of gaps in memory by imagined experiences.

Bibliography

Gloth, FM, et al: Vitamin D deficiency in homebound elderly persons. JAMA 254:1683–1686, 1995.
Goroll, A, et al: Primary Care Medicine Office Evaluation and Management of the Adult Patient, 4th ed. Lippincott Williams & Wilkins, Philadelphia, 2000.
Hooton, TM, and Stamm, WE: Diagnosis and treatment of uncomplicated urinary tract infections. Infect Dis Clin North Am 11:551–581, 1997.
Jones, JS: Elder abuse and neglect: Responding to a national problem. Ann Emerg Med 23: 845–848, 1994.

29

Transplantation

1 A 45-year-old man who had a bilateral lung transplant 2 months ago is being treated for an upper respiratory tract infection. He is on cyclosporine (Neoral), prednisone, and azathioprine (Imuran). Which of the following antibiotics should be avoided?

a Erythromycin (E-Mycin)
b Penicillin
c Vancomycin (Vancocin)
d Gentamicin (Garamycin)

2 Common side effects associated with cyclosporine (Neoral) are:

a abdominal pain, tremor, and dysphagia.
b headaches and fever.
c renal failure, headaches, and gingival hyperplasia.
d upper gastrointestinal bleeding, stroke, and hypertension.

3 The leading cause of death after lung transplantation is:

a rejection.
b infection.
c hypoxia.
d pulmonary embolus.

4 All of the following are indications for single lung transplantation **EXCEPT**:

a cystic fibrosis.
b emphysema.
c idiopathic pulmonary fibrosis.
d alpha 1-antitrypsin deficiency.

5 In a 55-year-old woman, which of the following complications would you expect 12 years after heart transplantation?

a Rejection
b Transplant arteriopathy
c Renal failure
d Infection

6 A 25-year-old man had a cardiac transplantation 4 weeks ago and is admitted to the telemetry floor with a severe rejection reaction. He is going to be started on OKT3. Which of the following should be done?

a Hydrate the patient with several liters of fluid before administration of OKT3.
b Hold all other immunosuppressants.
c Transfer the patient to the intensive care unit for pulmonary artery catheter placement.
d Put the patient in reverse isolation.

7 Which of the following factors may contribute to the development of cardiac transplant arteriopathy?

a Older donor age and hypertension
b Donor's smoking history
c Female donor
d Three to five cellular rejections the first year after transplant

8 Which of the following may represent cardiac allograft rejection?

a Hypertension
b Tachycardia
c Thrombocytopenia
d Atrial arrhythmia

9 A 50-year-old man who has had cardiac transplantation develops bradycardia with a heart rate of 30 and blood pressure of 100 systolic. All of the following medications can be used to treat the bradycardia **EXCEPT**:

a epinephrine.
b isoproterenol (Isuprel).
c atropine.
d dopamine (Intropin).

10 A 50-year-old man who had renal transplantation 2 months ago develops ureteral obstruction. Signs and symptoms of ureteral obstruction include:

a polyuria.
b lower abdominal pain.
c decreased creatinine level.
d weight loss.

11 *In reviewing discharge instructions with a patient 2 weeks after renal transplantation, the instructions should include all of the following* **EXCEPT:**

a monitoring of daily weights.
b monitoring of temperature daily.
c monitoring of intake and output.
d monitoring of urine specific gravity.

12 *A 35-year-old woman underwent a bone marrow transplantation (BMT) for treatment of leukemia. What is the most common fungal pathogen 2 months after BMT?*

a *Candida*
b *Aspergillus*
c Histoplasmosis
d Cytomegalovirus (CMV)

13 *The most common manifestation of cytomegalovirus (CMV) in the patient after BMT is:*

a retinitis.
b gastritis.
c pneumonitis.
d hepatitis.

14 *The most common bacterial pathogen occurring after BMT is:*

a *Streptococcus.*
b *Staphylococcus.*
c *Klebsiella.*
d *Enterococcus.*

15 *What is the most common viral infection occurring 6 months after BMT?*

a Cytomegalovirus (CMV)
b Varicella zoster virus (VZV)
c Epstein-Barr virus (EBV)
d Adenovirus

16 *Which of the following is an absolute contraindication to organ transplantation?*

a History of alcohol abuse
b Current cigarette smoking
c Diabetes mellitus
d Acquired immunodeficiency syndrome (AIDS)

17 *Which of the following solid organ recipients have the highest rate of infection?*

a Kidney transplant recipients
b Pancreatic transplant recipients

c Liver transplant recipients
d Heart-lung transplant recipients

18 *Evaluation of the potential cardiac transplantation recipient should include:*

a an echocardiogram.
b human immunodeficiency virus (HIV) serology testing.
c a social worker consultation.
d all of the above.

19 *Which of the following medications prescribed before heart transplantation may cause bradycardia in the patient after heart transplantation?*

a Milrinone (Primacor)
b Amiodarone (Cordarone)
c Digoxin (Lanoxin)
d Dobutamine (Dobutrex)

20 *Common side effects associated with corticosteroids include all of the following* **EXCEPT:**

a hyperlipidemia.
b glucose intolerance.
c weight gain.
d headaches.

21 *Liver transplantation may be indicated for all of the metabolic liver diseases* **EXCEPT:**

a primary sclerosing cholangitis.
b hemochromatosis.
c Wilson's disease.
d alpha 1-antitrypsin deficiency.

22 *Common clinical manifestations in patients with end-stage liver disease include:*

a headache and vomiting.
b muscle wasting and poor appetite.
c chronic diarrhea and epigastric pain.
d dysphagia and petechiae.

23 *A 50-year-old woman with diabetes has received a pancreatic transplantation. What is the hallmark of acute pancreatic graft rejection?*

a Abdominal pain
b Fever
c Abdominal bloating
d Hypoamylasuria

24 *A 45-year-old patient who had a heart transplantation 2 years ago presents with complaints of shortness of breath, abdominal bloating, and lower extremity edema for the past week. An endomyocardial biopsy is performed and is negative for rejection. What is the most likely cause of the patient's symptoms?*

a Pulmonary embolus
b Tricuspid regurgitation
c Vascular rejection
d *Pneumocystis carinii* pneumonia (PCP)

25 *Which of the following symptoms are rarely seen in cardiac transplantation recipients?*

a Shortness of breath
b Angina
c Paroxysmal nocturnal dyspnea
d Syncope

26 *Common indications for kidney transplantation include all of the following* **EXCEPT:**

a hypertension.
b diabetes.
c renal cell carcinoma.
d polycystic kidney disease.

27 *Which of the following therapies may be used as a bridge to liver transplantation?*

a Intra-aortic balloon pump (IABP)
b Hemodialysis
c Ultrafiltration
d Transjugular intrahepatic portosystemic shunts (TIPS)

28 *The most common indication for heart-lung transplantation is:*

a ischemic cardiomyopathy.
b primary pulmonary hypertension.
c hypertrophic cardiomyopathy.
d emphysema.

29 *The most common early complication after lung transplantation is:*

a myocardial infarction.
b pulmonary embolus.
c surgical healing defects at the anastomosis.
d bronchiolitis obliterans.

30 *Which of the following parameters are suggestive of rejection in lung transplantation recipients?*

a Palpitations
b Decreased exercise tolerance
c Elevated white blood cell count
d Tachycardia

31 *All of the following patients are considered candidates for lung transplantation* **EXCEPT:**

a a 60-year-old man who has been ventilator dependent for the past 2 years.
b a 35-year-old woman with cystic fibrosis.
c a 65-year-old man with emphysema.
d a 40-year-old man with idiopathic pulmonary fibrosis.

32 *All of the following statements concerning lung transplantation are true* **EXCEPT:**

a transbronchial biopsy is useful in detecting rejection.
b patients with cystic fibrosis have the best prognosis after lung transplantation.
c bronchiolitis obliterans is a late complication after lung transplantation.
d cardiopulmonary bypass is routinely used in double lung transplantation.

33 *Lung volume reduction surgery (LVRS) may be beneficial to all of the following patients awaiting lung transplantation* **EXCEPT:**

a those with pulmonary hypertension.
b those with emphysema.
c those with alpha 1-antitrypsin deficiency.
d those with idiopathic pulmonary fibrosis.

34 *A 1-year survival rate after liver transplantation is:*

a 20%.
b 80% to 90%.
c 50%.
d 70%.

35 *A 50-year-old woman with dilated cardiomyopathy awaiting a heart transplantation has deteriorated, requiring increasing doses of inotropic medications to maintain blood pressure. Which of the following measures may help to support the patient until a donor heart becomes available?*

a Permanent pacemaker implantation
b Ventricular assist device
c Angioplasty
d Emergency coronary artery bypass graft (CABG) surgery

36 *A 60-year-old man who had a heart transplantation 2 years ago develops histoplasmosis. What is the preferred treatment?*

a Cytomegalovirus immune globulin (CytoGam)
b Acyclovir (Zovirax)
c OKT3
d Amphotericin B

Answers

1 Answer a
The antibiotic erythromycin should be avoided in patients following transplantation. Erythromycin inhibits the CYP 3A4 system and increases the cyclosporine levels, which may lead to toxicity.

2 Answer c

Common side effects associated with cyclosporine are renal failure, headaches, gingival hyperplasia, hirsutism, tremors, and paresthesias.

3 Answer b

The leading cause of death after lung transplantation is infection, which commonly may be bacterial or fungal.

4 Answer a

Indications for single lung transplantation include emphysema, idiopathic pulmonary fibrosis, alpha 1-antitrypsin deficiency, and primary pulmonary hypertension. Cystic fibrosis is treated with double lung transplantation because of the chronic infection in the lungs of these patients.

5 Answer b

The most likely complication in a patient 12 years after heart transplantation is transplant coronary artery disease (such as transplant arteriopathy). Over half of all patients with heart transplants will have coronary disease 5 years after the transplant.

6 Answer c

The patient that is going to receive OKT3 should be in the intensive care unit for monitoring. Potential complications after the administration of OKT3 include pulmonary edema and fever.

7 Answer a

Risk factors associated with the development of cardiac transplant arteriopathy are older donor age, donor hypertension, and male gender.

8 Answer d

Cardiac allograft rejection may be manifested by an atrial arrhythmia.

9 Answer c

Atropine is contraindicated in the treatment of bradycardia in transplant patients because the denervation of the transplanted heart renders atropine ineffective.

10 Answer b

Signs and symptoms of ureteral obstruction include lower abdominal pain, pain over the transplanted kidney, decreased urine output, and elevated blood urea nitrogen (BUN) and creatinine levels.

11 Answer d

Discharge instructions for the patient after renal transplantation should include instructions about daily weight, monitoring temperature, monitoring intake and output, blood pressure, about activity precautions, diet, signs and symptoms of infection and rejection, and emergency contact numbers. The monitoring of urine specific gravity is not indicated.

12 Answer b

The most common fungal pathogen 2 months after bone marrow transplantation (BMT) is aspergillus. *Candida* is most prevalent in the first 30 days. Cytomegalovirus (CMV) is a viral infection. Histoplasmosis is rare.

13 Answer c

The most common manifestation of cytomegalovirus (CMV) in the patient after bone marrow transplantation (BMT) is pneumonitis, and it is usually associated with a high rate of mortality and morbidity. Other manifestations may include gastritis and retinitis.

14 Answer b

The most common bacterial pathogen after bone marrow transplantation (BMT) is *Staphylococcus.* The major source of the bacterial pathogens is central intravascular catheters.

15 Answer b

The most common viral infection 6 months after bone marrow transplantation (BMT) is varicella zoster virus (VZV). Prior to that time, cytomegalovirus (CMV) is the most common viral pathogen.

16 Answer d

An absolute contraindication to organ transplantation is acquired immunodeficiency syndrome (AIDS). AIDS remains an absolute contraindication because of the limited life expectancy in patients with the disease. History of alcohol abuse may be a relative contraindication to liver transplantation. History of current cigarette smoking is a relative contraindication to heart and lung transplantation. Diabetes mellitus is a relative contraindication because of the worsening of glucose control in patients after receiving corticosteroids.

17 Answer d

Heart-lung transplant recipients have the highest rate of infection and mortality associated with infection. The reasons for infection include immunosuppression, allograft rejection, anastomotic leak, tracheal anastomosis, and blunting of the cough reflex.

18 Answer d

Evaluation of the potential cardiac transplantation recipient should include an ECG; exercise stress test; cardiac catheterization; serologies for hepatitis, HIV, CMV, and EBV; and psychological and social worker consultations.

19 Answer b

Amiodarone (Cordarone) may produce bradycardia in the period after cardiac transplantation.

20 Answer d

Common side effects associated with corticosteroids include hyperlipidemia, glucose intolerance, hirsutism, weight gain, mood swings, and osteopenia; headaches are not common side effects.

21 Answer a

Liver transplantation may be indicated for hemochromatosis, Wilson's disease, and alpha 1-antitrypsin deficiency, which are all metabolic liver diseases. Primary sclerosing cholangitis is a chronic cholestatic disease and is an indication for liver transplantation.

22 Answer b

Common clinical manifestations in patients with end-stage liver disease include muscle wasting, poor appetite, encephalopathy, jaundice, pruritus, gastrointestinal bleeding, ascites, lower extremity edema, and coagulopathy.

23 Answer d

The hallmark of pancreatic graft rejection is hypoamylasuria, defined as a 30% decrease in urine amylase below baseline. Other factors, such as dehydration and anorexia, may also lead to a decrease in urine amylase.

24 Answer b

The most likely cause of the patient's symptoms is tricuspid regurgitation (TR). TR may develop secondary to the endomyocardial biopsy. Symptoms of TR are reflective of right heart dysfunction, such as ascites, elevated jugular venous pressure (JVP), and edema.

25 Answer b

Angina is rarely observed in patients after cardiac transplantation because of denervation of the heart.

26 Answer c

Common indications for kidney transplantation include hypertension, diabetes, polycystic kidney disease, and glomerulonephritis; renal cell carcinoma is not an indicator.

27 Answer d

Transjugular intrahepatic portosystemic shunts (TIPS) may be used as a bridge to liver transplantation and is effective in controlling portal hypertension.

28 Answer b

The most common indication for heart-lung transplantation is primary pulmonary hypertension. Other indications may include cystic fibrosis and congenital defects. Emphysema is one of the indications for double or single lung transplantation. Ischemic and hypertrophic cardiomyopathy are treated with cardiac transplantation.

29 Answer c

The most common early complication after lung transplantation is surgical healing defects at the anastamosis. Myocardial infarction and pulmonary embolus are not commonly associated with lung transplantation. Bronchiolitis obliterans is a late complication and may occur months to years after transplantation.

30 Answer b

Parameters suggestive of rejection in lung transplantation recipients include decreased exercise tolerance, fever, decreased oxygen saturation, and infiltrates on chest x-ray.

31 Answer a

A 60-year-old man who has been ventilator dependent for the past 2 years would not be a candidate for lung transplantation.

32 Answer b

Patients with emphysema and alpha 1-antitrypsin deficiency have the best prognosis after lung transplantation. Patients with cystic fibrosis are at increased risk for infection after transplantation.

33 Answer a

Lung volume reduction surgery (LVRS) is contraindicated for patients with pulmonary hypertension. The purpose of LVRS is to remove nonfunctional lung tissue to assist in the maximization of the residual lung tissue.

34 Answer b

The 1-year survival rate after liver transplantation is 80% to 90%.

35 Answer b

The patient deteriorating prior to heart transplantation may be supported with a ventricular assist device. The patient can be supported with right- and left-sided assist devices. The patient has dilated cardiomyopathy rather than ischemic cardiomyopathy, so angioplasty and emergency cardiac surgery would not be indicated. A pacemaker may be implanted if control of the patient's rhythm is an issue.

36 Answer d

The preferred treatment for histoplasmosis is amphotericin B. Cytomegalovirus immune globulin (CytoGam) may be used in prophylaxis for CMV. Acyclovir is used for herpes infections. OKT3 is used to treat rejections.

Bibliography

Bartucci, M: Kidney transplantation: State of the art. AACN Clin Issues 10:2, 153–163, May 1999.

Duke, T, and Perna, J: The ventricular assist device as a bridge to cardiac transplantation, AACN Clin Issues 10:2, 217–227, May 1999.

Maddrey, WC, and Sorrell, MF: Transplantation of the Liver. 2nd ed. Appleton & Lange, Norwalk, CT, 1995.

Ochoa, L, and Richardson, G: The current status of lung transplantation: A nursing perspective. AACN Clin Issues 10:2, 229–239, May 1999.

Rourke, T, et al: Heart Transplantation: State of the art. AACN Clin Issues 10:2, 185–201, May 1999.

UNIT FOUR

ISSUES IN ACUTE CARE

30
.

Issues in Acute Care

1 *The acute care nurse practitioner (ACNP) is a:*

a registered nurse with a bachelor's degree in nursing.
b registered nurse with expanded knowledge in a specialty area of practice, including graduate education.
c role designed for hospital care only.
d role that evolved as a result of physician shortages in pediatrics.

2 *The first state to recognize prescriptive authority for nurse practitioners was:*

a Pennsylvania.
b Washington.
c North Carolina.
d Ohio.

3 *Standards of care are:*

a peer review organizations.
b criteria to measure against to determine whether or not negligence occurred.
c descriptions of steps to be taken for a specific disease process.
d protocols.

4 *An ACNP notices a motor vehicle accident and stops at the scene to offer assistance. Which of the following statutes protects the ACNP from malpractice suits in this situation?*

a Good Samaritan statute
b Confidentiality
c Duty to warn
d Do no harm

5 *The American Academy of Nurse Practitioners (AANP) state entry-level preparation for nurse practitioner education is a:*

a bachelor's degree.
b certificate program.

c master's degree.
d doctoral degree.

6 *The Federal 1999 Balanced Budget Act allowed for:*

a nurse practitioner reimbursement to provide primary care services to the indigent.
b Medicare reimbursement for advanced practice nurse services.
c nurse practitioners to write prescriptions.
d nurse practitioners to be reimbursed from commercial insurers.

7 *Roles for the ACNP include:*

a educator.
b expert clinician.
c consultant.
d all of the above.

8 *The ACNP is involved in outcomes research. All of the following are examples of patient outcomes* **EXCEPT:**

a patient satisfaction.
b length of stay.
c mortality statistics.
d peer review.

9 *Clinical protocols are:*

a guidelines in providing patient care.
b privileges to perform independent skills.
c health-promotion practices.
d guidelines to develop research projects.

10 *The nurse practitioner role in research includes:*

a identifying the study population only.
b utilizing research findings in implementation of guidelines for patient care.
c performing teaching activities to promote health.
d providing continuing education to staff members.

11 *Certification is the:*

a monitoring of laws and regulations that affect nurse practitioner practice.

b agency that grants permission to individuals accountable for the practice of a profession and prohibits all others from doing so.

c process by which a nongovernmental agency certifies that an individual licensed to practice as a professional has met certain predetermined standards specified by that profession.

d monitoring of quality in health-care practice.

12 *Licensure is:*

a the granting of permission by an agency to individuals accountable for the practice of a profession and forbidding all others from doing so legally.

b not necessary to obtain certification.

c needed for the primary care exam certification only.

d defining the domains of nurse practitioner practice.

13 *The Patient Self-Determination Act:*

a requires every person to have a living will.

b provides for confidentiality of all patient records.

c assures patients' rights to participate in and direct their health-care decisions.

d is none of the above.

14 *The ethical principle of "first do no harm" is called:*

a beneficence.

b nonmaleficence.

c autonomy.

d utilitarianism.

15 *As the ACNP, you are caring for a 45 year-old woman with metastatic breast cancer, and she refuses further treatment. Which of the ethical principles does this represent?*

a Nonmaleficence

b Beneficence

c Autonomy

d Utilitarianism

16 *A 35-year-old man is admitted to the hospital with viral pneumonia. During the hospitalization, a human immunodeficiency virus (HIV) test is drawn, and it is positive. The patient is married and has two small children. He refuses to tell his wife or have you inform her. What is the most appropriate next step in the management of this issue?*

a Contact the local health department and have them inform the wife.

b Notify the wife and set up an office visit to discuss her husband's condition.

c Explain to him the importance of informing his wife and offer support.

d Confront the patient about his HIV status with the wife present.

17 *Quality assurance is:*

a a medical audit.

b the manner in which health professionals diagnose disease.

c the review of nurse practitioner services to Medicare patients.

d a program that evaluates care and implements programs to improve care where needed.

18 *Continuous quality improvement includes which of the following domains?*

a Structure

b Outcome

c Process

d All of the above

19 *All of the statements concerning clinical practice guidelines are true EXCEPT:*

a they are based on clinical research, literature, and judgment of expert physicians.

b they should be written and presented in a manner that can be easily accessed and understood.

c their main purpose is to legislate the certificate of need process.

d they may help to decrease health-care cost.

20 *Euthanasia is:*

a the active role of doing good by intervention.

b a patient-appointed decision maker.

c the active role in assisting in the death of a patient.

d all of the above.

21 *The role of a hospital ethics committee includes all of the following EXCEPT:*

a education of hospital staff.

b review of all do not resuscitate (DNR) orders.

c to provide consultation as needed.

d to create policy.

22 *Futile treatment is:*

a treatment that cannot achieve the stated goals.

b the designation of a health-care proxy.

c choosing alternatives to traditional care.

d placing a value on the life of the elderly patient.

23 *The only state in the nation in which physician-assisted suicide is legal is:*

a Michigan.

b Pennsylvania.

c California.

d Oregon.

24 *Evidence-based practice is:*

a the use of clinical guidelines.
b the care of patients using the best available evidence from the results of research to guide clinical decision making.
c a newsletter designed to update health-care providers.
d a quality-improvement program.

25 *Barriers to the use of evidence-based practice in daily decision making include:*

a lack of education.
b lack of available resources.
c lack of ability to generalize the results from large studies to practice populations.
d all of the above.

26 *Evidence-based guidelines for the use of fibrinolytic therapy in the treatment of pulmonary embolus (PE) include:*

a patients at risk for recurrent pulmonary emboli.
b patients with hypotension or hemodynamic compromise.
c patients with limited cardiac reserve.
d all of the above.

27 *Which of the following medications have been proven to be effective in the management of acute myocardial infarction?*

a Nitrates
b Calcium channel blockers
c Aspirin
d Heparin

28 *Healthy People 2010 is a:*

a national health plan for elderly patients.
b government-sponsored focus group.
c statement of national health objectives designed to identify the most significant preventable threats to health and to establish national goals for reduction of these threats.
d plan to have health insurance for all children by the year 2010.

29 *Managed care refers to:*

a fee for service.
b techniques employed by third-party payers to control health benefit expenditures.
c peer and utilization review programs.
d review of medical necessity by hospital admissions departments.

30 *Health-care proxy refers to:*

a a do not resuscitate (DNR) order.
b the designation of a person to carry out health-care wishes or make health-care decisions for you if you are unable to communicate.
c a decision to prolong life when death is imminent.
d a health-care liaison.

31 *Which of the following statements concerning do not resuscitate (DNR) orders is correct?*

a A DNR order means that the patient is abandoned.
b DNR status need only be reviewed with health-care team members.
c The DNR order only encompasses an order to not resuscitate if cardiopulmonary arrest occurs.
d The Joint Commission for the Accreditation of Healthcare Organizations (JCAHO) requires hospitals to have written guidelines and policies for DNR orders.

32 *A 25-year-old person involved in a diving accident is declared brain dead by defined criteria. Who is the best person to approach the family about possible organ donation?*

a The health-care provider (nurse practitioner or physician)
b The chaplain
c The organ procurement coordinator
d The health-care provider and the organ procurement coordinator

33 *Bronchiectasis is:*

a irreversible dilatation of the bronchi caused by destruction of the bronchial wall.
b an autosomal recessive disease characterized by exocrine gland dysfunction.
c a reversible airway obstruction.
d a localized area of infection in the lung.

34 *A positive sweat test in combination with pancreatic insufficiency is diagnostic of:*

a asthma.
b bronchitis.
c cystic fibrosis.
d chylothorax.

35 *Which of the following issues is the health-care provider under obligation to report?*

a Deaths
b Child abuse
c Accidental injuries involving firearms
d All of the above

36 *A 50-year-old man who has had a lung transplant has developed complications including respiratory failure, sepsis, and renal failure. As the ACNP, you are discussing the case with the intensivist and have expressed concern that the care seems futile.*

Which of the following factors should be taken into consideration when discussing futility of care?

a Expected quality of life
b Patient preferences
c Economics of continuing care
d All of the above

37 *Evidence-based medicine is:*

a enrolling patients in clinical trials to evaluate new treatment modalities.
b a health-maintenance schedule for individuals.
c the utilization of the best available evidence from research to guide clinical decision making.
d the practice of defensive medicine.

38 *Barriers associated with the application of evidence-based medicine include:*

a generalizability of research results.
b internal validity of research results.
c knowledge deficit.
d all of the above.

39 *The nurse practitioner who testifies as an expert witness:*

a reviews the records and provides an opinion.
b usually interviews the claimant.
c may not review the medical record involved.
d must have at least 10 years of practice.

40 *The duty to observe the pledges made by one's profession is referred to as:*

a autonomy.
b nonmaleficence.
c fidelity.
d justice.

41 *A 70-year-old woman is admitted to the hospital for the treatment of pneumonia. During the course of the hospitalization she develops an upper gastrointestinal bleed with a hemoglobin count of 5 g/dL. She is a Jehovah Witness and is refusing blood transfusions. You discuss the situation with the patient's family, and they are requesting that blood transfusions be given. The patient is deemed competent. What should you do next?*

a Transfuse the patient based upon the family's wishes.
b Explain to the patient the life-threatening nature of her condition and abide by her wishes.
c Obtain a court order for transfusion.
d Consult with the hospital ethics committee.

42 *The study of meaning and justification of ethical discourse and nature of moral concepts is:*

a philosophy.
b meta-ethics.
c personal value.
d theology.

43 *Components of informed consent include:*

a the nature and purpose of the proposed treatment.
b treatment alternatives.
c prognosis without treatment.
d all of the above.

44 *The National Practitioner Data Bank is a:*

a listing of all health-care practitioners in the United States.
b national registry that tracks malpractice claims against health-care providers.
c listing of nurse practitioners.
d listing of impaired health-care practitioners.

45 *Disclosure of information about a patient's case without the patient's permission is:*

a breach of confidentiality.
b informed consent.
c invasion of privacy.
d fraud.

46 *Certification of need laws require:*

a hospitals to seek approval for new capital expenditures.
b approval for renovations and hospital construction.
c that mobile computed tomography (CT) scanners be approved.
d all of the above.

47 *Medicare provides insurance coverage to:*

a persons aged 65 and older.
b pregnant women.
c persons with low income over age 65.
d none of the above.

48 *Medicare part B covers:*

a private-duty nursing.
b outpatient prescription plans.
c nursing home care.
d all of the above.

49 *The Medicare program is administered by the:*

a Department of Health and Human Services.
b Social Security administration.
c Health Care Financing Agency.
d Veteran's Administration.

50 *All of the statements concerning health maintenance organizations (HMOs) are true* **EXCEPT:**

a they restrict patient referrals to participating providers.
b they have unlimited fee schedules for participating providers.
c they emphasize low-cost alternative to inpatient care.
d they require each HMO member to select a primary care physician.

51 *The diagnosis-related group (DRG) payment system:*

a is a treatment classification system that assigns a fixed hospital payment rate.
b is a predetermined percentage of health-benefit cost paid by the patient.
c is a payment system for the medically indigent.
d are benefits not covered by a given insurance plan.

52 *A health-care plan in which nurse practitioners and physicians are employed directly by the health plan is:*

a a staff-model health maintenance organization (HMO).
b a preferred provider organization (PPO) plan.
c a commercial health plan.
d none of the above.

53 *Capitation is a:*

a fee-for-service charge.
b flat rate for each day in the hospital.
c fixed fee paid to the provider per patient per month for patients enrolled in the insurance plan.
d threshold amount allowed in an insurance policy.

54 *Which of the following services are reimbursed by Medicare?*

a Home-health aids
b Physical therapy
c Skilled nursing services
d All of the above

55 *Results from clinical research trials may be invalid if:*

a there is an inadequate sample.
b the study design is flawed.
c the clinical observations are biased.
d all of the above.

56 *The certificate of death may be certified by all of the following* **EXCEPT:**

a the physician.
b the nurse practitioner.
c the medical examiner.
d the coroner.

Answers

1 Answer b
The ACNP is a registered nurse with expanded knowledge in a specialty area of practice, including graduate education. The primary care role evolved as a result of physician shortages in the area of pediatrics.

2 Answer c
The first state to recognize prescriptive authority for nurse practitioners was North Carolina in 1975.

3 Answer b
Standards of care are criteria against which to measure whether or not negligence has occurred. Such knowledge of standards of care may help minimize malpractice claims.

4 Answer a
The Good Samaritan statute protects medical professionals from malpractice suits when they stop at an emergency scene to provide medical expertise.

5 Answer c
The AANP state entry-level preparation for nurse practitioner education is a master's degree.

6 Answer b
The Federal 1999 Balanced Budget Act allowed for Medicare reimbursement for advance practice nurse services.

7 Answer d
Roles for the ACNP include educator, expert clinician, consultant, and researcher.

8 Answer d
Patient satisfaction, length of stay, and mortality statistics are all examples of patient outcomes; peer review is not a patient outcome.

9 Answer a
Clinical protocols are guidelines in providing patient care.

10 Answer b
The nurse practitioner role in research includes using research findings in the implementation of guidelines for patient care.

11 Answer c
Certification is the process by which a nongovernmental agency certifies that an individual licensed to practice as a professional has met certain predetermined standards specified by that profession.

12 Answer a
Licensure is the granting of permission by an agency to individuals accountable for the practice of a profession and the forbidding of all others from doing so legally.

13 Answer c
The Patient Self-Determination Act assures that patients will have the right to participate in and direct their health-care decisions. This law makes it mandatory for health-care facilities to provide patients with written information about their health-care options and the availability of an advance directive.

14 Answer b

The ethical principle of "first do no harm" is nonmaleficence.

15 Answer c

The ethical principle used by the patient described is one of autonomy. Autonomy is the competent person's right to select his or her own course of action.

16 Answer c

The most appropriate next step in the management of the issue described is to explain to the patient the importance of informing his wife and to offer support. As the health-care provider, your informing the wife would be a breach of confidentiality.

17 Answer d

Quality assurance is a program that evaluates care and implements programs to improve care where needed.

18 Answer d

Continuous quality improvement includes structure, outcome, and process as its domains.

19 Answer c

The main purpose of clinical practice guidelines is to develop standards for the delivery of health care, not to legislate the certificate of need process. Clinical practice guidelines are based on clinical research, literature, and judgment of expert physicians; should be written and presented in a manner that can be easily accessed and understood; and may help to decrease health-care cost.

20 Answer c

Euthanasia is the active role in assisting in the death of a patient.

21 Answer b

The role of a hospital ethics committee is to educate hospital staff, provide consultation as needed, and create policies. It is not the role of the ethics committee to review all DNR orders.

22 Answer a

Futile treatment is treatment that cannot achieve the stated goals. Some health-care providers believe that futile treatment is treatment that is physiologically incapable of achieving the stated goal, whereas others believe that it is statistically unlikely to achieve the stated goal.

23 Answer d

Oregon is the only state in the nation in which physician-assisted suicide is legal.

24 Answer b

Evidence-based practice is the care of patients using the best available evidence from the results of research to guide clinical decision making.

25 Answer d

Barriers to the use of evidence-based practice in daily decision making are the lack of education, available resources, and ability to generalize the results from large studies to practice populations.

26 Answer d

Evidence-based guidelines for the use of fibrinolytic therapy in the treatment of pulmonary embolus (PE) are patients at risk of recurrent PE, patients with hemodynamic compromise, and patients with limited cardiac reserve.

27 Answer c

Aspirin has been proven to be effective in the management of acute myocardial infarction.

28 Answer c

Healthy People 2010 is a statement of national health objectives designed to identify the most significant preventable threats to health and to establish national goals for reduction of these threats.

29 Answer b

Managed care refers to techniques employed by third-party payers to control health benefit expenditures.

30 Answer b

Health-care proxy refers to the designation of a person to carry out health-care wishes or make health-care decisions for you if you are unable to communicate effectively for yourself.

31 Answer d

The Joint Committee for the Accreditation of Healthcare Organizations (JCAHO) mandates that hospitals have written guidelines and policies for do not resuscitate (DNR) orders. The decision for DNR must be discussed with the patient, when possible; the family; and health-care team members. The DNR order may encompass an order to not resuscitate in the event of cardiopulmonary arrest, but also may limit treatments or additions of treatments.

32 Answer d

The best approach to families concerning organ donation is to use a combined team including the organ procurement coordinator and health-care provider.

33 Answer a

Bronchiectasis is irreversible dilatation of the bronchi caused by destruction of the bronchial wall. Cystic fibrosis is an autosomal recessive disease with exocrine gland dysfunction. A localized area of infection in the lung is lung abscess. A reversible airway obstruction is asthma.

34 Answer c

A positive sweat test in combination with pancreatic insufficiency is diagnostic of cystic fibrosis.

35 Answer d

The health-care provider is under obligation to report deaths, child abuse, and accidental injuries involving firearms.

36 Answer d

The discussion of futility should involve discussion of the expected quality of life, patient preferences, and the economics of continuing care.

37 Answer c

Evidence-based medicine is the utilization of the best available evidence from research to guide clinical decision making.

38 Answer d

The application of evidence-based medicine to practice may be impeded by lack of ability to generalize results of large research studies to a specific population. There may also be some concerns about internal validity of research and lack of knowledge of the latest research studies.

39 Answer a

The nurse practitioner who testifies as an expert witness reviews the records and provides an opinion. The expert witness usually has no contact with the claimant and has to review the record to provide an opinion. Years of experience are not a criterion for one to be an expert witness.

40 Answer c

The duty to observe the pledges made by one's profession is referred to as fidelity.

41 Answer b

The approach to this patient would be to explain the medical condition and the life-threatening nature of the situation, and to then respect her wishes. The patient is deemed competent, and the family can not overrule her wishes. You can consult with the ethics committee, but the patient's wishes must be respected. A court order cannot impose transfusion on this competent patient.

42 Answer b

Meta-ethics is the study of meaning and justification of ethical discourse and nature of moral concepts.

43 Answer d

Components of informed consent include the nature and purpose of the proposed treatment, treatment alternatives, and prognosis without treatment.

44 Answer b

The National Practitioner Data Bank is a national registry that tracks malpractice claims against health-care providers.

45 Answer a

The disclosure of information about a patient's case without his or her permission is breach of confidentiality.

46 Answer d

The certification of need law requires that hospitals seek approval for new capital expenditures, hospital renovations, and mobile CT scanners.

47 Answer a

Medicare provides insurance coverage for all persons aged 65 and older.

48 Answer b

Medicare part B covers outpatient prescription plans. Other covered services include dental care, routine physical exams, preventive care, health-care provider charges, and eye care. Nursing home care and private duty nursing is covered under Medicare part A.

49 Answer c

The Medicare program is administered by the Health Care Financing Agency.

50 Answer b

Health Maintenance Organizations (HMOs) restrict patient referrals to participating providers, emphasize low-cost alternatives to inpatient care, and require each HMO member to select a primary care physician. HMOs employ maximum fee schedules for participating providers to control the cost of health benefits.

51 Answer a

The diagnosis-related group (DRG) payment system is a treatment classification system that is assigned a fixed hospital payment rate.

52 Answer a

A health-care plan in which nurse practitioners and physicians are employed directly by the health plan is a staff-model HMO.

53 Answer c

Capitation is a fixed fee paid to a provider per patient per month for patients enrolled in the insurance plan. A fee-for-service charge is billed on an itemized service. Per diem is a flat rate fee paid to providers per patient per month for patients enrolled in the insurance plan. Deductible is a threshold amount allowed in an insurance policy.

54 Answer d

Medicare reimburses for skilled nursing services, physical therapy, and home health aids.

55 Answer d

Results from clinical trials may be invalid if there is an inadequate sample, the study design is flawed, and the observations are biased.

56 Answer b

The physician, medical examiner, and coroner may certify the certificate of death. The nurse practitioner cannot certify the death certificate.

Bibliography

Ahronheim, JC, et al: Ethics in Clinical Practice. Little Brown, Boston, 1994.

American Academy of Nurse Practitioners: Scope of Practice for Nurse Practitioners. Revised 1998.

American Nurses Association and the American Association of Critical Care Nurses: Standards of Clinical Practice and Scope of Practice for Acute Care Nurse Practitioners. Washington, DC, 1995.

Calkins, D, et al: Health Care Policy. Blackwell Science, Cambridge, Mass., 1995.

Chin, A, et al: Legalized physician-assisted suicide in Oregon: The first year's experience. N Engl J Med 340:577, 1999.

Danis, M, et al: Stability of choices about life-sustaining treatments. Ann Intern Med 120:567, 1994.

Fletcher, RH, and Fletcher, SW: Evidence-based approach to the medical literature. J Gen Intern Med 12:S5, 1997.

Goolsby, M: Understanding nurse practitioner preparation. J Am Academy Nurs Practit 12:2, 43–48, Feb 2000.

Menikoff, JA, et al: Beyond advance directives: Health care surrogate laws. N Engl J Med 322:1165, 1992.

Molloy, DW, et al: Systematic implementation of an advance directive program in nursing homes. A randomized controlled trial. JAMA 283:1437, 2000.

Pearson, L: Annual update of how each state stands on legislative issues affecting advanced nursing practice. Nurs Practit 25:1, 16–68, Jan 2000.

Pozgar, GD: Legal Aspects of Health Care Administration. Aspen, Rockville, Md., 1995.

HEALTH PROMOTION AND RISK ASSESSMENT

31

Health Promotion and Risk Assessment

1 *Which of the following is an example of primary prevention?*

a Mammogram screening
b Pneumococcal vaccination
c Pap smear testing
d Controlling hypertension

2 *Influenza vaccine is given:*

a annually.
b once every 10 years.
c to prevent streptococcal infections.
d once every 5 years.

3 *A 25-year-old woman is 4 months pregnant, and you suspect partner abuse. Which of the questions should you NOT ask the patient?*

a Do you want to talk about it?
b What did you do to make him/her so angry?
c Does your partner ever keep you from seeing friends or family?
d Does your partner humiliate you?

4 *Barriers to screening for domestic violence may include:*

a discomfort with the topic.
b time constraints.
c perceived powerlessness to change problems.
d all of the above.

5 *The infant mortality rate is highest in those infants born to:*

a Japanese mothers.
b Puerto Rican mothers.
c African-American mothers.
d Cuban mothers.

6 *The leading cause of African-American infant death is:*

a sudden infant death syndrome (SIDS).
b a congenital anomaly.
c related to low birth weight.
d respiratory distress syndrome.

7 *The best way to detect breast cancer is by:*

a obtaining a computed tomography (CT) scan.
b performing an ultrasound of the breast.
c performing a breast self-exam.
d obtaining a mammogram.

8 *The leading cause of injury-related deaths in adolescents is:*

a gun violence.
b motor vehicle accidents.
c drowning.
d falls.

9 *A 65-year-old woman has been diagnosed with breast cancer. Risk factors associated with the development of breast cancer include all of the following EXCEPT:*

a late age of menopause (after age 55 years).
b menarche before age 12 years.
c having children before age 20 years.
d nulliparity.

10 *Carcinoembryonic antigen (CEA) is most useful for monitoring the activity of:*

a breast cancer.
b melanoma.
c thyroid cancer.
d colorectal cancer.

11 *All of the statements concerning menopause are true* **EXCEPT:**

a   it usually occurs between the ages of 44 and 55 years.
b   it may be associated with osteoporosis.
c   it may lead to an increased incidence of anxiety.
d   it is associated with an increased incidence of breast and cervical cancers.

12 *Screening is defined as:*

a   a method to monitor the status of a disease.
b   the likelihood of having an abnormal test result.
c   identification of the incidence of a disease state.
d   detection of a disease process before occurrence of symptoms in attempts to alter the natural history.

13 *Sensitivity of a test is defined as the:*

a   probability that a test will be positive if the disease state is present.
b   probability that a test will be negative if the disease is absent.
c   false-positive of a test.
d   negative predictive value of a test.

14 *Factors important to consider in screening for a disease process include:*

a   the frequency of the disease.
b   that the identification of the disease will alter the natural history.
c   the sensitivity and specificity of the screening tool.
d   all of the above.

15 *Which of the following patients should be treated with a cholesterol-lowering agent?*

a   A 40-year-old man with a low-density lipoprotein (LDL) cholesterol level of 100
b   A 55-year-old post-menopausal woman with an LDL cholesterol level of 170 despite diet and exercise.
c   A 60-year-old man with a high-density lipoprotein (HDL) cholesterol level of 35.
d   A 25-year-old man with a family history of coronary artery disease.

16 *A 35-year-old man is having a routine physical exam. Which of the following tests have been proven effective for cancer screening?*

a   Chest x-ray
b   Sputum cytology
c   Prostate-specific antigen (PSA)
d   Fecal occult blood testing

17 *How often should a 68-year-old woman have a Pap smear?*

a   Annually.
b   Every 2 years.

c   There is no need for her to have a Pap smear if three previous smears have been negative.
d   Every 5 years.

18 *The most effective method of preventing lung cancer is:*

a   counseling patients against the use of tobacco.
b   performing annual chest x-rays.
c   using nicotine patches.
d   avoiding second-hand smoke.

19 *Which of the following patients has an increased risk for colorectal cancer?*

a   A patient with ulcerative colitis
b   A patient with a history of peptic ulcer disease
c   A patient taking nonsteroidal anti-inflammatory drugs (NSAIDs)
d   A patient with a spousal history of colorectal cancer

20 *Which of the following may produce a false-positive fecal occult blood test result?*

a   High-dose aspirin
b   Ferrous sulfate
c   Vitamin C
d   All of the above

21 *All of the statements concerning testicular cancer are true* **EXCEPT:**

a   the overall cure rate is more than 90%.
b   it is a relatively uncommon cancer.
c   a patient with a history of undescended testes is at an increased risk.
d   it is very common in men ages 50 to 65.

22 *Oropharyngeal cancers have been associated with:*

a   alcohol and tobacco use.
b   oral intercourse.
c   alcohol and foods high in protein.
d   snuff and foods high in sugar.

23 *The American Heart Association's (AHA) recommended diet for the general population is to limit:*

a   fat intake to 50% of calories per day.
b   cholesterol to 500 mg/d.
c   30% of calories to carbohydrates.
d   polyunsaturated fat intake to 10% of calories.

24 *A 30-year-old healthy man with no cardiac risk factors wants to enroll in an exercise program. Which of the following tests should be performed to clear him for participation?*

a   Exercise electrocardiogram (ECG)
b   Echocardiogram

c None indicated
d Baseline cholesterol level and ECG

25 *The beneficial effects of exercise include all of the following* **EXCEPT:**

a increased serum lipid levels.
b improved mental well-being.
c protection against osteoporosis.
d lowered blood pressure.

26 *Preventive measures indicated in patients after myocardial infarction include:*

a use of aspirin and beta blockers.
b increase in vitamin E and beta carotene.
c screening of all siblings.
d reduction of cholesterol and use of vitamin C supplements.

27 *Hepatitis A vaccine is recommended for all of the following groups* **EXCEPT:**

a food handlers.
b bisexual men.
c international travelers.
d persons with chronic heart and lung diseases.

28 *Which of the following immunizations is an attenuated vaccine?*

a Diphtheria
b *Haemophilus influenzae*
c Varicella
d Hepatitis B

29 *A tetanus and diphtheria booster is recommended:*

a every 5 years.
b every 10 years after the primary series is completed.
c once in a lifetime.
d every 20 years.

30 *Which of the following diseases has been associated with the influenza vaccine?*

a Guillain-Barré syndrome
b Lyme disease
c Multiple sclerosis
d Meningitis

31 *Which of the following persons should receive the influenza vaccine?*

a A 20-year-old pregnant woman who will be in the second or third trimester during the influenza season
b A 25-year-old man with hypertension who is taking no medications
c A 30-year-old man following knee surgery
d A 40-year-old woman with no health problems

32 *Which of the following antiviral medications have been shown to be effective in the prevention and treatment of influenza?*

a Acyclovir (Zovirax)
b Zidovudine (Retrovir)
c Amantadine (Symmetrel) and rimantadine (Flumadine)
d Varicella vaccine (Varivax)

33 *The recommended dosage of amantadine (Symmetrel) for patients with influenza and renal insufficiency is:*

a 100 mg/d.
b 200 mg/d.
c 200 mg twice daily.
d 100 mg three times daily.

34 *Which of the following may be barriers to immunization in adults?*

a Patient and provider fears about adverse effects of vaccinations
b Lack of vaccine delivery systems
c Provider concern about efficacy of vaccinations
d All of the above

35 *The single most important infection control measure is:*

a wearing gloves.
b hand washing.
c immunizations.
d use of private rooms.

36 *Contraindications to the administration of pneumococcal vaccine include all of the following* **EXCEPT:**

a Hodgkin's disease.
b active infection.
c pregnancy.
d human immunodeficiency virus (HIV) infection.

37 *The influenza vaccine has been associated with false-positive assays for:*

a hepatitis A.
b human immunodeficiency virus (HIV).
c Epstein-Barr virus (EBV).
d hepatitis B.

38 *A 55-year-old man is having a routine physical exam, and you are reviewing his immunizations. He tells you he is unsure if he received the primary series of tetanus and diphtheria immunizations. What would you do?*

a Administer one dose of diphtheria and tetanus now, the next dose in 4 weeks, and the last dose in 6 to 12 months.

b   Administer one dose of tetanus and diphtheria now, and give the subsequent dose 2 months later.
c   Administer all three doses of tetanus and diphtheria over a 4-month period.
d   There is no need to administer any immunizations at this time.

39   *Systemic reactions that may occur after the tetanus and diphtheria vaccine include:*

a   acute renal failure.
b   anaphylaxis.
c   Guillain-Barré syndrome.
d   meningitis.

40   *Which of the following groups of persons are at the highest risk for developing tetanus and diphtheria?*

a   Elderly adults
b   Persons with human immunodeficiency virus (HIV) infection
c   Intravenous drug users
d   Persons who have not completed their primary immunization series

41   *Which of the following persons should be screened for tuberculosis (TB)?*

a   Health-care workers
b   Persons with human immunodeficiency virus (HIV) infection
c   Medically underserved, low-income populations
d   All of the above

42   *Which diagnostic test should be used in screening for syphilis in the asymptomatic person?*

a   Fluorescent treponemal antibody (FTA-ABS)
b   Rapid plasma reagin (RPR)
c   Microhemagglutination test (MHA-TP)
d   Western blot

43   *Which of the following is considered a positive Mantoux test in a patient with human immunodeficiency virus (HIV) infection?*

a   Induration of 5 mm or more
b   Induration of 20 mm or more
c   Induration of 15 mm or more
d   Induration of 10 mm or more

44   *Risk factors associated with a stroke include:*

a   diastolic hypertension only.
b   atrial fibrillation and advancing age.
c   mitral valve prolapse.
d   hypothyroidism.

45   *Routine screening should be done for all of the following EXCEPT:*

a   asymptomatic carotid disease.
b   hyperlipidemia.
c   breast cancer.
d   cervical cancer.

46   *All of the statements concerning ovarian cancer are true EXCEPT:*

a   the incidence of ovarian cancer increases with age.
b   there is an increased risk in patients with a positive family history.
c   an elevated CA-125 is diagnostic of ovarian cancer.
d   low parity may be a risk factor for ovarian cancer.

47   *Prevalence is defined as the:*

a   probability of not having disease in a patient with a positive test result.
b   proportion of people with a disease who have a positive test result.
c   proportion of people without a disease that have a negative test result.
d   proportion of a group possessing a clinical condition at a given point in time.

48   *Traveler's disease is most commonly caused by:*

a   *Haemophilus influenzae.*
b   *Escherichia coli.*
c   hepatitis A
d   *Staphylococcus.*

49   *A 55-year old woman is planning a trip to South Africa. Which of the following immunizations are recommended for this patient before departure?*

a   Hepatitis A and C
b   Yellow fever and poliomyelitis
c   Smallpox
d   Pneumococcal vaccine

50   *What is the medication of choice for the malaria prophylaxis?*

a   Trimethoprim sulfamethoxazole (Bactrim DS).
b   Cephalexin (Keflex)
c   Ampicillin (Omnipen)
d   Chloroquine (Aralen)

51   *An infection of the teeth is known as:*

a   dental caries.
b   gingivitis.
c   plaque.
d   periodonitis.

52   *Healthy People 2010 is a:*

a   hospital quality assurance program.
b   national health-promotion and disease-prevention initiative.

c program to provide health care to the elderly.
d plan for national health insurance.

53 *The best intervention for elder abuse is:*

a prevention.
b education for the abuser and the victim.
c institutionalization of all elders.
d a social worker referral.

54 *The most common site of nosocomial infections is the:*

a blood.
b urinary tract.
c respiratory tract.
d gastrointestinal tract.

55 *Which of the following persons is more likely to commit suicide?*

a A 40-year-old married woman with two children
b A 75-year-old man married for 50 years whose wife died 2 months ago
c A 30-year-old unmarried woman
d A 25-year-old married man

56 *Crude death rate is defined as the:*

a number of deaths assigned to a specified cause during a given time interval.
b number of deaths assigned to a specific disease.
c total number of deaths reported during a given interval divided by the estimated midinterval population.
d number of new cases of specific disease during a given time interval.

57 *A case-control study is a(n):*

a observational study in which exposed and nonexposed populations are identified and followed prospectively over time to determine the rate of a specific disease.
b observational study in which affected and unaffected persons are identified after the fact and then compared regarding specific characteristics to determine possible association or risk factors for the disease.
c report of clinical outcomes.
d experimental study used to assess differences between two or more groups receiving different interventions.

58 *In clinical research, a systemic error that is unintentionally made is known as:*

a causality.
b validity.
c bias.
d efficacy.

59 *All of the statements concerning institutional review boards (IRBs) are true EXCEPT:*

a IRBs are federally mandated.
b the purpose of the IRB is to review research proposals for scientific value and ethical concerns.
c IRBs are composed of only physicians.
d IRB approval requires an informed consent form.

60 *Which of the following vaccines should not be given to persons with an egg allergy?*

a Pneumococcal vaccine
b Influenza vaccine
c Tetanus toxoid
d Hepatitis B

61 *Which of the following interventions may help to decrease dental caries?*

a Reduction of sugar in the diet
b Topical fluoride applications
c Community fluoridation of the water supply
d All of the above

62 *Repetitive tasks may produce which of the following occupational disorders?*

a Back pain
b Carpal tunnel syndrome
c Eye strain
d Depression

63 *Human immunoglobulins are available for preventing all of the following diseases EXCEPT:*

a Hepatitis B
b Tetanus
c Rabies
d Hepatitis A

64 *Which of the following immunizations are contraindicated during pregnancy?*

a Influenza vaccine
b Varicella vaccine
c Hepatitis B
d None of the above

65 *Pneumococcal vaccine is recommended in all the following persons EXCEPT:*

a a 30-year-old with idiopathic thrombocytopenia purpura (ITP) who is scheduled for a splenectomy.
b a 45-year-old healthy woman.
c a 70-year-old healthy man.
d a 20-year-old woman with sickle cell disease.

66 *Which of the following factors is associated with cervical cancer?*

a Early menarche

b Menopause before age 50
c Alcohol use
d First coitus before age 20

67 *Which of the following groups has the lowest suicide rate?*

a Married individuals
b Divorced men
c Unemployed individuals
d Alcohol users

68 *A high maternal alpha fetal protein (AFP) level may be seen in:*

a Down's syndrome.
b Marfan's syndrome.
c spina bifida.
d lead poisoning.

69 *Ergonomics is the:*

a study of mechanical interactions between people and their living or work environment for the purpose of tailoring workplace design for better well-being.
b diagnosis and treatment of disease caused by one's work environment.
c study of environmental toxins.
d study of disease in populations.

70 *An influenza-like illness that affects pet shop owners and individuals who raise and process poultry is:*

a tetanus.
b anthrax.
c brucellosis.
d psittacosis.

71 *The Americans with Disabilities Act (ADA) of 1990 includes all of the following* **EXCEPT:**

a it prohibits an agency from discriminating against a qualified individual with a disability.
b it prevents agencies from hiring persons with human immunodeficiency virus (HIV) infection.
c it helps to secure access to health-care services.
d it covers employment agencies, labor organizations, and employers.

72 *The accreditation of hospitals is carried out by the:*

a American Association of Medical Colleges.
b Joint Commission on Accreditation of Health Care Organizations (JCAHO).
c American Board of Internal Medicine (ABIM).
d American Medical Association (AMA).

73 *The most common cause of post-transfusion hepatitis is:*

a Hepatitis C.
b Hepatitis A.
c Hepatitis E.
d Hepatitis D.

74 *Which of the following forms of hepatitis can be prevented with immunization?*

a Hepatitis A
b Hepatitis C
c Hepatitis B
d Hepatitis D

75 *The incubation period for chickenpox is:*

a 7 days.
b 10 to 21 days.
c 30 days.
d 7 to 10 days.

76 *Occult blood stool testing is recommended:*

a yearly for persons over age 50.
b yearly for persons over age 40.
c every 3 years for persons over age 70.
d at no specific time—there is no specific recommendation.

77 *A 55-year-old man with emphysema and a 40-pack-per-year smoking history has quit smoking for the past month. Which form of prevention does this represent?*

a Primary prevention
b Secondary prevention
c Tertiary prevention
d None of the above

78 *Which of the following is a form of primary prevention?*

a Routine immunizations
b Mammography
c Tuberculin skin testing
d Pap smears

79 *The upper limit of acceptable noise exposure in the work place is:*

a 50 dB.
b 90 dB.
c 100 dB.
d 75 dB.

80 *The leading cause of blindness in the United States is:*

a hypertension.
b retinal detachment.
c carotid artery stenosis.
d diabetes.

81 *A 28-year-old woman in her second trimester of pregnancy asks about the benefits of folate. You tell her that it:*

a increases blood volume.
b reduces the incidence of fetal anomalies.
c decreases birth weight.
d decreases the need to take iron during pregnancy.

82 *The incidence of nosocomial (hospital-associated) infection is:*

a less than 1%.
b 5% to 10%.
c 20%.
d 40%.

83 *The most commonly reported sexually transmitted disease (STD) is:*

a syphilis.
b *Chlamydia.*
c herpes.
d gonorrhea.

84 *A 45-year-old man is admitted with acute exacerbation of asthma. All of the following are associated with acute exacerbations* **EXCEPT:**

a caffeinated coffee.
b aspirin use.
c upper respiratory infections.
d dust.

85 *The most closely correlated risk factor for the development of osteoporosis is:*

a age.
b steroid use.
c family history.
d smoking.

86 *A 65-year-old man had surgery for gastric carcinoma 1 week ago. Which of the following statements concerning gastric carcinoma is true?*

a Gastric carcinoma is higher in smokers.
b Gastric carcinoma is higher in persons with a history of gastric ulcers.
c Gastric carcinoma is more common in men than women.
d Gastric carcinoma is more common in the United States than other countries.

87 *Risk factors associated with development of colon cancer include:*

a a diet high in fiber.
b a diet high in animal fat.
c cholelithiasis.
d gastritis.

88 *Symptoms associated with lead poisoning include:*

a headache.
b abdominal pain.
c memory loss.
d all of the above.

89 *Clinical features associated with fetal alcohol syndrome (FAS) include:*

a hydrocephalus.
b abdominal hernias.
c esophageal fistulas.
d microcephaly.

90 *Prevention of fetal alcohol syndrome (FAS) may be done by:*

a education of the public regarding the dangers of drinking during pregnancy.
b maternal alcohol abstinence during pregnancy.
c identification of women at greatest risk.
d all of the above.

91 *All of the statements concerning fetal alcohol syndrome (FAS) are true* **EXCEPT:**

a the infant mortality rate is approximately 20%.
b the mental retardation associated with FAS is reversible.
c binge drinking increases the risk of FAS.
d the incidence is less than 1%.

92 *Down syndrome is:*

a associated with abnormalities of the thyroid gland.
b an alteration in chromosome 21.
c most commonly associated with births to mothers younger than 20 years.
d associated with mitral valve prolapse.

93 *A 75-year-old man presents for an annual physical exam, and you want to assess his functional status. Functional status provides information about:*

a general physical health.
b overall quality of life.
c the ability to perform activities of daily living.
d all of the above.

94 *Which of the following women should not breast-feed?*

a A 20-year-old multiparous woman
b A 25-year-old woman with human immunodeficiency virus (HIV) infection
c A 30-year-old woman who delivers 2 months early
d A 16-year-old healthy woman

95 *All of the following should be done at the first prenatal visit* **EXCEPT:**

a hemoglobin and hematocrit level.
b a breast examination.
c a mammogram.
d a Pap smear.

96 *Polio is associated with which of the following complications?*

a Pneumonia
b Paralysis
c Encephalitis
d Mental retardation

97 *Epidemiology is:*

a the application of preventive medicine techniques.
b the science that forms the basis for public health actions.
c the early detection and prompt treatment of disease.
d a state of complete physical, mental, and social well-being.

98 *A group of 1000 newly diagnosed men with lung cancer are to be treated with surgical resection and radiation, or with radiation alone. This is an example of a:*

a clinical trial.
b cohort study.
c case report.
d primary prevention trial.

99 *Hepatocellular carcinoma is associated with which of the following viruses?*

a Cytomegalovirus (CMV)
b Herpes simplex virus (HSV)
c human immunodeficiency virus (HIV)
d Hepatitis B virus

100 *A 55-year-old male smoker presents for a routine examination. He states he is afraid he will die from lung cancer because his brother died from lung cancer and was a heavy smoker. He smokes two packs of cigarettes a day and states he has no intentions of quitting smoking. Which of the approaches should you take to help this patient?*

a Refer him to smoking cessation classes.
b Provide self-help materials and reassess him in 6 months.
c Give a concise, personalized message concerning smoking cessation, and reassess him at the next visit.
d Start him on a nicotine patch.

101 *The National Cholesterol Education Program (NCEP) guidelines recommend pharmacologic therapy for which of the following patients?*

a A 30-year-old woman with an LDL cholesterol level of 120
b A 55-year-old man with an LDL cholesterol level of 140 and history of myocardial infarction
c A 60-year-old woman smoker with a total cholesterol level of 180
d A 45-year-old male smoker with an LDL cholesterol level of 110

102 *A 75-year-old woman has a blood pressure of 190/78 mm Hg and is currently not taking medications. She has a past medical history significant for hypothyroidism, renal insufficiency, and gastroesophageal reflux disease (GERD). Which of the following statements is true concerning her blood pressure?*

a There is no need to treat isolated systolic hypertension.
b All elderly persons have systolic hypertension.
c Isolated systolic hypertension is a risk factor for stroke.
d Isolated systolic hypertension is more common in women.

103 *Which of the following tests is the most reliable screening test for detection of lead poisoning?*

a Hemoglobin
b Complete blood cell count
c Ferritin level
d Serum lead level

104 *The most effective method for screening for alcohol abuse is to:*

a obtain liver function tests.
b check the blood alcohol level.
c administer a standardized questionnaire.
d check a liver ultrasound for evidence of cirrhosis.

105 *Poor bone mineralization and osteoporosis are associated with a deficiency in:*

a calcium.
b sodium.
c phosphorus.
d vitamin E.

106 *Niacin deficiency is associated with:*

a neuropathy.
b petechiae.
c dermatitis, diarrhea, and delirium.
d edema.

107 *Tay-Sachs disease is more common in which population?*

a Ashkenazic Jews
b Asian-Americans
c African-Americans
d Italians

108 *Typhoid fever may be controlled by:*

a immunization.
b proper sanitation.
c control of the rodent population.
d control of the snake population.

109 *All of the statements concerning botulism are true* **EXCEPT:**

a visual disturbances and sore throat are early symptoms.
b it should be treated with an antitoxin.
c most cases result from improper handling of meat.
d the incubation period is 12 to 36 hours.

110 *If the positive predictive value of a given disease is 5%, how many true positives are in a sample of 100 positive test results?*

a 20
b 5
c 40
d 10

111 *Prevalence of a disease is the:*

a proportion of a group possessing a clinical condition at a given point in time.
b proportion of people with a disease that have a positive test.
c true negative rate.
d probability of not having the disease in a person with a negative test.

112 *A 40-year-old college professor is going to Africa to teach a 6-month course and is leaving in 4 days. Which of the following immunizations should he receive before his trip?*

a Smallpox
b Yellow fever
c Hepatitis A
d Pneumococcal

113 *The leading cause of food poisoning in the United States is:*

a *Staphylococcus aureus.*
b *Clostridium perfringens.*
c *Salmonella.*
d *Streptococcus viridans.*

114 *Risk factors associated with* **Salmonella** *food poisoning include:*

a human immunodeficiency virus (HIV) infection.
b antacid use.
c diabetes mellitus.
d all of the above.

115 *Which of the following medications may be prescribed as prophylaxis for malaria?*

a Penicillin
b Ceclor (Cefaclor)
c Doxycycline (Vibramycin)
d Prednisone

116 *The epidemic period for influenza is:*

a August to November.
b October to December.
c December to March.
d January to March.

117 *Elevated levels of homocystine are associated with:*

a acute renal failure.
b pneumonia.
c premature coronary artery disease.
d gastroesophageal reflux disease (GERD).

118 *Leading health indicators identified by the Healthy People 2010 agenda include all of the following* **EXCEPT:**

a tobacco use.
b environmental quality.
c access to health care.
d combating anorexia nervosa.

119 *Screening for diabetes is recommended in all of the following persons* **EXCEPT:**

a those with a family history of diabetes.
b those with anemia.
c those who are obese.
d those with glucose abnormalities during pregnancy.

120 *The most common risk factor associated with hepatic cirrhosis is:*

a alcohol consumption.
b diabetes.
c hepatitis.
d cigarette smoking.

121 *Which of the following types of hepatitis is common in day-care centers?*

a Hepatitis B
b Hepatitis C
c Hepatitis A
d Hepatitis D

122 *All of the following animals are common carriers of rabies* **EXCEPT:**

a cats.
b bats.
c raccoons.
d skunks.

123 *When individuals are immunized with vaccines, the type of immunity is called:*

a natural immunity.
b artificially acquired immunity.
c passive immunity.
d none of the above.

124 *Which of the following is a contraindication to receiving the influenza vaccine?*

a Having an allergy to penicillin
b Being pregnant
c Having an immunocompromised condition
d Having an allergy to eggs

125 *All of the following statements concerning pertussis are true* **EXCEPT:**

a it is highly communicable.
b it is more prevalent in adults.
c permanent neurologic damage may occur.
d it is associated with elevated temperatures and seizures.

126 *Potential complications of mumps include:*

a deafness.
b orchitis.
c encephalitis.
d all of the above.

127 *Which of the following persons should receive the hepatitis B vaccine?*

a A 78-year-old nursing home patient
b A 50-year-old man on hemodialysis for the past year
c A 68-year-old man with renal insufficiency
d An 80-year-old woman with osteoporosis and hypertension

128 *All of the statements concerning pelvic inflammatory disease (PID) are true* **EXCEPT:**

a it may lead to infertility.
b it may lead to an increased frequency of ectopic pregnancies.
c it has been associated with Kaposi's sarcoma.
d it may be caused by *Neisseria gonorrheae* or *Chlamydia*.

129 *Which of the following measures may potentially decrease the incidence of sexually transmitted diseases (STDs)?*

a Limiting the number of sexual partners
b Having multiple sexual partners
c Administering prophylactic antibiotics
d Avoiding barrier methods of contraception

130 *An untreated syphilis infection may lead to:*

a aortic aneurysms.
b diabetes mellitus.
c hypothyroidism.
d chronic renal failure.

131 *Which of the following persons should be screened for syphilis?*

a A 25-year-old pregnant woman
b A 40-year-old woman with a monogamous relationship for the past 10 years
c An 85-year-old woman admitted to a nursing home
d A 45-year-old man with hypertension

132 *The United States Preventive Services Task Force (USPSTF) recommends an exercise ECG for which of the following persons?*

a A 25-year-old woman with fibromyalgia prior to her joining a health club
b A 60-year-old male smoker with hypertension prior to his beginning an exercise program
c A 40-year-old diabetic man
d A 45-year-old healthy woman

133 *The American Cancer Society (ACS) recommends prostate cancer screening with a prostate-specific antigen (PSA) test:*

a annually after age 50.
b twice yearly after age 60.
c every 2 years after age 50.
d every 3 to 5 years after age 65.

134 *Which of the following statements concerning the rubella vaccine is true?*

a Persons with neomycin allergy should not receive the rubella vaccine.
b It is indicated for all adults over age 65 years.
c It should be repeated every 5 years.
d Women should avoid pregnancy for 3 months after immunization.

135 *The benefits of exercise include all of the following* **EXCEPT:**

a reduced blood pressure.
b a reduced HDL level.
c increased insulin sensitivity.
d a reduced triglyceride level.

136 *Which of the following persons are at increased risk for skin cancer?*

a A 60-year-old sunbather with a family history of melanoma
b A 50-year-old woman who uses SPF 15 sunscreen when exposed to the sun

c A 25-year-old woman who avoids the sun between the hours of 11 AM and 3 PM

d All of the above

137 *An 85-year-old woman is being admitted to your service at a long-term-care facility. Which of the following tools would you use to assess her cognitive function?*

a MAST questionnaire

b CAGE questionnaire

c Mini-Mental State Examination (MMSE)

d None of the above

138 *Prevention of falls in the elderly may include:*

a removing throw rugs from the home.

b using assistive devices.

c installing safety bars in bathrooms.

d all of the above.

139 *A 45-year-old woman with no previous health problems is admitted for pneumonia. She states that she has not seen a health-care provider in 20 years. Which of the following preventive health measures should be recommended after the acute illness has resolved?*

a Colonoscopy

b Mammogram and Pap smear

c Computed tomography (CT) scan of the chest

d Hepatitis B immunization

140 *Health-care workers are at increased risk for which of the following disorders?*

a Pneumococcal pneumonia

b Cytomegalovirus (CMV)

c Hepatitis

d Brucellosis

141 *Which of the statements concerning human immunodeficiency virus (HIV) infection is true?*

a Female heterosexuals are the fastest growing group of people infected with HIV.

b A woman infected with HIV has approximately a 10% chance of transmitting HIV to the fetus.

c Male homosexuals represent the fastest growing group of people infected with HIV.

d Infants infected with HIV will usually die in the first year of life.

142 *All of the following can be transmitted via blood-bank blood* **EXCEPT:**

a cytomegalovirus (CMV).

b human immunodeficiency virus (HIV).

c hepatitis C.

d syphilis.

143 *Foundry workers are at an increased risk for developing:*

a asbestosis.

b stomach cancer.

c bone cancer.

d cardiomyopathy.

144 *Crisis intervention is a form of:*

a primary prevention.

b secondary prevention.

c tertiary prevention.

d none of the above.

145 *Medicare part A covers:*

a physician services.

b inpatient services.

c outpatient services.

d durable medical supplies.

146 *Risk factors for the development of diabetes mellitus include:*

a obesity.

b age over 30 years.

c Caucasian race.

d male gender.

147 *The United States Preventive Services Task Force (USPSTF) recommendations for smoking cessation counseling include:*

a the use of nicotine gum while decreasing the number of cigarettes.

b tobacco cessation counseling at each visit.

c the use of nicotine patches for persons anticipating smoking cessation.

d all of the above.

148 *Symptoms of nicotine withdrawal include:*

a irritability.

b restlessness.

c anger.

d all of the above.

149 *The average age for a person to begin smoking today is:*

a 20 years.

b 15 years.

c 10 years.

d 25 years.

150 *Which of the following tests may be used to screen for syphilis?*

a vitamin B_{12} level.

b Venereal Disease Research Laboratories (VDRL) or rapid plasma reagin (RPR).

c Computed tomography (CT) scan of the head.
d electroencephalogram (EEG).

151 *Side effects associated with hormone replacement therapy (HRT) include:*

a vaginal bleeding.
b ascites.
c peptic ulcer disease.
d peripheral neuropathy.

152 *Which of the following persons should have a baseline colonoscopy to screen for colon cancer?*

a A 55-year-old woman with ulcerative colitis
b A 60-year-old man with no known health history
c A 75-year-old man with a negative colonoscopy 2 years ago
d A 25-year-old woman with irritable bowel syndrome (IBS)

153 *The second leading cause of cancer-related deaths in men is:*

a lung cancer.
b colorectal cancer.
c prostate cancer.
d testicular cancer.

154 *A 35-year-old woman has had two abnormal Pap smears with atypical cells. What is the next appropriate step?*

a Perform a colposcopy.
b Repeat the Pap smear.
c Order an abdominal ultrasound.
d Order a computed tomography (CT) scan of the abdomen.

155 *The leading cause of cancer deaths in men and women is:*

a colorectal cancer.
b brain cancer.
c lung cancer.
d bone cancer.

156 *On admission to the nursing care facility, an 80-year-old woman has a purified protein derivative (PPD) test done to screen for tuberculosis (TB). The PPD is negative. How should you proceed?*

a Order a chest x-ray.
b Repeat the PPD in 2 to 4 weeks.
c Order a CT scan of the chest.
d Start the patient on a medication regime that includes isoniazid (INH) and rifampin.

157 *The primary goal of screening is to:*

a identify persons at risk for developing a disease.

b detect a disease process.
c identify the natural history of a disease process.
d increase public health awareness.

158 *A 55-year-old healthy man presents for an annual physical exam. Which of the following should be obtained as part of the health screening?*

a Chest x-ray
b ECG
c Thyroid stimulating hormone (TSH) level
d Stool for occult blood

159 *Health Maintenance Organizations (HMOs):*

a are for preventive health services only.
b provide only inpatient services.
c are primary care practices.
d provide both inpatient and outpatient services through a referral system.

160 *A healthy 65-year-old man should receive which of the following?*

a Annual influenza vaccine
b Hepatitis B vaccine
c Annual chest x-ray
d Prostate ultrasound

161 *Radon exposure is a risk factor for:*

a vision loss.
b lung cancer.
c colorectal cancer.
d coronary artery disease.

162 *Initial management of spousal abuse includes:*

a a prescription for narcotics.
b a prescription for sedatives.
c placing the abused spouse in protective custody.
d a nonjudgmental inquiry about the possibility of abuse.

163 *A normal grief reaction may include:*

a weight loss.
b insomnia.
c periods of crying.
d all of the above.

164 *Which of the following is a primary prevention measure?*

a Mammography
b Immunizations
c Occult blood test of stool
d Testing for human immunodeficiency virus (HIV)

165 *Typhoid fever vaccinations should be administered:*

a after an earthquake.
b when traveling to countries with endemic typhoid.
c after a hurricane.
d once yearly.

166 *The organism usually responsible for traveler's diarrhea is:*

a *Escherichia coli.*
b *Salmonella.*
c *Pseudomonas.*
d *Streptococcus.*

167 *The total daily iron requirement for a woman with a normal pregnancy is:*

a 100 to 200 mg.
b 800 to 1000 mg.
c 1500 to 2000 mg.
d 200 to 400 mg.

168 *Which of the following antibiotics should be used to treat traveler's diarrhea?*

a Ciprofloxacin (Cipro)
b Erythromycin (E-Mycin)
c Amoxicillin (Amoxil)
d Metronidazole (Flagyl)

169 *Meningococcal meningitis outbreaks may be treated with:*

a rifampin (Rifadin).
b meningococcal vaccine.
c nothing; there is no effective treatment.
d penicillin.

170 *The most common mental illness in young adults is:*

a depression.
b mania.
c schizophrenia.
d delirium.

Answers

1 Answer b

Pneumococcal vaccination is a form of primary prevention. Primary prevention is aimed at the prevention of disease occurrence and includes immunizations, exercising, and eating properly. Mammogram and Pap smear screening and testing are forms of secondary prevention, which is early detection of a disease state. Control of hypertension is tertiary prevention, which is the stopping or slowing of disease progression.

2 Answer a

Influenza vaccine is given annually.

3 Answer b

The question you should not ask the patient to whom you suspect partner abuse is, "What did you do to make him/her so angry?" This statement suggests that the patient did something to provoke the partner.

4 Answer d

Barriers to screening for domestic violence may include discomfort with the topic, time constraints, and perceived powerlessness to change the problem.

5 Answer c

The infant mortality rate is highest in those infants born to African-American mothers with a rate of 13.8 deaths per 1000 live births. The mortality of Japanese-born infants is 3.5 per 1000 live births. The mortality rate for infants born to Puerto Rican mothers is 7.8 per 1000 live births, and the mortality rate for Cuban infants is 3.6 per 1000 live births.

6 Answer c

The leading cause of African-American infant death is related to low birth weight.

7 Answer d

The best way to detect breast cancer is by obtaining a mammogram. A mammogram may be able to detect masses that are too small to be felt during self-breast examination.

8 Answer b

The leading cause of injury-related deaths in adolescents is motor vehicle accidents.

9 Answer c

Risk factors related to the development of breast cancer may include early menarche, late age of menopause, nulliparity, and pregnancy after the age of 30 years. Childbirth before the age of 20 years has not been linked to the development of breast cancer.

10 Answer d

Carcinoembryonic Antigen (CEA) is a useful serum marker in monitoring the activity of colorectal cancer.

11 Answer d

Menopause has not been associated with an increased incidence of breast and cervical cancers. Menopause usually occurs between the ages of 44 and 55 years, may be associated with osteoporosis, and may lead to an increased incidence of anxiety.

12 Answer d

Screening is defined as detection of a disease process before occurrence of symptoms in attempts to alter the natural history.

13 Answer a

Sensitivity of a test is the probability that a test will be positive if the disease state is present. Specificity is the probability that a test will be negative if the disease is absent. Negative predictive value is the probability that the disease is absent given a negative test result.

14 Answer d

Factors important to consider in screening for a disease process include the frequency of the disease, that the identification of the disease will alter the natural history, and the sensitivity and specificity of the screening tool.

15 Answer b

The patient that should be treated with a cholesterol-lowering agent is the 55-year-old post-menopausal woman with an LDL cholesterol level of 170 despite diet and exercise. Evidence from clinical trials suggests those patients without known coronary heart disease and an LDL cholesterol level more than 160 should be treated with medication if diet and exercise do not lower cholesterol. Evidence supports the use of cholesterol-lowering medications in patients with known coronary artery disease and an LDL cholesterol level more than 130. There is no evidence to support the use of cholesterol-lowering agents in patients with an HDL cholesterol level less than 35, although low levels of HDL cholesterol and high levels of triglycerides have been linked epidemiologically to an increased risk of coronary artery disease.

16 Answer d

Fecal occult blood testing has been shown in several randomized controlled studies to reduce mortality from colorectal cancer. This has been associated with an early detection and improved survival. The United States Preventive Services Task Force has proposed the use of chest x-ray and sputum cytology for the early detection of lung cancer. Several clinical trials have not demonstrated a reduction in lung cancer mortality from frequent screening with chest x-ray and sputum cytology. Widespread screening with prostate-specific antigen (PSA) has not been shown to reduce morbidity and mortality from prostate cancer.

17 Answer c

A 68-year-old woman does not need a Pap smear after the age of 65 if multiple smears have been negative.

18 Answer a

The most effective method of preventing lung cancer is counseling patients against the use of tobacco. More than 80% of all lung cancers are related to smoking.

19 Answer a

The patient that has an increased risk for colorectal cancer is the person with ulcerative colitis. Other risk factors for colorectal cancer include previous history of cancer, family history of cancer, and history of adenomatous polyps.

20 Answer d

The intake of high-dose aspirin, ferrous sulfate, and vitamin C may all produce a false-positive fecal occult blood test. Other factors include foods with a high peroxidase content, red meats, and nonsteroidal anti-inflammatory drugs (NSAIDs).

21 Answer d

Testicular cancer is a relatively uncommon cancer and may affect men in the age range of 20 to 35 years (not 50 to 65 years). It has an overall cure rate of more than 90%, and patients with a history of undescended testes are at increased risk of developing it.

22 Answer a

Oropharyngeal cancers have been associated with alcohol and tobacco use. The use of snuff and chewing tobacco, but not snuff and food high in sugar, has been associated with oropharyngeal cancers.

23 Answer d

The American Heart Association's (AHA) recommended diet for the general population is to limit polyunsaturated fatty intake to 10% of calories, achieve ideal body weight, limit fat intake to 30%, limit cholesterol to 300 mg/d, and limit carbohydrate intake to 50% to 60% of calories.

24 Answer c

A 30-year-old man with no cardiac risk factors does not need clearance to enroll in an exercise program. An exercise ECG may be indicated in older patients with identified risk factors.

25 Answer a

The beneficial effects of exercise include improved mental well-being, protection against osteoporosis, lowered blood pressure, decreased weight, altered glucose metabolism, and decreased (not increased) serum lipid levels.

26 Answer a

Preventative measures indicated in patients post–myocardial infarction include the use of antiplatelet therapy with aspirin and the use of beta blockers. Both of these measures have been shown to reduce the incidence of subsequent infarction or limit the size of infarction. Vitamin E has been shown in one clinical trial to reduce the incidence of fatal myocardial infarction. Beta carotene and vitamin C have not been shown to have beneficial effect. The information provided does not support the indication for screening of siblings.

27 Answer d

Hepatitis A vaccine is recommended for homosexual or bisexual men; food handlers; international travelers to parts of Eastern Europe, Asia, Africa, and South America; drug users; and persons with chronic liver disease. It is not recommended for persons with chronic heart and lung diseases.

28 Answer c

Varicella is an attenuated or live vaccine.

29 Answer b

A tetanus and diphtheria booster is recommended every 10 years after the primary series is completed.

30 Answer a

Guillain-Barré syndrome has been associated with the influenza vaccine and was first noted in 1976. During the 1993 and 1994 flu seasons, less than one case per million was reported in patients receiving the influenza vaccine.

31 Answer a

A woman who will be in the second or third trimester of pregnancy during the influenza season should have the influenza vaccine. The Advisory Committee on Immunizations Practices of the Centers for Disease Control and Prevention recommends influenza vaccination of women with chronic medical conditions regardless of the stage of pregnancy. Other indications for influenza vaccine include persons age 65 years, residents of nursing homes and chronic-care facilities, persons who are immunocompromised, and health-care providers.

32 Answer c

Amantadine (Symmetrel) and rimantadine (Flumadine) have been shown to be effective in the prevention and treatment of influenza. It needs to be administered daily throughout the period of highest risk for influenza. There have been clinical trials that have demonstrated the efficacy of amantadine and rimantadine in the treatment of influenza A when it is administered within 48 hours of the onset of illness.

33 Answer a

The recommended dosage of amantadine (Symmetrel) in the

treatment of patients with influenza and renal insufficiency is 100 mg daily. The dosage in the absence of renal insufficiency is 200 mg daily.

34 Answer d

Barriers to immunization in the adult are patient and provider fears about adverse effects of vaccinations, lack of vaccine delivery systems, and provider concern about efficacy of vaccinations.

35 Answer b

The single most important infection control measure is hand washing.

36 Answer d

The pneumococcal vaccine is contraindicated in patients with Hodgkin's disease, active infection, or pregnancy. It is recommended for patients who are immunocompromised, such as those with human immunodeficiency virus (HIV) infection.

37 Answer b

The influenza vaccine has been associated with false-positive assays for human immunodeficiency virus (HIV) and hepatitis C. The mechanism for these false-positive results is not known. If the test is initially positive, it usually reverts to negative within $2^{1}/_{2}$ months.

38 Answer a

A patient who has not received the primary series of tetanus and diphtheria vaccine should have three doses of diphtheria and tetanus to booster the immunity. The first dose can be given initially, the second dose should be administered 4 weeks later, and then the final dose should be administered 6 to 12 months later.

39 Answer b

Systemic reactions that may occur after the tetanus and diphtheria vaccine include anaphylaxis, generalized urticaria, and angioedema.

40 Answer d

The persons who are at the highest risk for developing tetanus and diphtheria are those who have not completed their primary immunization series.

41 Answer d

Tuberculosis (TB) screening should be performed on healthcare workers, persons with human immunodeficiency virus (HIV) infection, and medically underserved low-income populations. Other groups that should be screened include patients with chronic renal failure, foreign-born persons from countries with high rates of TB who arrived in the United States within the last 5 years, intravenous drug users, residents and employees of long-term-care facilities or correctional institutions, nursing home residents, homeless shelter persons, and household members with close contacts of persons with known or suspected TB.

42 Answer b

The diagnostic test that should be used for screening of syphilis in the asymptomatic person is the rapid plasma reagin (RPR). If the RPR is positive, then further confirmation is done with the fluorescent treponemal antibody test (FTA-ABS) or the microhemagglutination test (MHA-TP).

43 Answer a

A patient with human immunodeficiency virus (HIV) infec-

tion is considered to have a positive Mantoux test if the induration is 5 mm or greater.

44 Answer b

Risk factors associated with stroke include atrial fibrillation, advancing age, diastolic and systolic hypertension, diabetes, smoking, history of prior transient ischemic attack (TIA), and hyperlipidemia.

45 Answer a

Routine screening should be done for hyperlipidemia, breast cancer, and cervical cancer. There is no data to support the routine screening of patients with asymptomatic disease.

46 Answer c

Elevated CA-125 is not diagnostic of ovarian cancer. CA-125 may be elevated in healthy women and in women with benign cysts or with nongynecologic tumors, and the levels may vary with the stage of disease. The incidence of ovarian cancer increases with age and has a high incidence in patients with a positive family history and women who have low parity.

47 Answer d

Prevalence is defined as the proportion of a group possessing a clinical condition at a given point in time. Positive predictive value is the probability of a patient with a positive test result not having the disease. Sensitivity is the proportion of people with a disease that have a positive test result. Specificity is the proportion of people without a disease that have a negative test result.

48 Answer b

Traveler's disease is most commonly caused by *Escherichia coli.*

49 Answer b

Patients traveling to South Africa should have yellow fever and poliomyelitis immunizations before departure. They should also receive prophylaxis against hepatitis A.

50 Answer d

The treatment of choice for malaria prophylaxis is 500 mg/wk of chloroquine (Aralen) for 1 to 2 weeks prior to travel. It should be continued during the stay and for 6 weeks after return.

51 Answer a

An infection of the teeth is known as dental caries. Consumption of sugar and cooked starches is a leading risk factor for tooth decay. Gingivitis is an infection of the gums and characterized by bleeding gums, pain, and erythema of the gums. Plaque is a thin film that grows on the teeth. Periodontitis is an infection that breaks down the periodontal ligament and results in bone loss.

52 Answer b

Healthy People 2010 is a national health-promotion and disease-prevention initiative to improve the health of all Americans, eliminate disparities in health, and improve years and quality of healthy life.

53 Answer a

The best intervention for elder abuse is prevention. After elder abuse has been identified, it is important to comply with state regulations in regard to reporting abuse. Also the elderly person should be informed about available resources for assistance, such as social workers, and given education about abuse.

54 Answer b

The most common site of nosocomial infections is the urinary tract, accounting for approximately 30% to 40% of all nosocomial infections. Surgical incisions are the second most common source of nosocomial infection.

55 Answer b

The person more likely to commit suicide is the elderly man with a recent loss. Suicide is more common in older men.

56 Answer c

The crude death rate is defined as the total number of deaths reported during a given interval divided by the estimated mid-interval population.

57 Answer b

A case-control study is an observational study in which affected and unaffected persons are identified after the fact and then compared regarding specific characteristics to determine possible association or risk factors for the disease.

58 Answer c

Bias is a systematic error that is unintentionally made. Causality denotes direct effect. Validity is the accuracy and reliability of a test. Efficacy is the true treatment and its effect.

59 Answer c

An institutional review board (IRB) may be composed of nurses, physicians, attorneys, and some laypersons. IRBs are federally mandated institutional committees that review research proposals for scientific value and ethical concerns. Informed consent is part of the IRB application and approval process.

60 Answer b

Persons with allergies to eggs should not receive the influenza vaccine.

61 Answer d

The reduction of sugar in the diet, topical fluoride applications, and community fluoridation of the water supply may all lead to a reduction of dental caries.

62 Answer b

Repetitive tasks may produce carpal tunnel syndrome, which is an occupational disorder.

63 Answer d

Human immunoglobulins are available for preventing hepatitis B, tetanus, and rabies. There are no immunoglobulins for the prevention of hepatitis A.

64 Answer b

The varicella vaccine, which is a live attenuated vaccine, should not be administered during pregnancy because of the risk of infecting the fetus and causing congenital abnormalities. Hepatitis B and influenza vaccines are inactivated and can be safely administered to pregnant women.

65 Answer b

Pneumococcal vaccine is not recommended for healthy persons younger than age 65. Indications for the pneumococcal vaccine include persons older than age 65 and those with anatomic or functional asplenia, nephrotic syndrome, sickle cell disease, chronic cardiac and pulmonary diseases, cirrhosis, and diabetes mellitus.

66 Answer d

First coitus before age 20 correlates highly with the development of cervical cancer. Research studies have shown a progressive increase in risk the earlier the first coitus, even if there are no other sexual partners. Early menarche, menopause before age 50, and achohol (ETOH) use have not been associated with cervical cancer.

67 Answer a

Married individuals have the lowest suicide rate.

68 Answer c

A high maternal AFP level may be seen in spina bifida.

69 Answer a

Ergonomics is the study of mechanical interactions between people and their living or work environments for the purposes of tailoring workplace design for better well-being. Occupational medicine is the diagnosis and treatment of disease caused by one's work environment. Environmental epidemiology is the study of environmental toxins and their effects on populations. Epidemiology is the study of disease in populations.

70 Answer d

Psittacosis is an influenza-like illness that affects pet shop owners and individuals who raise and process poultry. Tetanus is common in agricultural workers and may present with muscle spasms. Anthrax is an infection that manifests as skin ulcerations and is seen in handlers of imported hides and goat hair. Brucellosis is a bacterial infection that causes weight loss, fever, and malaise, and may affect packing-house workers, veterinarians, and laboratory workers.

71 Answer b

The American with Disabilities Act (ADA) of 1990 covers employment agencies, labor organizations, and employers. The Act prevents agencies from discriminating against a qualified individual with a disability and persons with human immunodeficiency virus (HIV) infection. The Act also helps secure access to health care.

72 Answer b

The accreditation of hospitals is carried out by the Joint Commission on Accreditation of Health Care Organizations (JCAHO).

73 Answer a

Hepatitis C is the most common cause of post-transfusion hepatitis.

74 Answer c

Hepatitis B can be prevented with immunizations.

75 Answer b

The incubation period for chickenpox is 10 to 21 days.

76 Answer a

Occult blood stool testing is recommended yearly for persons older than 50 years.

77 Answer c

In the person with an established disease process, measures taken to control the disease, such as stopping smoking, would be considered tertiary prevention because the disease process is still present.

78 Answer a

Routine immunizations are a form of primary prevention because the goal of immunizations is to prevent disease.

79 Answer b

The upper limit of acceptable noise exposure in the work place is 90 dB, as established by the Occupational Safety and Health Administration (OSHA).

80 Answer d

The leading cause of blindness in the United States is diabetes.

81 Answer b

Folate has been shown to decrease the risk of fetal anomalies, particularly neural tube defects. Folate should be taken prior to conception.

82 Answer b

The incidence of nosocomial (hospital-associated) infection is 5% to 10% with the incidence higher in chronic settings.

83 Answer b

The most commonly reported sexually transmitted disease is *Chlamydia.*

84 Answer a

Acute exacerbations of asthma have been linked to aspirin use, upper respiratory infections, dust, animal dander, environmental allergens, and stress. Caffeine has not been associated with asthma exacerbations. Caffeine is a methylxanthine and has bronchodilator properties.

85 Answer a

The development of osteoporosis is most closely correlated with age. It is more prevalent as women age, particularly in the postmenopausal period.

86 Answer c

Gastric carcinoma is more common in men than women. There is no increased risk of gastric carcinoma in smokers and persons with a history of gastric ulcers. Gastric carcinoma is more common in Japan than in other countries.

87 Answer b

Risk factors associated with development of colon cancer include a diet high in animal fat, a history of IBD or Crohn's disease, and a diet low in fiber.

88 Answer d

Symptoms of lead poisoning include headache, abdominal pain, memory loss, ataxia, anemia, renal toxicity, and peripheral neuropathy.

89 Answer d

Clinical features associated with fetal alcohol syndrome include microcephaly, mild to moderate mental retardation, cleft palate, congenital cardiac defects, and joint deformities.

90 Answer d

Prevention of fetal alcohol syndrome may be done through education of the public regarding the dangers of drinking during pregnancy, maternal alcohol abstinence during pregnancy, and identification of women at greatest risk.

91 Answer b

The mental retardation associated with fetal alcohol syndrome (FAS) is not reversible. The incidence of FAS is less than 1%; however, the infant mortality rate is 20% in affected infants and usually occurs in the first 2 weeks of life. Binge drinking increases the risk of FAS.

92 Answer b

Down syndrome is an alteration in chromosome 21. The types of Down syndrome may be trisomy 21, translocation, and trisomy mosaic 21.

93 Answer d

Functional status provides information about general physical health, overall quality of life, and the ability to perform activities of daily living. An assessment of functional status should be done during all health-care visits.

94 Answer b

A woman with human immunodeficiency virus (HIV) infection should not breastfeed because of the possibility of HIV transmission via breast milk.

95 Answer c

The first prenatal visit should include a breast exam, hemoglobin and hematocrit levels to check for anemia, and a Pap smear. A mammogram is not indicated.

96 Answer b

Polio is associated with paralysis. Measles may be associated with pneumonia, encephalitis, and mental retardation.

97 Answer b

Epidemiology is the science that forms the basis for public health action. Public health is the application of preventive medicine techniques. Secondary prevention is the early detection and prompt treatment of disease. Health is a state of complete physical, mental, and social well-being.

98 Answer a

The information provided is an example of a clinical trial. A clinical trial is an experimental study design used to assess differences in groups receiving different treatment modalities or interventions. A cohort study is an observational study in which populations are identified and followed prospectively. A case report is an objective report of a clinical event or outcome. The patients are already diagnosed with lung cancer, so this is not a primary prevention trial.

99 Answer d

Hepatocellular carcinoma is associated with the hepatitis B virus.

100 Answer c

The approach to the patient described should include a personalized message concerning smoking cessation and reassessment at the next visit. It is important to assess smoking status at each visit and advise patients to quit smoking to help motivate them. You should focus on the death of the patient's sibling, which was smoking related. Smoking cessation classes, self-help materials, and use of a nicotine patch are only effective when the person is committed to smoking cessation.

101 Answer b

The National Cholesterol Education Program (NCEP) guidelines recommend pharmacologic therapy for patients despite dietary intervention if the LDL level remains more than 190 in the absence of coronary heart disease and the patient has fewer than two risk factors, the LDL level is more than 160 in the absence of coronary heart disease and two or more risk factors, and the LDL level is more than 130 in the presence of coronary heart disease.

102 Answer c

Isolated systolic hypertension, which is as serious as diastolic hypertension, is a risk factor for stroke and should be aggressively treated.

103 Answer d

The most reliable screening test for the detection of lead poisoning is a serum lead level. The hemoglobin, ferritin level, and complete blood cell count are all usually abnormal in persons with lead poisoning, but are not diagnostic.

104 Answer c

The most effective method for screening for alcohol abuse is to administer a standardized questionnaire such as the CAGE questionnaire.

105 Answer a

Poor bone mineralization and osteoporosis are associated with a deficiency in calcium and vitamin D.

106 Answer c

Niacin deficiency causes pellagra, which is associated with dermatitis, diarrhea, and delirium.

107 Answer a

Tay-Sachs disease is more common in Ashkenazic Jews.

108 Answer b

Typhoid fever may be controlled by proper sanitation. Typhoid fever is caused by *Salmonella typhi* and is excreted in the feces of the human carrier.

109 Answer c

Botulism is an intoxication produced by *Clostridium botulinum*. Cases of botulism are associated with improper handling of home-canned vegetables, fish, and fruits. Early symptoms include visual disturbances and sore throat, it has an incubation period of 12 to 36 hours, and an antitoxin should be administered to treat it.

110 Answer b

If the positive predictive value of a given disease is 5%, then in a sample of 100 positive results there would be 5 persons who are true positives.

111 Answer a

Prevalence is the proportion of a group possessing a clinical condition at a given point in time. Sensitivity is the proportion of people with a disease who have a positive test. Specificity is the true negative rate. Negative predictive value is the probability of not having the disease in a person with a negative test.

112 Answer b

Yellow fever and polio immunizations should be given prior to travel to Africa. Smallpox immunization is no longer recommended. Immunoglobulin can be given for hepatitis A, but should be given 2 weeks before travel to be effective. Pneumococcal vaccine is not indicated.

113 Answer c

The leading cause of food poisoning in the United States is *Salmonella.*

114 Answer d

Risk factors associated with salmonella food poisoning include human immunodeficiency virus (HIV) infection, antacid use, diabetes mellitus, decreased gastrointestinal motility, altered intestinal flora, and history of gastrectomy.

115 Answer c

Doxycycline (Vibramycin) may be prescribed as a prophylaxis for malaria.

116 Answer b

The epidemic period for influenza is October to December.

117 Answer c

Elevated levels of homocystine are associated with thrombosis and the development of premature coronary artery disease.

118 Answer d

Leading health indicators identified by the Healthy People 2010 agenda include physical activity, obesity, tobacco use, substance abuse, sexual behavior, mental health, injuries and violence, environmental quality, immunizations, and access to health care. Combating anorexia nervosa is not one of the indicators.

119 Answer b

Screening for diabetes is recommended in persons with a family history of diabetes and those who are obese or have glucose abnormalities during pregnancy. Screening is not recommended in persons with anemia.

120 Answer a

The most common risk factor associated with hepatic cirrhosis is alcohol consumption.

121 Answer c

Hepatitis A is common in day-care centers and institutions where people are crowded together and sanitation is poor.

122 Answer a

Cats are generally not carriers of rabies. Raccoons, bats, foxes and skunks may be carriers of rabies.

123 Answer b

Artificially acquired immunity is when individuals are immunized with vaccines. Natural immunity is acquired immunity. Passive immunity is antibody protection received from the mother early in life.

124 Answer d

Persons with an allergy to eggs should not receive the influenza vaccine.

125 Answer b

Pertussis is highly contagious and communicable, is more prevalent in children (not adults), and is usually associated with elevated temperatures, shock, and seizures. Permanent neurologic damage and death may occur.

126 Answer d

Potential complications of mumps include deafness, orchitis, and encephalitis.

127 Answer b

The Centers for Disease Control and Prevention (CDC) recommends that all dialysis patients receive the hepatitis B vaccine. However, despite these recommendations, fewer than 30% of all hemodialysis patients have received the vaccine.

128 Answer c

Pelvic Inflammatory Disease (PID) may be caused by *Neiserria gonorrhea* or *Chlamydia*. It may lead to infertility and is associated with an increased frequency of ectopic pregnancies. It has not been associated with Kaposi's sarcoma.

129 Answer a

The incidence of sexually transmitted diseases (STDs) may be decreased by limiting the number of sexual partners.

130 Answer a

An untreated syphilis infection may lead to aortitis, with aortic aneurysms. Other complications include psychosis and blindness.

131 Answer a

A 25-year-old pregnant woman should be screened for syphilis as a means of preventing congenital syphilis. Other persons who should be screened are those with multiple sexual partners and those who have other STDs.

132 Answer b

The United States Preventive Services Task Force (USPSTF) recommends an exercise electrocardiogram (ECG) for men over age 40 who have two or more risk factors for heart disease and who are about to begin a vigorous exercise program.

133 Answer a

The American Cancer Society (ACS) recommends that prostate cancer screening with a prostate-specific antigen (PSA) test be performed annually in men over age 50.

134 Answer d

Women should avoid pregnancy for 3 months after immunization with the rubella vaccine because of the potential risk to the fetus. Fetal abnormalities associated with rubella include blindness, deafness, mental retardation, and congenital cardiac anomalies. Persons with neomycin allergy should receive the oral polio vaccine.

135 Answer b

The benefits of exercise include a decrease in LDL cholesterol level, blood pressure, and triglyceride level. HDL cholesterol is increased with exercise. Exercise improves glucose metabolism and increases insulin sensitivity.

136 Answer a

A 60-year-old sunbather with a family history of melanoma is at increased risk for skin cancer. Persons with a family history of melanoma, increased exposure to the sun, and a personal history of precancerous skin lesions are all at risk for the development of skin cancer. Preventive measures include avoiding sun exposure between the hours of 11 AM and 3 PM and use of sunscreen and protective clothing.

137 Answer c

The Folstein Mini-Mental State exam is a well-recognized tool for assessing cognitive function. The MAST and CAGE questionnaires assess for alcohol abuse.

138 Answer d

Prevention of falls in the elderly may include removing throw rugs from the home, using assistive devices, installing safety bars in bathrooms, and keeping areas well lighted, particularly at night.

139 Answer b

The preventive health measures of a mammogram and Pap smear should be recommended for the patient described. Colonoscopy is a recommended screening, not preventive measure, unless the patient has a family history of ulcerative colitis. A computed tomogrpahy (CT) scan of the chest is not a preventive health measure. There is no information that would support immunization for hepatitis B.

140 Answer c

Health-care workers are at risk for the development of hepatitis.

141 Answer a

Female heterosexuals (not male homosexuals) are the fastest growing group of people infected with human immunodeficiency virus (HIV). A woman has approximately a 50% (not 10%) chance of transmitting HIV to the fetus.

142 Answer d

Syphilis is not transmitted via blood-bank blood because the spirochete responsible for the disease is killed by the 24- to 48-hour refrigeration process before transfusion. Blood-bank blood is screened for cytomegalovirus (CMV), human immunodeficiency virus (HIV), and hepatitis C; however, it is possible to transmit each of these viruses during transfusion.

143 Answer a

Foundry workers are at an increased risk for developing asbestosis, silicosis, lung cancer, and pleural disease. Hazardous exposures include aromatic hydrocarbons, metal dust, and fumes.

144 Answer b

Crisis intervention is a form of secondary prevention. Secondary prevention is provision of treatment to minimize sequelae and disability.

145 Answer b

Medicare part A covers inpatient services, limited skilled nursing facility care, and home care. Medicare part B covers physician services, outpatient services, and medical supplies.

146 Answer a

Risk factors for the development of diabetes mellitus include obesity, age older than 45 years, hypertension, and being African-American, Hispanic, or Asian-American.

147 Answer b

The United States Preventive Services Task Force (USPSTF) recommendations for smoking-cessation counseling include tobacco-cessation counseling at each visit.

148 Answer d

Symptoms of nicotine withdrawal include irritability, restlessness, anger, anxiety, inability to concentrate, and increased appetite.

149 Answer b

The average age for a person to begin smoking today is 15 years.

150 Answer b

Nontreponemal Venereal Disease Research Laboratories

(VDRL) or rapid plasma reagin (RPR) may be used to screen for syphilis. If the test is positive, then fluorescent treponemal antibody absorption (FTA-ABS) or microhemagglutination–Treponema pallidum (MHA-TP) is used.

151 Answer a

Side effects associated with hormone replacement therapy include vaginal bleeding, bloating, breast tenderness, irritability, depression, and headaches.

152 Answer a

A 55-year-old woman with ulcerative colitis should have a baseline colonoscopy to screen for colon cancer.

153 Answer c

The second leading cause of cancer-related deaths in men is prostate cancer; the first is lung cancer.

154 Answer a

The next step in a patient with two abnormal Pap smears is to perform a colposcopy.

155 Answer c

The leading cause of cancer deaths in men and women is lung cancer.

156 Answer b

For the patient described, the PPD should be repeated in 2 to 4 weeks to allow for anamnestic response in an attempt to prevent a false diagnosis.

157 Answer b

The primary goal of screening is to detect a disease process in the hopes of altering the natural history of a given disease process.

158 Answer d

Stool for occult blood should be done as part of health screening in the patient described.

159 Answer d

Health Maintenance Organizations (HMOs) provide both inpatient and outpatient services through a referral system.

160 Answer a

A healthy 65-year-old man should receive an annual influenza vaccine.

161 Answer b

Radon exposure is a risk factor for lung cancer.

162 Answer d

The initial management of spousal abuse includes a nonjudgmental inquiry about the possibility of abuse.

163 Answer d

A normal grief reaction may include weight loss, insomnia, and periods of crying.

164 Answer b

Immunizations are a primary prevention measure. Mammography and occult blood testing of stool are secondary prevention measures. HIV testing is a secondary prevention measure.

165 Answer b

Typhoid fever vaccinations should be administered to persons who are traveling to countries with endemic typhoid. There is no evidence that immunizations after earthquakes or disasters are effective.

166 Answer a

The organism usually responsible for traveler's diarrhea is *Escherichia coli.*

167 Answer b

The total daily iron requirement for a woman with a normal pregnancy is 800 to 1000 mg.

168 Answer a

The antibiotic of choice to treat traveler's diarrhea is ciprofloxacin (Cipro).

169 Answer a

Meningococcal meningitis outbreaks may be treated with rifampin (Rifadin) and ceftriaxone (Rocephin).

170 Answer c

The most common mental illness in young adults is schizophrenia.

Bibliography

Dunphy, L: Management Guidelines for Adult Nurse Practitioners. FA Davis, Philadelphia, 1999.

Gardner, P, et al: Adult immunizations. Ann Intern Med 12:35, 1996.

Goroll, A, et al: Primary Care Medicine Office Evaluation and Management of the Adult Patient, 4th ed. Lippincott Williams & Wilkins, Philadelphia, 2000.

Gross, PA, et al: The efficacy of the influenza vaccine in elderly persons: A meta-analysis and review of the literature. Ann Intern Med 125:518, 1975.

Portaels, F: Epidemiology of mycobacterial diseases. Clin Dermatol 13:207, 1995.

Prevention of pneumococcal disease. Recommendations of the Advisory Committee on Immunization Practices. MMWR Morb Mortal Wkly Rep 46(RR-8):1, 1997.

Saag, MS: Candidate antiretroviral agents for use in postexposure prophylaxis. Am J Med 102 (supplement 5B):25, 1997.

PRACTICE EXAMINATIONS

Examination 1

1 *A heart transplantation recipient develops bradycardia. What is the best medication to treat this problem?*

a Dopamine (Intropin)
b Metoprolol (Lopressor)
c Isoproterenol (Isuprel)
d Atropine

2 *A 35-year-old woman has been positive for human immunodeficiency virus (HIV) for the past 5 years, and within the past 3 months she developed acquired immunodeficiency syndrome (AIDS). Which of the following is an AIDS-defining illness?*

a Herpes simplex
b Epstein-Barr virus (EBV)
c Peripheral neuropathy
d Invasive cervical cancer

3 *The most common cause of chronic pancreatitis is:*

a alcohol abuse.
b cholecystitis.
c pancreatic cancer.
d diabetes mellitus.

4 *All of the following are clinical manifestations of right ventricular failure* **EXCEPT:**

a edema.
b ascites.
c jugular vein distention.
d crackles.

5 *A 48-year-old woman is seen in your clinic with complaints of hot flashes, irritability, and weight gain. You suspect menopause. Which of the following test results would confirm your diagnosis?*

a Low estrogen level
b High follicle-stimulating hormone (FSH) and lutenizing hormone (LH) levels

c Normal estrogen level
d Normal prolactin level

6 *The most common cause of bacterial pneumonia in persons infected with human immunodeficiency virus (HIV) is:*

a *Pneumococcus.*
b *Staphylococcus.*
c *Pneumocystis carinii.*
d *Histoplasma.*

7 *The initial therapy of choice in patients with acute pulmonary embolus is:*

a warfarin (Coumadin).
b heparin.
c aspirin.
d an inferior vena cava filter.

8 *Disseminated intravascular coagulopathy (DIC) is characterized by:*

a normal prothrombin time (PT) and activated partial thromboplastin time (APTT).
b an elevated platelet count.
c a decreased fibrinogen level.
d anemia.

9 *At what age should all women have a baseline mammogram?*

a 50
b Between 35 and 40
c 45
d 30

10 *The diagnostic gold standard for the detection of prostate cancer is a(n):*

a prostate-specific antigen (PSA) level.
b alkaline phosphatase level.

c transrectal ultrasound.
d digital rectal examination.

11 *A 70-year-old man has prostatitis. The duration of antibiotic treatment should be:*

a 3 days.
b 14 days.
c 1 day.
d 7 days.

12 *Treatment of uric acid stones includes:*

a diuretics.
b a parathyroidectomy.
c allopurinol (Zyloprim).
d potassium citrate.

13 *A 45-year-old nurse is seen with a complaint of weakness and fatigue for the past 2 months. She is able to work for 8 hours, but is exhausted by the end of the day. She is unable to find a comfortable position to rest. She has lost 10 lb over the past 2 months. Her physical exam is normal. What is the most likely diagnosis?*

a Hyperthyroidism
b Polymyalgia rheumatica
c Rheumatoid arthritis
d Depression

14 *A 35-year-old secretary in a busy law firm complains of a 4-week history of awakening at night with left hand discomfort that spontaneously resolves. Physical exam reveals limited thumb abduction and decreased pain response on the palmar aspect of the thumb and left index finger. What is the most likely diagnosis?*

a Carpal tunnel syndrome
b Left wrist fracture
c Arthritis
d Transient ischemic attack (TIA)

15 *The initial mainstay of treatment for Parkinson's disease is:*

a amantadine (Symmetrel).
b carbidopa/levodopa combinations.
c steroids.
d bromocriptine (Parlodel).

16 *Which of the following is a contraindication to renal allograft transplantation?*

a Diabetes mellitus
b Previous steroid use
c AIDS
d Hypertension

17 *Which of the following abnormalities would you expect in a patient after partial gastric resection?*

a Vitamin B_{12} deficiency
b Iron-deficiency anemia
c Anemia of chronic disease
d Vitamin B_6 deficiency

18 *Total lung capacity is the:*

a amount of functional residual capacity that can be expelled by maximal respiratory effort.
b volume of air in the lungs after a maximal inspiratory effort.
c volume of air in one breath during normal quiet breathing.
d volume of air forcefully expired during the first second after a deep breath.

19 *Which of the following physical findings would you expect in a person admitted with congestive heart failure exacerbation?*

a Normal heart sounds
b A fourth heart sound
c A diastolic murmur
d A third heart sound

20 *Which of the following may cause a reversible form of cardiomyopathy?*

a Alcohol abuse
b Doxorubicin (Adriamycin) therapy
c Amyloidosis
d Myocardial infarction

21 *The most common presenting symptom in patients with esophageal cancer is:*

a weight loss.
b cough.
c dysphagia.
d hoarseness.

22 *A 25-year-old man having a routine physical exam is noted to have xanthomas on his neck and forehead. Xanthomas are associated with:*

a diabetes mellitus.
b peptic ulcer disease.
c hypertension.
d hyperlipidemia.

23 *The most common cause of pulsus paradoxus is:*

a right ventricular infarction.
b cardiac tamponade.
c constrictive pericarditis.
d mitral stenosis.

24 *The upper quadrant of the liver is located on examination by:*

a palpation.
b percussion.

c the scratch test.
d auscultation.

25 *Which of the following conditions is associated with a fixed split of the second heart sound?*

a Atrial septal defect
b Ventricular septal defect
c Aortic stenosis
d Mitral valve prolapse

26 *Which of the following nerves supply the lateral rectus muscle of the eye?*

a Trochlear nerve
b Oculomotor nerve
c Abducens nerve
d Olfactory nerve

27 *Dorsiflexion or extension of the great toe in response to stroking the lateral aspect of the sole of the foot is:*

a Kernig's sign.
b Romberg's sign.
c Tinel sign
d Babinski's sign

28 *Tophi are found in patients with:*

a rheumatoid arthritis.
b gouty arthritis.
c Lyme disease.
d sarcoidosis.

29 *A 70-year-old woman had a tracheotomy 3 days ago, and the staff nurse notifies you that there is a large amount of bright red blood coming from the tracheotomy site. What is the most likely cause of this finding?*

a Erosion of the carotid artery
b Tracheal fistula
c Erosion of the subclavian artery
d Erosion of the innominate artery

30 *The electrolyte imbalance seen in patients with chronic hypoxia is:*

a hyperkalemia.
b hypochloremia.
c acidosis.
d hypocalcemia.

31 *Which of the following is a contraindication to heart transplantation?*

a Irreversible pulmonary hypertension
b Hepatitis B infection
c Diabetes mellitus
d Ventricular assist device longer than 120 days

32 *Which of the following medications are routinely used after coronary stenting?*

a Isosorbide mononitrate (Imdur)
b Nifedipine (Procardia)
c Clopidogrel (Plavix)
d Diltiazem (Cardizem)

33 *Which of the following conditions is a contraindication to intra-aortic balloon pump (IABP) placement?*

a Coronary ischemia
b Severe aortic insufficiency
c Myocardial infarction
d Mitral regurgitation

34 *All of the following are diastolic murmurs EXCEPT:*

a mitral stenosis.
b aortic regurgitation.
c tricuspid stenosis.
d pulmonic stenosis.

35 *The cardiac valve most frequently affected by rheumatic fever is the:*

a pulmonic valve.
b mitral valve.
c aortic valve.
d tricuspid valve.

36 *The most common type of vaginal infection is:*

a *Trichomonas.*
b *Candida.*
c bacterial vaginosis.
d syphilis.

37 *What is the best indicator of renal function?*

a Blood urea nitrogen (BUN) level
b Creatinine level
c Urine output.
d Glomerular filtration rate (GFR)

38 *The owner of a deli reported that one of his workers, who prepares all the sandwiches, was just diagnosed with hepatitis A. Recommendations to prevent further spread of the hepatitis A virus include:*

a giving immunoglobulin G (IgG) to all family members of the worker.
b giving IgG to all persons who ate sandwiches at the deli during the last 3 weeks.
c advising the worker not to return to work until he is over the acute illness.
d closing the deli for 2 weeks.

39 *All of the following are risk factors for lung cancer EXCEPT:*

a family history.
b smoking.
c air pollution.
d occupational exposure.

40 *Medicaid was designed to serve persons who are:*

a unemployed.
b indigent.
c chronically ill.
d over the age of 65.

41 *Vitamin A deficiency is associated with:*

a night blindness.
b hearing loss.
c osteoporosis.
d gastric ulcers.

42 *The most common adverse effect associated with cyclosporine is:*

a headache.
b nephrotoxicity.
c anemia.
d syncope.

43 *A 40-year-old man is brought to the emergency department in a comatose state after an overdose of poison. The patient has a strong odor of almonds present on his body. What is the most likely cause of his poisoning?*

a Acetaminophen (Tylenol)
b Aspirin
c Methanol
d Cyanide

44 *A 35-year-old woman is receiving a blood transfusion secondary to an upper gastrointestinal bleed. The staff nurse notifies you that the patient is complaining of chills and has a temperature of 102°F. What is the most appropriate recommendation?*

a Notify the transfusion medicine department.
b Stop the transfusion.
c Continue the transfusion and monitor for increasing temperatures.
d Give 650 mg of acetaminophen and continue the transfusion.

45 *A patient with type 2 diabetes who requires insulin is suspected of having the Somogyi effect. What is the most appropriate treatment?*

a Decrease the insulin dose.
b Increase the insulin dose.
c Tell the patient to have a nighttime snack.
d Increase the insulin dose and add an oral antihypoglycemic agent.

46 *Laboratory findings in a patient with diabetes insipidus include a(n):*

a increased urinary osmolarity.
b decreased urinary osmolarity and increased urinary specific gravity.
c decreased serum osmolarity.
d decreased urine osmolarity and increased serum osmolarity.

47 *Azidothymidine (AZT) is commonly used to treat HIV infection. Common side effects associated with this medication include:*

a diarrhea.
b hypotension.
c peripheral neuropathy.
d bradycardia.

48 *Which of the following medications is used acutely to treat aortic dissection?*

a Dopamine (Inotropin)
b Nitroprusside (Nipride)
c Dobutamine (Dobutrex)
d Epinephrine

49 *Which of the following statements concerning burn injuries is correct?*

a Burns are more common in elderly patients.
b Most burns require inpatient care.
c Mortality is increased in elderly patients if the burn exceeds 25% of body surface area.
d Most burn-related deaths are the result of a motor vehicle accident.

50 *Which of the following is the most reliable physical finding in appendicitis?*

a Localized right lower quadrant pain
b Tenderness on rectal examination
c Right upper quadrant pain
d Diarrhea

51 *The most common tumor of the anterior mediastinal compartment in adults is:*

a lymphoma.
b substernal thyroid.
c thymoma.
d teratoma.

52 *A 50-year-old woman is seen in your clinic complaining of an acute onset of visual loss in the right eye. She states she felt like a curtain was being lowered as she was watching television. She denies pain or any trauma to the eye. What is the most likely diagnosis?*

a Glaucoma
b Retinitis

c Central retinal artery occlusion
d Retinal detachment

53 *A 50-year-old man has complaints of severe headache in the temporal area and blurred vision. He has pain upon palpation of the temporal area, without erythema. What is the most likely diagnosis?*

a Temporal arteritis
b Migraine headache
c Sinusitis
d Transient ischemic attack (TIA)

54 *A 25-year-old woman is involved in a motor vehicle accident and has suffered a closed head injury. In the intensive care unit, she is unresponsive, and her urine output has been 30 cc/h for the past 2 hours with a serum sodium level of 124. The most likely cause of this clinical scenario is:*

a syndrome of inappropriate antidiuretic hormone (SIADH).
b diabetes mellitus.
c stroke.
d adrenal crisis.

55 *Symptoms of a subarachnoid hemorrhage include all of the following* **EXCEPT:**

a headache.
b hypotension.
c photophobia.
d fever.

56 *A 55-year-old woman has suffered a massive cerebral hemorrhage after abdominal aortic aneurysm surgery. She is declared brain dead by the neurologist and identified as a potential organ donor. She is married, but legally separated, and has two daughters ages 18 and 24. Her mother is 78 and is still living. Who can give permission for organ donation in this case?*

a Her children
b Her mother
c Her husband
d Her 24-year-old child

57 *Neuropathy associated with diabetes may cause:*

a orthostatic hypotension.
b gastroparesis.
c sexual dysfunction.
d all of the above.

58 *Risk factors for type 2 diabetes include all of the following* **EXCEPT:**

a obesity.
b male sex.
c family history.
d ancestry.

59 *The leading cause of blindness in the adult in the United States is:*

a glaucoma.
b retinal detachment.
c diabetes mellitus.
d hypertension.

60 *Which of the following may lead to hypoglycemia in a patient with type 2 diabetes?*

a Excessive alcohol intake
b Fever
c Stress
d Lack of exercise

61 *Which of the following findings would you expect in a patient with adrenal insufficiency?*

a Hypertension
b Hypernatremia
c Hypokalemia
d Hyperkalemia

62 *What is the most common cause of Cushing's syndrome?*

a Hypertension
b Type 2 diabetes
c Pituitary adenoma
d Osteoporosis

63 *The most common arrhythmia associated with myocardial contusion is:*

a complete heart block.
b supraventricular tachycardia.
c ventricular fibrillation.
d sinus arrhythmia.

64 *A 20-year-old woman is seen with increasing obesity, amenorrhea, hypertension, and abdominal striae. Which of the following tests should be performed to support your diagnosis?*

a Thyroid function test
b Cortisol level
c Follicle stimulating hormone (FSH) and luteinizing hormone (LH) levels
d Overnight dexamethasone suppression test

65 *A 50-year-old woman was prescribed diazepam three times daily for anxiety. She decided to double her dose because she thinks it is not effective at the current dose. She is found by her daughter and is lethargic with shallow breathing. She is taken to the emergency department. Which of the following medications should be given as an antidote?*

a Naloxone (Narcan)
b Acetylcysteine (Mucomyst)

c Flumazenil (Romazicon)
d Activated charcoal

66 *Which of the following medications may cause hearing loss?*

a Penicillin
b Gentamicin (Garamycin)
c Acetaminophen (Tylenol)
d Toradol (Ketorolac)

67 *A 25-year-old man is involved in an altercation and suffers a human bite on the hand. What is the appropriate management of this wound?*

a Perform primary closure and start broad-spectrum antibiotics.
b Obtain a surgical consultation with a plastic surgeon.
c Leave the wound open for 24 hours and have the patient return in 24 hours for primary closure.
d Thoroughly irrigate the wound, and do not close.

68 *A 50-year-old woman complains of left-sided chest discomfort for the past week. She noted a group of vesicles in the same location 2 days ago. What is the most likely diagnosis?*

a Herpes zoster
b Pneumothorax
c Pulmonary embolus
d Pericarditis

69 *Stevens-Johnson syndrome is commonly caused by the use of:*

a trimethoprim sulfamethoxazole (Bactrim DS).
b aspirin.
c penicillin.
d erythromycin (E-Mycin).

70 *A 25-year-old woman is seen with complaints of headache, pressure sensation, and facial pain under the right eye, which is worst with bending forward, for 1 week. What is the most likely diagnosis?*

a Frontal sinusitis
b Ethmoid sinusitis
c Maxillary sinusitis
d None of the above

71 *The most common cause of home accidents is:*

a a fire.
b a fall.
c medication overdose.
d violence.

72 *Which of the following patients should receive prophylactic antibiotics prior to dental procedures?*

a A 50-year-old woman with no known health problems
b A 55-year-old man with a holosystolic murmur at the apex
c An 18-year-old man with a third heart sound
d A 70-year-old man with diabetes mellitus and coronary artery disease

73 *Which of the following is a sign of hepatic encephalopathy?*

a Hematemesis
b Dullness on abdominal examination
c Icteric sclera
d Asterixis of the hands

74 *A 90-year-old woman had a left total hip replacement 3 days ago and complains of shortness of breath. Physical exam reveals an elderly woman in moderate distress, with a respiratory rate of 40, heart rate of 128 and blood pressure of 80/60 mm Hg. The lung sounds are decreased at the base, and the heart tones are normal. An electrocardiogram (ECG) reveals atrial fibrillation with a ventricular rate of 130. What is the most likely diagnosis?*

a Pulmonary embolus
b Aspiration pneumonia
c Myocardial infarction
d Postoperative atelectasis

75 *All of the following statements concerning migraine headaches are true* **EXCEPT:**

a migraines are usually unilateral temporal headaches.
b attacks may be precipitated by stress and foods that contain tyramine.
c migraines are usually bilateral and viselike headaches.
d propranolol (Inderal) may be used as a prophylactic medication to treat migraines.

76 *A 55-year-old woman is on peritoneal dialysis. Which of the following indicate normal peritoneal dialysate drainage?*

a Mucoid drainage
b Clear and straw-colored fluid
c Cloudy fluid
d None of the above

77 *A 30-year-old woman is being treated with methotrexate for psoriatic arthritis. What are some of the potential side effects of methotrexate?*

a Hematemesis
b Dermatitis
c Bone marrow suppression
d Hemorrhagic cystitis

78 *Which of the following medications should be prescribed to treat side effects associated with the use of isoniazid (INH) and rifampin (Rifadin)?*

a Vitamin B$_{12}$
b Vitamin B$_6$
c Magnesium oxide
d Calcium

79 *Which of the following types of breath sounds may be heard over pleural effusions?*

a Vesicular
b Bronchial
c Absent
d All of the above

80 *The bleating and goatlike sound produced by the patient's voice when heard over the chest is known as:*

a normal breath sounds.
b bronchophony.
c egophony.
d pectoriloquy.

81 *Stretch marks that are located either on the flanks or lateral aspects of the abdomen are called:*

a striae.
b ecchymosis.
c petechiae.
d angiomas.

82 *A firm liver on physical exam is usually associated with:*

a ascites.
b passive congestion.
c cirrhosis.
d hepatic carcinoma.

83 *A 35-year-old obese woman is seen with complaints of abdominal pain and nausea for the past 2 months associated with fatty food ingestion. On physical exam, she has a positive Murphy's sign. What is the most likely diagnosis?*

a Acute appendicitis
b Pancreatitis
c Cholecystitis
d Hepatitis

84 *What is the best modality for assessing renal size?*

a Palpation
b Percussion
c Abdominal computed tomography (CT) scan
d Ultrasound

85 *The most common cause of unilateral scrotal swelling is:*

a congestive heart failure.
b a variocele.
c a spermatocele.
d a hydrocele.

86 *Fixed or matted axillary nodes are usually associated with a(n):*

a malignancy.
b local infection.
c sebaceous cyst.
d upper arm ischemia.

87 *A 70-year-old man complains of dizziness and the inability to hear. Which cranial nerve has been affected?*

a Cranial nerve II
b Cranial nerve IV
c Cranial nerve VIII
d Cranial nerve V

88 *The American Heart Association (AHA) recommends a baseline resting ECG for:*

a no one; there is no recommendation for screening.
b all persons over age 60.
c all men over age 50.
d all men and women over age 40.

89 *A 65-year-old man with diabetes is recovering in a rehabilitation setting after having an above-the-knee amputation performed 6 weeks ago. Which of the following types of pain may he experience?*

a Phantom pain
b Neuropathic pain
c Visceral pain
d Somatic pain

90 *All of the following are risk factors for the development of endometrial cancer* **EXCEPT:**

a pelvic irradiation.
b early menopause.
c a history of breast cancer.
d a history of diabetes mellitus.

91 *A 50-year-old woman is admitted for elective thyroid surgery. The preoperative lab work revealed an abnormal white blood cell count, and you suspect leukemia. As the acute care nurse practitioner (ACNP), what is the next most appropriate step?*

a Consult with the surgeon, and plan for a bone marrow biopsy.
b Refer the patient to an oncologist for evaluation.
c Discuss a bone marrow transplantation with the patient.
d Order chest and abdominal computed tomography (CT) scans.

92 *Which of the following medications may be used in an induction protocol for a patient with acute lymphocytic leukemia (ALL)?*

a Prednisone
b Vincristine (Oncovin)
c Doxorubicin (Adriamycin)
d All of the above

93 *The presence of Reed-Sternberg cells on biopsy is diagnostic of:*

a non-Hodgkin's lymphoma.
b chronic lymphocytic leukemia.
c metastatic cancer.
d Hodgkin's disease.

94 *The reticulocyte count indicates the:*

a size of the red blood cell.
b distribution of the red blood cells.
c bone marrow's response to anemia.
d morphology of the red blood cells.

Questions 95–98 refer to the following scenario:

A 45-year-old woman with uterine fibroids is seen complaining of increased fatigue and shortness of breath over the last 6 weeks. Her hemoglobin is 8.5 g/dL. Physical exam is normal. You suspect iron-deficiency anemia.

95 *Which of the following laboratory findings would you expect in this patient?*

a Decreased ferritin level and increased total iron-binding capacity (TIBC)
b Elevated mean corpuscle volume (MCV)
c Elevated reticulocyte count
d Decreased red blood cell distribution width (RDW)

96 *The appropriate management of this patient is to:*

a arrange for a transfusion of 2 units of packed red blood cells.
b start intravenous iron therapy.
c refer for a bone marrow biopsy.
d start oral iron supplements.

97 *Which of the following dietary recommendations should be made to increase iron levels?*

a Green leafy vegetables
b Organ meats
c Apricots
d All of the above

98 *The patient is seen 3 months later with persistent complaints of fatigue. The hemoglobin is 9.0 g/dL. She has been taking iron supplements three times a day for the past 3 months. As the ACNP, what is your next step in the plan of care?*

a Continue the iron therapy for another 3 months.
b Refer the patient to a hematologist for evaluation.
c Order a bleeding scan.
d Start erythropoietin (Epogen).

99 *Acute tumor lysis syndrome is characterized by which of the following electrolyte abnormalities?*

a Hypouricemia and hypercalcemia
b Hypocalcemia and hypokalemia
c Hyperphosphatemia and hypercalcemia
d Hyperkalemia and hypocalcemia

100 *The most common cause of intestinal obstruction is a(n):*

a adhesion.
b tumor.
c ischemic bowel.
d umbilical hernia.

101 *A 30-year-old woman is admitted to the hospital with an acute exacerbation of asthma. What is the most appropriate treatment regime?*

a Intravenous theophylline and inhaled corticosteroids
b An oral beta-2 agonist
c Inhaled corticosteroids
d An inhaled beta-2 agonist and oral corticosteroids

102 *The most common cause(s) of blood transfusion reaction is(are):*

a clerical error.
b prior antibodies.
c massive transfusion.
d all of the above.

103 *Serum carcinoembryonic antigen (CEA):*

a is a good screening tool for colon cancer.
b may be used to follow the progression of breast cancer.
c is usually elevated in metastatic colon cancer.
d is a marker for prostate cancer.

104 *Which of the following intravenous fluids is similar to plasma composition?*

a Lactated Ringer's injection
b Total parenteral nutrition (TPN)
c 5% dextrose in normal saline (D5NS)
d Normal saline solution

105 *A 40-year-old carpenter accidentally amputated his thumb with a power saw. The amputated thumb should be transported to the emergency department:*

a in a clean plastic bag filled with Betadine.
b in a sterile gauze dressing.

c in a clean sealed plastic bag and placed in a cooler with crushed ice.
d in no particular fashion because there is no need to transport the thumb because the rate of re-implantation is low.

106 *What is the most common cause of hypoparathyroidism?*

a Carcinoma of the parathyroid
b Altered calcium metabolism
c Chronic renal failure
d Previous thyroid surgery

107 *Which of the following statements concerning adult respiratory distress syndrome (ARDS) is true?*

a Patients with ARDS initially have metabolic acidosis.
b Peak inspiratory pressures are usually low.
c The initial chest x-ray may be normal.
d The respiratory effort decreases.

108 *Which of the following treatments may slow the progression of diabetic nephropathy in patients with concomitant hypertension and diabetes?*

a Angiotensin-converting enzyme (ACE) inhibitors and calcium channel blockers
b ACE inhibitors and liberalizing protein in the diet
c Beta blockers and diuretics
d ACE inhibitors and diuretics

109 *A 50-year-old woman has received a living-related renal transplantation 2 months ago. Which of the following opportunistic infections occurs more frequently during this time period?*

a Histoplasmosis
b Cytomegalovirus (CMV)
c Herpes simplex
d *Pneumocystitis carnii*

110 *Which of the following medications administered in the post-transplantation period may contribute to the development of hyperlipidemia?*

a Corticosteroids
b Tacrolimus (FK-506)
c Trimethoprim sulfamethoxazole
d Azathioprine

Questions 111–115 refer to the following scenario:

A 25-year-old obese woman is admitted to the intensive care unit after having a syncopal episode while having dinner. She lost consciousness for approximately 1 minute, with no loss of bowel or bladder control. In the emergency department, she has a blood pressure of 220/110 mm Hg, and a heart rate of 96. Physical exam reveals no papilledema. The heart exam reveals normal

first and second heart sounds with a S_4 gallop. The lungs are clear. The abdomen is without bruits. The peripheral pulses are all palpable and strong. She has no previous health history, no known allergies, and is currently taking an oral contraceptive.

111 *As the ACNP, which of the following medications should you initiate to treat this patient's hypertension?*

a Sodium nitroprusside (Nitropress)
b Enalapril (Vasotec)
c Nitroglycerin (Tridil)
d Dobutamine (Dobutrex)

112 *The initial goal in lowering blood pressure in this patient should be to:*

a abruptly lower the blood pressure to prevent stroke.
b slowly reduce the blood pressure to minimize precipitating cerebral ischemia.
c rapidly reduce the blood pressure with intravenous medications, then switching to oral medications.
d prevent renal failure.

113 *Which of the following conditions should be listed in the differential diagnosis for this patient?*

a Pheochromocytoma
b Aortic dissection
c Arrhythmia
d All of the above

114 *The S_4 on physical exam in this patient indicates:*

a left atrial enlargement.
b left ventricular hypertrophy.
c right ventricular hypertrophy.
d pericardial constriction.

115 *Features of hypertensive encephalopathy include:*

a headache and seizures.
b nausea and vomiting.
c flank pain and renal failure.
d somnolence and flank pain.

116 *In patients with chronic respiratory acidosis, how does the serum bicarbonate change in response to increases in partial pressure of carbon dioxide ($Paco_2$)?*

a It increases.
b It decreases.
c There is no change.
d It initially decreases, then increases.

117 *A 55-year-old man is admitted to your service with hypervolemic hyponatremia. What is the most appropriate treatment?*

a Liberalize fluid intake.
b Order vasopressin (Pitressin).
c Give intravenous normal saline.
d Restrict water intake.

118 *Symptoms associated with hypernatremia include:*

a nausea.
b vomiting.
c coma.
d all of the above.

119 *Which of the following is a cause of central diabetes insipidus?*

a Lithium
b Head trauma
c Hypercalcemia
d Acute tubular necrosis

120 *Causes of renovascular hypertension include all of the following* **EXCEPT:**

a coarctation of the aorta.
b vasculitis.
c fibromuscular dysplasia.
d atherosclerosis.

121 *The most common finding in the urinalysis of patients with diabetic nephropathy is:*

a white blood cells.
b casts.
c hematuria.
d proteinuria.

122 *An 85-year-old nursing home resident has a chronic indwelling urinary (Foley) catheter and develops a* **Candida** *urinary tract infection. She is asymptomatic. What is the most appropriate treatment?*

a Removal of the catheter
b Amphotericin B (Fungizone) bladder washes
c Intravenous amphotericin B
d All of the above

123 *A 30-year-old man develops a urinary tract infection. Which of the following medication regimes should be used?*

a Single-dose antibiotic
b 3-day course of antibiotics
c 7- to 10-day course of antibiotics
d 14-day course of antibiotics

124 *Impetigo is commonly associated with:*

a systemic lupus erythematosus (SLE).
b an acute interstitial nephritis.
c poststreptococcal glomerulonephritis.
d vasculitis.

125 *Which of the following medications have been proven to be effective in treating congestive heart failure?*

a Enalapril (Vasotec)
b Nifedipine (Procardia)
c Verapamil (Calan)
d Doxazosin (Cardura)

126 *Chronic bronchitis is described as:*

a the permanent destruction of the alveolar walls.
b the presence of a cough for at least a year.
c a precursor to chronic obstructive pulmonary disease (COPD).
d the presence of cough and sputum production on most days for at least 3 months of the year and for a minimum of 2 years.

127 *Which of the following laboratory tests should be ordered in a patient with suspected fibromyalgia?*

a Erythrocyte sedimentation rate (ESR)
b Antinuclear antibody (ANA)
c Complete blood cell count (CBC)
d All of the above

128 *All of the statements concerning fibromyalgia are true* **EXCEPT:**

a it is characterized by chronic, diffuse achiness affecting three or more areas for more than 3 months.
b it is more common in men.
c it may be associated with chronic headache and sleep disturbances.
d it is associated with tender points.

129 *A 25-year-old woman presents with complaints of bloody diarrhea for the past month associated with a 20-lb weight loss. Which of the following conditions usually presents with bloody diarrhea?*

a Crohn's disease
b Diverticulitis
c Colon cancer
d Ulcerative colitis

130 *Kerley B lines on chest x-ray are most consistent with:*

a aortic stenosis.
b adult respiratory distress syndrome (ARDS).
c pulmonary edema.
d pneumonia.

131 *Which of the following disorders is commonly associated with Raynaud's disease?*

a Lyme disease
b Multiple sclerosis
c Myasthenia gravis
d Systemic lupus erythematosus (SLE)

132 *Which of the following certifying bodies offers a certification examination for the acute care nurse practitioner (ACNP)?*

a American Academy of Nurse Practitioners
b American Association of Critical Care Nurses
c American Nurses Credentialing Center
d National League of Nursing

133 *The purpose of certification is to:*

a negotiate employment contracts.
b influence legislation concerning health-care reform.
c ensure the public that an individual has mastered a certain body of knowledge and acquired skills in a particular specialty.
d market the nurse practitioner role to the public.

134 *The scope of practice for the acute care nurse practitioner (ACNP) may be described as:*

a independent.
b interdependent.
c dependent.
d all of the above.

135 *Federal oversight of the Medicaid program is done by the:*

a Health Care Financing Administration (HFCA).
b state.
c Social Security administration.
d National Board of Medicine.

136 *A health maintenance organization (HMO) is a(n):*

a fee-for-service organization.
b health-care system for the retired veterans of the United States military.
c organized health-care system that focuses on health promotion and maintenance.
d health-care plan for the indigent population.

137 *The ethical principle of do no harm reflects the principle of:*

a fidelity.
b beneficence.
c nonmaleficence.
d autonomy.

138 *The acute care nurse practitioner (ACNP) is a member of the heart transplantation candidacy committee. A patient is presented who had a heart transplantation 2 years ago, but continued to smoke and drink after the transplantation. He has developed severe transplant arteriopathy and needs another transplantation. Which of the following ethical principles may help in the decision making of this patient and the allocation of organs?*

a Fidelity
b Beneficence
c Autonomy
d Nonmaleficence

139 *The purpose of the Agency for Healthcare Research and Quality (AHRQ) is to:*

a enhance quality, appropriateness, and effectiveness of health-care services.
b define recommendations for clinical care.
c decrease malpractice claims.
d study the quality of care provided to Medicare recipients.

140 *Which of the following infections may lead to dementia, blindness, and aortic insufficiency?*

a Acquired immunodeficiency syndrome (AIDS)
b Herpes simplex virus infection
c Epstein-Barr virus infection
d Syphilis

141 *All of the following are "B" symptoms of Hodgkin's disease* **EXCEPT:**

a drenching night sweats.
b unexplained fever of 101°F or higher.
c dysphagia.
d loss of more than 10% of body weight in the last 6 months.

142 *The most common form of leukemia is:*

a Acute lymphoblastic leukemia (ALL).
b Chronic lymphocytic leukemia (CLL).
c Chronic myelogenous leukemia (CML).
d Acute myelogenous leukemia (AML).

143 *A 45-year-old woman is admitted to the intensive care unit with hemoptysis. You suspect vitamin K deficiency. What is the initial treatment of choice for vitamin K deficiency?*

a Protamine
b Intravenous vitamin K
c Fresh frozen plasma (FFP)
d Cryoprecipitate

144 *All of the following are treatments for idiopathic thrombocytopenia purpura (ITP)* **EXCEPT:**

a total lymphoid irradiation.
b corticosteroids.
c splenectomy.
d high-dose gamma globulin.

145 *A positive Schilling test is diagnostic of:*

a pernicious anemia.
b hemolytic anemia.

c iron-deficiency anemia.
d folate deficiency.

146 *The most common side effect(s) associated with oral iron therapy is(are):*

a an ileus.
b constipation and abdominal pain.
c paresthesias.
d abdominal bloating.

147 *Depression may be associated with:*

a weight changes.
b sleep disturbances.
c feelings of worthlessness.
d all of the above.

148 *Which of the following diseases may produce chronic monoarticular arthritis?*

a Gonococcal arthritis
b Rheumatoid arthritis
c Reiter's syndrome
d Osteoarthritis

149 *Which of the following classically produces a migratory pattern of arthritis?*

a Paget's disease
b Rheumatoid arthritis
c Gonococcal arthritis
d Systemic lupus erythematosus (SLE)

150 *Electrocardiogram (ECG) manifestations of pericarditis include:*

a flat P waves.
b diffuse ST elevation.
c ST depression.
d peaked T waves.

Answers

1 Answer c
Content area: Chapter 3, Cardiovascular Problems

2 Answer d
Content area: Chapter 10, Immunology Problems

3 Answer a
Content area: Chapter 8, Gastrointestinal Problems

4 Answer d
Content area: Chapter 3, Cardiovascular Problems

5 Answer b
Content area: Chapter 5, Endocrine Problems

6 Answer a
Content area: Chapter 10, Immunology Problems

7 Answer b
Content area: Chapter 4, Pulmonary Problems

8 Answer c
Content area: Chapter 9, Hematology and Oncology Problems

9 Answer b
Content area: Chapter 31, Health Promotion and Risk Assessment

10 Answer d
Content area: Chapter 31, Health Promotion and Risk Assessment

11 Answer b
Content area: Chapter 7, Renal, Genitourinary, and Gynecologic Problems

12 Answer c
Content area: Chapter 7, Renal, Genitourinary, and Gynecologic Problems

13 Answer b
Content area: Chapter 5, Endocrine Problems

14 Answer a
Content area: Chapter 6, Neurologic Problems

15 Answer b
Content area: Chapter 6, Neurologic Problems

16 Answer c
Content area: Chapter 29, Transplantation

17 Answer a
Content area: Chapter 8, Gastrointestinal Problems

18 Answer b
Content area: Chapter 4, Pulmonary Problems

19 Answer d
Content area: Chapter 3, Cardiovascular Problems

20 Answer a
Content area: Chapter 3, Cardiovascular Problems

21 Answer c
Content area: Chapter 9, Hematology and Oncology Problems

22 Answer d
Content areas: Chapter 22, Comorbidities and Chapter 25, Dermatologic Problems

23 Answer b
Content area: Chapter 3, Cardiovascular Problems

24 Answer b
Content area: Chapter 8, Gastrointestinal Problems

25 Answer a
Content area: Chapter 3, Cardiovascular Problems

26 Answer c
Content area: Chapter 6, Neurologic Problems

27   Answer d
Content area: Chapter 6, Neurologic Problems

28   Answer b
Content area: Chapter 11, Musculoskeletal Problems

29   Answer d
Content area: Chapter 12, Head, Ear, Nose, and Throat Problems

30   Answer b
Content area: Chapter 19, Fluid, Electrolyte, and Acid-Base Imbalances

31   Answer a
Content area: Chapter 29, Transplantation

32   Answer c
Content area: Chapter 3, Cardiovascular Problems

33   Answer b
Content area: Chapter 3, Cardiovascular Problems

34   Answer d
Content area: Chapter 3, Cardiovascular Problems

35   Answer b
Content area: Chapter 3, Cardiovascular Problems

36   Answer c
Content area: Chapter 7, Renal, Genitourinary, and Gynecologic Problems

37   Answer d
Content area: Chapter 7, Renal, Genitourinary, and Gynecologic Problems

38   Answer c
Content area: Chapter 8, Gastrointestinal Problems

39   Answer a
Content area: Chapter 4, Pulmonary Problems

40   Answer b
Content area: Chapter 30, Issues in Acute Care

41   Answer a
Content area: Chapter 18, Nutritional Imbalances

42   Answer b
Content area: Chapter 20, Poisoning and Drug Toxicities

43   Answer d
Content area: Chapter 20, Poisoning and Drug Toxicities

44   Answer b
Content area: Chapter 27, Management of Rapidly Changing Situations

45   Answer a
Content area: Chapter 5, Endocrine Problems

46   Answer d
Content area: Chapter 5, Endocrine Problems

47   Answer c
Content area: Chapter 10, Immunology Problems

48   Answer b
Content area: Chapter 3, Cardiovascular Problems

49   Answer c
Content area: Chapter 21, Wound Management

50   Answer a
Content area: Chapter 8, Gastrointestinal Problems

51   Answer c
Content area: Chapter 9, Hematology and Oncology Problems

52   Answer d
Content area: Chapter 6, Neurology Problems

53   Answer a
Content area: Chapter 6, Neurology Problems

54   Answer a
Content area: Chapter 6, Neurology Problems

55   Answer b
Content area: Chapter 6, Neurology Problems

56   Answer c
Content area: Chapter 30, Issues in Acute Care

57   Answer d
Content area: Chapter 5, Endocrine Problems

58   Answer b
Content area: Chapter 5, Endocrine Problems

59   Answer c
Content area: Chapter 12, Head, Ear, Nose, and Throat Problems

60   Answer d
Content area: Chapter 5, Endocrine Problems

61   Answer d
Content area: Chapter 5, Endocrine Problems

62   Answer c
Content area: Chapter 5, Endocrine Problems

63   Answer b
Content area: Chapter 3, Cardiovascular Problems

64   Answer d
Content area: Chapter 5, Endocrine Problems

65   Answer c
Content area: Chapter 16, Altered Mental State

66   Answer b
Content area: Chapter 12, Head, Ear, Nose, and Throat Problems

67   Answer d
Content area: Chapter 20, Poisoning and Drug Toxicities

68   Answer a
Content area: Chapter 25, Dermatologic Problems

69   Answer a
Content area: Chapter 25, Dermatologic Problems

70 Answer b
Content area: Chapter 12, Head, Ear, Nose, and Throat Problems

71 Answer b
Content area: Chapter 31, Health Promotion and Risk Assessment

72 Answer b
Content area: Chapter 24, Infections

73 Answer d
Content area: Chapter 8, Gastrointestinal Problems

74 Answer a
Content area: Chapter 4, Pulmonary Problems

75 Answer c
Content area: Chapter 6, Neurologic Problems

76 Answer b
Content area: Chapter 7, Renal, Genitourinary, and Gynecologic Problems

77 Answer c
Content area: Chapter 10, Immunology Problems

78 Answer b
Content area: Chapter 4, Pulmonary Problems

79 Answer d
Content area: Chapter 4, Pulmonary Problems

80 Answer c
Content area: Chapter 4, Pulmonary Problems

81 Answer a
Content area: Chapter 5, Endocrine Problems

82 Answer b
Content area: Chapter 8, Gastrointestinal Problems

83 Answer c
Content area: Chapter 8, Gastrointestinal Problems

84 Answer d
Content area: Chapter 7, Renal, Genitourinary, and Gynecologic Problems

85 Answer b
Content area: Chapter 7, Renal, Genitourinary, and Gynecologic Problems

86 Answer a
Content area: Chapter 22, Comorbidities

87 Answer c
Content area: Chapter 6, Neurology Problems

88 Answer d
Content area: Chapter 31, Health Promotion and Risk Assessment

89 Answer a
Content area: Chapter 14, Pain

90 Answer b
Content area: Chapter 9, Hematology and Oncology Problems

91 Answer b
Content area: Chapter 9, Hematology and Oncology Problems

92 Answer d
Content area: Chapter 9, Hematology and Oncology Problems

93 Answer d
Content area: Chapter 9, Hematology and Oncology Problems

94 Answer c
Content area: Chapter 9, Hematology and Oncology Problems

95 Answer a
Content area: Chapter 7, Renal, Genitourinary, and Gynecologic Problems

96 Answer d
Content area: Chapter 7, Renal, Genitourinary, and Gynecologic Problems

97 Answer d
Content area: Chapter 18, Nutritional Imbalances

98 Answer b
Content area: Chapter 27, Management of Rapidly Changing Situations

99 Answer d
Content area: Chapter 9, Hematology and Oncology Problems

100 Answer a
Content area: Chapter 8, Gastrointestinal Problems

101 Answer d
Content area: Chapter 4, Pulmonary Problems

102 Answer a
Content area: Chapter 10, Immunology Problems

103 Answer c
Content area: Chapter 31, Health Promotion and Risk Assessment

104 Answer a
Content area: Chapter 19, Fluid, Electrolyte, and Acid-Base Imbalances

105 Answer c
Content area: Chapter 27, Management of Rapidly Changing Situations

106 Answer d
Content area: Chapter 5, Endocrine Problems

107 Answer c
Content area: Chapter 4, Pulmonary Problems

108 Answer a
Content area: Chapter 22, Comorbidities

109 Answer b
Content area: Chapter 24, Infections

110 Answer a
Content area: Chapter 22, Comorbidities

111 Answer a
Content area: Chapter 27, Management of Rapidly Changing Situations

112 Answer b
Content area: Chapter 27, Management of Rapidly Changing Situations

113 Answer d
Content area: Chapter 27, Management of Rapidly Changing Situations

114 Answer b
Content area: Chapter 27, Management of Rapidly Changing Situations

115 Answer a
Content area: Chapter 27, Management of Rapidly Changing Situations

116 Answer a
Content area: Chapter 19, Fluid, Electrolyte, and Acid-Base Imbalances

117 Answer d
Content area: Chapter 19, Fluid, Electrolyte, and Acid-Base Imbalances

118 Answer d
Content area: Chapter 19, Fluid, Electrolyte, and Acid-Base Imbalances

119 Answer b
Content area: Chapter 19, Fluid, Electrolyte, and Acid-Base Imbalances

120 Answer a
Content area: Chapter 7, Renal, Genitourinary, and Gynecologic Problems

121 Answer d
Content area: Chapter 7, Renal, Genitourinary, and Gynecologic Problems

122 Answer a
Content area: Chapter 28, Age- and Culture-Related Considerations

123 Answer c
Content area: Chapter 28, Age- and Culture-Related Considerations

124 Answer c
Content area: Chapter 24, Infections

125 Answer a
Content area: Chapter 3, Cardiovascular Problems

126 Answer d
Content area: Chapter 4, Pulmonary Problems

127 Answer d
Content area: Chapter 10, Immunology Problems

128 Answer b
Content area: Chapter 10, Immunology Problems

129 Answer d
Content area: Chapter 8, Gastrointestinal Problems

130 Answer c
Content area: Chapter 3, Cardiovascular Problems

131 Answer d
Content area: Chapter 11, Musculoskeletal Problems

132 Answer c
Content area: Chapter 30, Issues in Acute Care

133 Answer c
Content area: Chapter 30, Issues in Acute Care

134 Answer d
Content area: Chapter 30, Issues in Acute Care

135 Answer a
Content area: Chapter 30, Issues in Acute Care

136 Answer c
Content area: Chapter 30, Issues in Acute Care

137 Answer c
Content area: Chapter 30, Issues in Acute Care

138 Answer b
Content area: Chapter 30, Issues in Acute Care

139 Answer a
Content area: Chapter 30, Issues in Acute Care

140 Answer d
Content area: Chapter 24, Infections

141 Answer c
Content area: Chapter 9, Hematology and Oncology Problems

142 Answer b
Content area: Chapter 9, Hematology and Oncology Problems

143 Answer c
Content area: Chapter 27, Management of Rapidly Changing Situations

144 Answer a
Content area: Chapter 9, Hematology and Oncology Problems

145 Answer a
Content area: Chapter 9, Hematology and Oncology Problems

146 Answer b
Content area: Chapter 9, Hematology and Oncology Problems

147 Answer d
Content area: Chapter 15, Psychosocial Issues

148 Answer d
Content area: Chapter 11, Musculoskeletal Problems

149 Answer c
Content area: Chapter 11, Musculoskeletal Problems

150 Answer b
Content area: Chapter 3, Cardiovascular Problems

Examination 2

1 *The most common organism responsible for brain abscess is:*

a *Proteus.*
b *Streptococcus.*
c *Candida.*
d herpes.

2 *Innocent cardiac murmurs are usually:*

a holosystolic murmurs.
b early- to mid-systolic murmurs.
c more common in women
d commonly heard in older patients.

3 *Complications that may be associated with mitral valve prolapse (MVP) include all of the following* **EXCEPT:**

a ventricular septal defect.
b severe mitral regurgitation.
c transient ischemic attacks (TIAs).
d arrhythmias.

4 *Alcoholic cardiomyopathy may:*

a cause a dilated left ventricle.
b cause arrhythmias.
c be reversible.
d be all of the above.

5 *A 70 year-old man is seen in your office with complaints of abdominal bloating and lower extremity edema. On physical exam, the patient is noted to have elevated neck veins, liver span two finger breadths below the right costal margin, and a grade II/VI holosystolic murmur heard at the left sternal border that increases with inspiration. What is the most likely diagnosis?*

a Atrial septal defect
b Ventricular septal defect
c Mitral regurgitation
d Tricuspid regurgitation

6 *A 25 year-old woman with no known health history is seen in your office for an employment exam. On physical exam, she is found to be a very thin woman in no acute distress with stable vital signs. Positive physical exam findings include a pectus excavatum chest wall deformity, mid-systolic click, and a late musical systolic murmur. What is the most likely diagnosis?*

a Mitral regurgitation
b Aortic stenosis
c Hypertrophic cardiomyopathy
d MVP

Questions 7–9 refer to the following scenario:

A 50-year-old man who has been on chronic hemodialysis for the past year is admitted to the hospital with complaints of lower extremity edema, palpitations, and shortness of breath. He has been unable to sleep for the past two nights because of shortness of breath. He was last dialyzed 2 days ago. The physical exam reveals he is tachypneic with a respiratory rate of 32 using accessory muscles and has equal chest excursions with bibasilar crackles. The heart exam reveals distant heart tones with a heart rate of 110, a ventricular gallop, and elevated neck veins. Peripheral pulses are weak. A chest x-ray reveals a widened mediastinum.

7 *What is the most likely diagnosis?*

a Cardiac tamponade
b Pulmonary embolus
c Congestive heart failure
d Aortic dissection

8 *Which of the following physical exam findings supports your diagnosis?*

a Use of accessory respiratory muscles and tachypnea
b Distant heart tones and neck vein distention
c Lower extremity edema and weak peripheral pulses
d Ventricular gallop and crackles

9 *Which of the following diagnostic tools should be used to confirm your diagnosis?*

a ECG
b Chest x-ray
c Echocardiogram
d Thoracentesis

10 *The most important clinical manifestation of acute rheumatic fever is:*

a complete heart block.
b polyarthritis.
c carditis.
d lymph node enlargement.

11 *Causes of sudden cardiac death may include all of the following* **EXCEPT:**

a prolonged QT syndrome.
b myocardial infarction.
c Lyme disease.
d aortic stenosis.

12 *The physiologic effects of intra-aortic balloon counterpulsation (IABC) include:*

a improved contractility.
b increased afterload.
c decreased organ perfusion.
d increased preload.

13 *A patient is seen with acute myocardial infarction with blood pressure of 80/60 mm Hg, a heart rate of 92, a cardiac index of 1.7, and a wedge pressure of 24. The pharmacologic agent of choice would be:*

a epinephrine.
b dopamine (Intropin).
c nitroglycerin.
d milrinone (Primacor).

14 *The* Streptococcus *most frequently associated with subacute bacterial endocarditis (SBE) is:*

a *Streptococcus bovis.*
b *Streptococcus viridans.*
c *Streptococcus pneumoniae.*
d *Streptococcus pyogenes.*

15 *Components of a diet history include all of the following* **EXCEPT:**

a physical activity and exercise.
b recent laboratory studies.
c current medications.
d food allergies.

16 *Which of the following fluids should be given to the patient in hemorrhagic shock?*

a Albumin.
b Fresh frozen plasma (FFP).
c Whole blood cells.
d Normal saline solution.

17 *Diastasis recti:*

a is a true hernia.
b is a separation of the two rectus abdominis muscles.
c is caused by heavy lifting.
d may cause intestinal obstruction.

18 *Causes of persistent hiccups include:*

a pericarditis.
b hiatal hernia.
c subdiaphragmatic abscess.
d all of the above.

19 *The major cause of mortality from influenza is:*

a pneumococcal pneumonia.
b streptococcal pharyngitis.
c rheumatic fever.
d viral meningitis.

20 *All of the statements concerning hyperglycemic hyperosmolar nonketotic (HHNK) coma are true* **EXCEPT:**

a osmotic diuresis occurs resulting in dehydration.
b ketogenesis does not occur.
c the symptoms are caused by an elevated serum potassium level.
d it may occur in association with pancreatitis.

21 *A 45-year-old woman is being treated with vancomycin (Vancocin) and gentamicin (Garamycin) for an osteomyelitis of the right ankle. On the 5th day of treatment, she develops oliguria. The patient has a serum potassium level of 6.5 mEq/L, blood urea nitrogen (BUN) level of 60 mg/dL, serum creatinine level of 4.5 mg/dL, and serum sodium level of 135 mEq/L. Which type of renal failure is this patient exhibiting?*

a Acute tubular necrosis (ATN)
b Intrarenal failure
c Postrenal failure
d Prerenal failure

22 *Which of the following should be administered after a splenectomy?*

a Influenza vaccine
b Tetanus toxoid
c Pneumococcal vaccine
d Hepatitis B vaccine

23 *Which of the following medications should be administered with activated charcoal?*

a Magnesium citrate
b Aluminum hydroxide (Amphojel)
c Psyllium (Metamucil)
d Polycarbophil (FiberCon)

24 *A 70-year-old woman is brought to the emergency department after being found in her home sitting unconscious by a wood-burning stove. You suspect carbon monoxide poisoning. Which of the following antidotes should be administered?*

a Naloxone (Narcan)
b Activated charcoal
c Sodium bicarbonate
d Oxygen

25 *The most common cause of otitis media and sinusitis is:*

a *Streptococcus bovis.*
b *Haemophilus.*
c *Streptococcus pneumoniae.*
d *Staphylococcus.*

26 *Which of the following conditions is a contraindication to palpation of the spleen?*

a Hepatitis
b Infectious mononucleosis
c Pneumonia
d Distended abdomen

27 *A hepatic venous hum indicates:*

a hepatic neoplasm.
b hepatitis.
c portal venous hypertension.
d hepatic cirrhosis.

28 *A 70-year-old man is hospitalized with pneumonia. Which of the following physical exam findings would you expect?*

a Bronchial breath sounds and dullness on percussion
b Vesicular breath sounds and hyper-resonant percussion note
c Absent breath sounds and tympanic percussion note
d Decreased breath sounds and hyper-resonant percussion note

29 *The second most common cause of cancer in women is:*

a breast cancer.
b colorectal cancer.
c thyroid cancer.
d lung cancer.

30 *Tumor lysis syndrome is usually associated with:*

a hypokalemia.
b hypocalcemia.
c elevated white blood cell count.
d thrombocytosis.

31 *All of the statements concerning breast cancer are true* **EXCEPT:**

a early menarche is associated with increased incidence of breast cancer.
b estrogen-receptor-positive tumors are more common in premenopausal women.
c most breast cancers are adenocarcinomas.
d all women should be taught breast self-examination.

32 *Which of the following statements concerning esophageal varices is true?*

a It is usually associated with portal hypertension.
b Medical management may include the use of vasopressin (Pitressin).
c Transjugular intrahepatic portocaval shunts (TIPS) may be used to manage esophageal varices.
d All of the above.

33 *Which of the following imaging modalities is most beneficial in evaluating shoulder pain?*

a Plain x-rays
b Magnetic resonance imaging (MRI)
c Computed tomography (CT) scan
d Bone scan

34 *Which of the following arteries supplies most of the blood to the hand?*

a Radial artery
b Brachial artery
c Ulnar artery
d Subclavian artery

35 *A patient is started on haloperidol (Haldol) for psychosis. Which of the following symptoms would you expect 7 days after initiation of this medication?*

a Tardive dyskinesis
b Delirium
c Muscle spasms
d Anorexia

36 *Which of the following medications is a selective serotonin reuptake inhibitor (SSRI)?*

a Paroxetine (Paxil)
b Amitriptyline (Elavil)
c Risperidone (Risperdol)
d Lorazepam (Ativan)

37 *A 40-year-old woman is taking methotrexate for treatment of arthritis. Which of the following is a side effect associated with methotrexate?*

a Acute renal failure
b Pancreatitis
c Bone marrow depression
d Exfoliative dermatitis

a 5:1.
b 20:1.
c 2:1.
d 10:1.

38 *An 80-year-old woman complains of hard stools and constipation. She states she has a bowel movement one to two times per week. She is currently taking the following medications: aspirin, ferrous sulfate, and nifedipine (Procardia). She has a history of hypertension and diverticulosis. All of the following factors may be contributing to her problem* **EXCEPT:**

a taking ferrous sulfate.
b taking nifedipine.
c age.
d diverticulosis.

39 *Causes of hypercalcemia include all of the following* **EXCEPT:**

a thiazide diuretic therapy.
b hyperthyroidism.
c primary hypoparathyroidism.
d immobilization.

40 *Glucocorticoids may lower serum calcium levels in all of the following patients* **EXCEPT** *those with:*

a sarcoidosis.
b vitamin D intoxication.
c hyperparathyroidism.
d multiple myeloma.

41 *Long-term administration of high-dose nitroprusside (Nipride) may lead to:*

a renal failure.
b cyanide toxicity.
c bradycardia.
d bronchospasm.

42 *A 30-year-old man is admitted to the intensive care unit 2 hours after repair of a left lung stab wound. You note that he has drained 500 cc of blood from the chest tube in the past 30 minutes. Vital signs are a heart rate of 120, blood pressure of 80/60 mm Hg, central venous pressure of 3, pulmonary artery pressure of 20/10, and cardiac index of 2.0. He is intubated. As the ACNP, which of the following actions is most appropriate for you to take?*

a Order 2 units of fresh frozen plasma.
b Order another chest x-ray.
c Notify the surgeon, and ask the staff nurse to autotransfuse the shed blood loss.
d Order 2 units of whole blood.

43 *Intrarenal acute renal failure is characterized by a blood urea nitrogen to creatinine ratio of:*

44 *Which of the following medications are not used in treating diastolic dysfunction?*

a Digoxin (Lanoxin)
b Diltiazem (Cardizem)
c Metoprolol (Lopressor)
d Carvedilol (Coreg)

45 *A 50-year-old man is involved in a motor vehicle accident and has a fractured pelvis. Two days after hospitalization, he complains of shortness of breath with a decrease in pulse oximetry. Vital signs are a heart rate of 140, a respiratory rate of 40, and blood pressure of 130/80 mm Hg. He is very agitated and confused. On physical exam you also note a petechial rash in the axillae and the anterior chest wall. These findings suggest:*

a pulmonary embolus.
b fat emboli.
c pneumonia.
d myocardial infarction.

46 *The most frequent complication after thoracoabdominal aneurysm repair is:*

a paralysis.
b myocardial infarction.
c pulmonary embolus.
d pulmonary insufficiency.

47 *Renal tubular acidosis is characterized by:*

a metabolic alkalosis.
b hypokalemia.
c hypernatremia.
d hypomagnesemia.

48 *A 55-year-old woman is being treated for osteomyelitis with oxacillin (Bactocill). You suspect that the patient may have acute interstitial nephritis. The typical presentation includes all of the following* **EXCEPT:**

a fever.
b rash.
c thrombocytopenia.
d eosinophilia.

49 *Carcinoembryonic antigen (CEA) is usually elevated in patients with:*

a metastatic lung cancer.
b testicular cancer.
c prostate cancer.
d metastatic or recurrent colon cancer.

50 *Human chorionic gonadotropin is a tumor marker for:*

a breast cancer.
b testicular cancer.
c prostate cancer.
d bone cancer.

51 *A 30-year-old man is involved in a minor traffic accident and is seen in the emergency department complaining of abdominal pain. A computed tomography (CT) scan of the abdomen is done. No injuries are noted, but a 3-cm solid adrenal mass is detected. All of the following studies should be done in the workup of this mass* **EXCEPT:**

a fine-needle aspiration of the mass.
b serum electrolyte level.
c serum aldosterone level.
d chest x-ray.

52 *Patients with primary adrenal insufficiency will have:*

a decreased adrenocorticotropic hormone (ACTH) levels.
b decreased aldosterone levels.
c decreased cortisol levels.
d normal skin pigmentation.

53 *Functions of the parathyroid hormone include:*

a increasing mobilization of calcium and phosphate from the bone.
b decreasing calcium reabsorption in the distal nephron.
c decreasing vitamin D absorption.
d regulating aldosterone metabolism.

54 *Treatment of Graves' disease includes all of the following* **EXCEPT:**

a propylthiouracil (PTU).
b levothyroxine (Synthroid).
c methimazole (Tapazole).
d radioactive iodine thyroid ablation.

55 *A 20-year-old woman is involved in a motor vehicle accident and requires a blood transfusion. The family inquires about the risk of contracting human immunodeficiency virus (HIV) from the blood transfusions. Which of the following risk ratios is true?*

a 1 in 100.
b 1 in 300,000.
c 1 in 1,000,000.
d 1 in 25,000.

56 *Which of the following ECG changes is associated with hypocalcemia?*

a Presence of U waves
b Elevated T waves
c Prolonged PR interval
d Shortened QT interval

57 *Which of the following is associated with a poor outcome in surgical patients?*

a Hypokalemia
b Severe hypoalbuminemia
c Elevated transferrin levels
d Normal prealbumin levels

58 *A 70-year-old man has a segment of the ileum resected because of a tumor. Which of the following nutritional disorders is associated with this procedure?*

a Pernicious anemia
b Iron-deficiency anemia
c Hypocalcemia
d Hypercalcemia

Questions 59–61 refer to the following scenario:

A 50-year-old woman is seen in the emergency department complaining of abdominal pain, nausea, and vomiting for the past 72 hours. Her past health history is significant for an abdominal hysterectomy done 10 years ago for uterine fibroids. On physical exam her abdomen is distended, but nontender without rebound. Vital signs include a temperature of 100°F, a pulse rate of 92, a respiratory rate of 20, and blood pressure of 110/60 mm Hg.

59 *Initial management of this patient should include:*

a a stat surgical consultation.
b placement of a nasogastric tube.
c administration of antiemetics and analgesics.
d an abdominal computed tomography (CT) scan.

60 *What is the most likely diagnosis in this patient?*

a Acute appendicitis
b Small-bowel obstruction
c Recurrent fibroids
d Acute cholecystitis

61 *The patient required abdominal surgery, and 2 days after surgery she develops a fever of 102°F. What is the most likely cause?*

a Pneumonia
b Wound infection
c Atelectasis
d Deep-vein thrombosis

62 *The most common serious complication after laparoscopic cholecystectomy is:*

a pneumonia.
b peritonitis.
c bile duct injury.
d hepatitis.

63 *The cardinal signs of polycythemia vera are increased:*

a red blood cell mass, oxygen saturation 92% or more, and splenomegaly.
b hemoglobin, thrombocytopenia, and hepatomegaly.
c hemoglobin, leukopenia, and splenomegaly.
d red blood cell mass, thrombocytopenia, and leukopenia.

64 *Treatment of polycythemia vera may include:*

a plasmapheresis.
b phlebotomy.
c steroids.
d bone marrow transplantation.

65 *The most definitive test to establish the diagnosis of sarcoidosis is a:*

a chest x-ray.
b chest computed tomography (CT) scan.
c tissue biopsy.
d sputum culture.

66 *Virchow's triad associated with pulmonary emboli consists of:*

a congestive heart failure, obesity, and trauma.
b stasis, hypercoagulability, and endothelial injury.
c hypocoagulability, malignancy, and extensive pelvic surgery.
d anemia, thrombocytosis, and hypercoagulability.

67 *The incidence of breast cancer in women is:*

a 1 in 200.
b 1 in 1000.
c 1 in 50.
d 1 in 10.

Questions 68–72 refer to the following scenario:

A 45-year-old man is seen in the emergency department complaining of a persistent nosebleed for the past hour. He has no other health problems. Physical exam reveals a well-nourished man in no acute distress. There is fresh blood noted in the nasal mucosa. Petechiae are noted on the forearms and anterior chest wall. The spleen is enlarged. Initial laboratory results reveal a white blood cell count of 7.8 with a normal differential, a hemoglobin of 13.5 g/dL, a hematocrit of 40%, a platelet count of 10,000, a prothrombin time (PT) of 10.5, an International Normalized Ratio (INR) of 1.0, and an activated partial thromboplastin time (aPTT) of 25 seconds.

68 *What should be included in the initial management of this patient?*

a Head computed tomography (CT) scan
b Consultation with otolaryngology
c Packed red blood cell transfusion
d Platelet transfusion

69 *What would be the next step in the management of this patient?*

a Platelet transfusion.
b Transfusion with platelets and fresh frozen plasma.
c Consultation with hematology for a bone marrow biopsy.
d No further treatment is indicated.

70 *The clinical scenario is most consistent with:*

a idiopathic thrombocytopenia purpura (ITP).
b iron-deficiency anemia.
c hemolytic anemia.
d von Willebrand's disease.

71 *Which of the following findings would you expect on bone marrow biopsy?*

a Increased number of megakaryocytes
b Sternberg-Reed cells
c Spherocytes
d Hypersegmented granulocytes

72 *The initial management of idiopathic thrombocytopenia purpura (ITP) is:*

a splenectomy.
b photopheresis.
c platelet transfusion.
d administration of corticosteroids.

73 *Which of the following immunizations should be given several weeks before an elective splenectomy?*

a *Haemophilus influenzae*
b Pneumococcal
c Meningococcal
d All of the above

74 *The most common presenting symptom in patients with multiple myeloma is:*

a back pain.
b headache.
c weight loss.
d polyuria.

75 *Epinephrine works in the treatment of anaphylaxis by:*

a lowering blood pressure.
b constricting bronchial smooth muscle.

c inhibiting mediator release from mast cells and basophils.

d decreasing heart rate.

76 *Which of the following medications may affect theophylline (Aminophylline) levels?*

a Rifampin (Rifadin)
b Cimetidine (Tagamet)
c Phenytoin (Dilantin)
d All of the above

77 *Which of the following is a symptom of biliary colic?*

a Dysphagia
b Weight loss
c Diarrhea
d Dyspepsia

Questions 78–80 refer to the following scenario:

A 28-year-old woman is seen in your clinic complaining of fullness in both breasts for the past 3 months, especially at the time of her menstrual cycle. She states she did a self-breast examination and the breast felt "knotty." Physical exam reveals a well-nourished woman in no acute distress. There is a 1-cm mass palpable in the left outer quadrant of the left breast and smaller lumps noted in both breasts. There is no supraclavicular or axillary adenopathy.

78 *What is the most likely diagnosis in this patient?*

a Carcinoma of the breast
b Fibrocystic breast changes
c Intraductal papilloma
d None of the above

79 *Which of the following is the most appropriate diagnostic procedure at this time?*

a Mammogram
b Ultrasound of the breast
c Biopsy
d Aspiration of breast cyst

80 *Which of the following may be a treatment option for this patient?*

a Oral progesterone
b Vitamin C supplements
c Folic acid
d Vitamin E supplements

81 *A 40-year-old woman is seen with a 3-month history of unilateral bloody nipple discharge and a small mass around the nipple. What is the most likely diagnosis?*

a Fibrocystic breast disease
b Intraductal papilloma

c Breast carcinoma
d Paget's disease

82 *All of the statements concerning fibroadenoma of the breast are true* **EXCEPT:**

a it is a painless, well-circumscribed, freely mobile lesion.
b it is common in young women.
c it is malignant and requires surgical resection.
d it is the most frequent solid benign tumor of the breast.

83 *The most common presenting symptom of breast cancer is:*

a breast pain.
b erythema of the breast.
c itching of the nipple.
d painless breast lump.

84 *A normal grief reaction includes:*

a decreased interest in personal life.
b resentment toward health-care providers who cared for the deceased.
c insomnia.
d all of the above.

85 *A 25-year-old woman in her 28th week of pregnancy is suspected of having gestational diabetes. All of the following statements are true concerning gestational diabetes* **EXCEPT:**

a management should include diabetic diet and oral hypoglycemics.
b patients with gestational diabetes are at high risk for fetal macrosomia.
c the American College of Obstetricians recommends screening for women over the age of 30 with a family history of diabetes.
d women who develop gestational diabetes are at increased risk for developing type 2 diabetes later in life.

86 *The most common form of anemia is:*

a iron-deficiency anemia.
b pernicious anemia.
c anemia of chronic disease.
d thalassemia.

Questions 87–90 refer to the following scenario:

A 60-year-old man is being evaluated for a 2-month history of epigastric pain that occurs 2 hours after meals and is relieved by either eating or taking antacids. The pain is dull and often wakes him up at night. There is no associated weight loss. Physical exam reveals mild tenderness in the epigastrium. The rest of the abdominal exam is normal.

87   *The most likely diagnosis is:*

a   gastric carcinoma.
b   gastric ulcer.
c   cholecystitis.
d   duodenal ulcer.

88   *Which of the following diagnostic modalities should be done initially in this patient?*

a   Abdominal computed tomography (CT) scan
b   Colonoscopy
c   Upper gastrointestinal series
d   Abdominal x-ray

89   *If the patient is found to have a gastric ulcer, which of the following tests should be ordered?*

a   Colonoscopy
b   Barium enema
c   Endoscopy
d   Abdominal computed tomography (CT) scan

90   *Treatment of peptic ulcer disease may include:*

a   antacids.
b   histamine-2 receptor antagonists.
c   avoidance of smoking.
d   all of the above.

91   *The most frequent complication of intubation and mechanical ventilation is:*

a   pneumothorax.
b   bronchopleural (BP) fistula.
c   laryngeal edema.
d   oral ulcers.

92   *Chronic hypoxia may lead to:*

a   increased erythropoiesis.
b   decreased cardiac output.
c   pulmonary hypertension.
d   anemia of chronic disease.

93   *A 50-year-old man has had abdominal and pelvic trauma. His mixed venous saturation is 40%. This indicates:*

a   high cardiac output.
b   alkalosis.
c   inadequate tissue perfusion.
d   hypercapnia.

94   *Which of the following patients may be most likely to develop hypercalcemia?*

a   A 30-year-old trauma patient who has received 10 units of blood
b   An 80-year-old patient with type 2 diabetes
c   A 50-year-old man with congestive heart failure

taking angiotensin-converting enzyme (ACE) inhibitors and diuretics
d   A 45-year-old woman with adenocarcinoma of the lung

95   *All of the following medications may be associated with hyperphosphatemia* **EXCEPT:**

a   Fleet's enema.
b   vitamin D supplements.
c   potassium and sodium phosphates (Neutra-Phos).
d   furosemide (Lasix).

96   *Signs and symptoms associated with hyperphosphatemia may include:*

a   muscle weakness.
b   polyuria.
c   hyporeflexia.
d   weight gain.

97   *Which of the following arterial blood gas (ABG) results indicate compensated respiratory alkalosis?*

a   pH of 7.45, $PaCO_2$ of 35, bicarbonate ion (HCO_3) of 22.
b   pH 7 of .2, $PaCO_2$ of 40, HCO_3 of 18
c   pH of 7.3, $PaCO_2$ of 30, HCO_3 of 28
d   None of the above

98   *Which of the following acid-base disturbances is likely to develop in a patient with nasogastric drainage greater than 2000 cc/d?*

a   Metabolic acidosis
b   Metabolic alkalosis
c   Respiratory alkalosis
d   None of the above

99   *Which of the following acid-base abnormalities would you expect in a patient with chronic obstructive pulmonary disease (COPD)?*

a   Metabolic acidosis
b   Metabolic alkalosis
c   Respiratory acidosis
d   Respiratory alkalosis

100   *A 65-year-old man is 2 days after hemicolectomy and complains of shortness of breath and bilateral leg pain. The results of his ABG are pH of 7.5, $PaCO_2$ of 28, and HCO_3 of 22. What is the most likely diagnosis based on the ABG result?*

a   Congestive heart failure
b   Pneumonia
c   Pulmonary embolus
d   Myocardial infarction

101   *Which of the following mechanisms may account for acute respiratory failure?*

a Alveolar hypoventilation
b Ventilation-perfusion mismatch
c Intrapulmonary shunting
d All of the above

102 *Which of the following patients is most likely to benefit from total parenteral nutrition (TPN)?*

a A 45-year-old otherwise healthy man 1 day after nephrectomy for polycystic kidney disease
b A 30-year-old man with acute pancreatitis not resolved after 1 week
c A patient 1 day after cholecystectomy
d A patient with a tracheostomy who is ventilator dependent

103 *A patient who is not actively bleeding receives 1 unit of blood. You would expect a(n):*

a increase in the hematocrit by 10%.
b increase in the hemoglobin by 3 g/dL.
c increase in the hematocrit by 3%.
d decrease in the hemoglobin by 1 g/dL.

104 *The most common blood type is type:*

a A.
b AB.
c B.
d O.

105 *Facial twitching that occurs when the facial nerve is tapped is called:*

a Tinel sign.
b Murphy's sign.
c Chvostek's sign.
d Battle sign.

Questions 106–109 refer to the following scenario:

A 60-year-old woman with a history of hypertension and hyperlipidemia is seen in the emergency department with complaints of a throbbing headache, visual changes, nausea, and vomiting. Physical exam reveals her blood pressure to be 180/110 mm Hg. She is agitated and disoriented to place and time. She has nuchal rigidity but no other neurologic signs.

106 *The most likely diagnosis based on the clinical history and findings is:*

a migraine headache.
b cerebral aneurysm.
c bacterial meningitis.
d transient ischemic attack.

107 *Which of the following diagnostic tests would confirm the diagnosis?*

a Lumbar puncture

b Transesophageal echocardiogram
c Carotid ultrasound
d computed tomography (CT) scan of the head and cerebral angiogram

108 *What is the next step in the management of this patient?*

a Neurosurgical consultation
b Anticoagulation
c Admission to the intensive care unit and aggressive management of her hypertension
d Repeat computed tomography (CT) scan of the head

109 *Which of the following may occur as a late complication of subarachnoid hemorrhage?*

a Meningitis
b Hydrocephalus
c Transient ischemic attack
d Blindness

Questions 110–113 refer to the following scenario:

A 50-year-old woman with no prior health history is seen by the nurse practitioner with complaints of insomnia. She states that for the past 3 months she has been unable to sleep at night, and sleeps for only 2 to 3 hours during the night. She complains of daytime fatigue and sadness, but it improves by the end of the day. She also complains of constipation and a 10-lb weight loss over the past 3 months. She states she has contemplated suicide. The physical exam is normal.

110 *The most likely diagnosis is:*

a depression.
b anxiety disorder.
c hypothyroidism.
d dementia.

111 *The most appropriate treatment for this patient is:*

a lithium (Eskalith).
b diazepam (Valium).
c paroxetine (Paxil).
d lorazepam (Ativan).

112 *Which of the following medical conditions may account for this patient's symptoms?*

a Congestive heart failure
b Thyroid disease
c Rheumatoid arthritis
d Renal failure

113 *The patient presents 3 weeks later with no improvement in symptoms. What is the appropriate intervention at this time?*

a Refer to psychiatry.
b Order a computed tomography (CT) scan of the head.
c Increase the dose of medication.
d Change to a new medication.

114 *Which of the following laboratory tests should be done before starting a patient on lithium?*

a Thyroid stimulating hormone (TSH) and thyroxine level
b Complete blood cell count
c Liver function test
d Echocardiogram

115 *A 20-year-old woman is 30 weeks pregnant and has a positive cervical culture for* Chlamydia trachomatis. *What is the most appropriate antibiotic choice?*

a Trimethoprim sulfamethoxazole (Bactrim DS).
b Ampicillin (Omnipen)
c Erythromycin (E-Mycin)
d Ciprofloxacin (Cipro)

116 *The most common cause of acute upper gastrointestinal hemorrhage is:*

a esophageal varices.
b peptic ulcer disease.
c ulcerative colitis.
d gastric carcinoma.

117 *The most frequently occurring symptom of ulcerative colitis is:*

a fever.
b bloody diarrhea.
c weight loss.
d abdominal pain.

118 *The most common cause of secondary amenorrhea in reproductive-age women is:*

a hypothyroidism.
b pituitary adenoma.
c pregnancy.
d ovarian failure.

119 *In which of the following women is the use of oral contraceptives contraindicated?*

a A 37-year-old female smoker
b A 25-year-old woman with diabetes
c A 30-year-old woman with polycystic ovary syndrome
d A 20-year-old woman 4 months postpartum

Questions 120–123 refer to the following scenario:

A 30-year-old woman is seen in the emergency depart-ment with a 2-day history of nausea, abdominal pain, and bloody diarrhea. She has a history of ulcerative colitis. Physical exam reveals a thin woman in moderate distress. Her abdomen is distended and tender to touch throughout. Vital signs reveal a pulse of 120 and blood pressure of 100/60 mm Hg. Laboratory tests reveal an elevated white blood cell count with a left shift and a hemoglobin 10 g/dL.

120 *As the ACNP caring for this patient, what is your next step in evaluation of this patient?*

a Abdominal x-ray
b Barium enema
c Surgical consultation
d Abdominal computed tomography (CT) scan

121 *What is a life-threatening complication of ulcerative colitis?*

a Toxic megacolon
b Diverticulitis
c Duodenal ulcer
d Ischemic bowel

122 *Which of the following interventions should be included in the management of this patient?*

a IV fluids
b Antibiotics
c Steroids
d All of the above

123 *The patient shows no clinical improvement in 72 hours. What is the next step in the management of this patient?*

a Surgical intervention
b Increased steroid doses
c Antibiotic therapy
d None of the above

Questions 124–129 refer to the following scenario:

A 40-year-old woman is seen in the emergency depart-ment with complaints of a swollen, painful right calf. She has just returned from a 20-hour flight from Hong Kong. She has no other health history, is not taking any med-ications, and smokes.

124 *Which of the following diagnostic modalities should be initially used in the evaluation of this patient?*

a Pulmonary angiogram
b Ventilation perfusion scan
c Duplex scanning of the lower extremities
d X-ray of right leg

125 *A decision is made to start heparin therapy on this patient. Which of the following should be checked before heparin is initiated?*

a   Computed tomography (CT) scan of the chest
b   Stool occult blood
c   Complete blood cell count
d   arterial blood gas

126   *The patient is started on heparin therapy. Which of the following laboratory tests should be monitored?*

a   aPTT and platelet count
b   Complete blood cell count and PT/INR.
c   Electrolytes
d   PT/INR and platelet count

127   *The patient is noted on day 3 of heparin therapy to have a drop in the platelet count from 140,000/mm³ at baseline to 60,000/mm³. What is the most likely diagnosis?*

a   Disseminated intravascular coagulopathy (DIC)
b   Idiopathic thrombocytopenia purpura (ITP)
c   Heparin-induced thrombocytopenia
d   Thrombocytosis

128   *Based on the decreased platelet count, what is the appropriate intervention?*

a   Stop the heparin.
b   Continue the heparin and start warfarin (Coumadin).
c   Stop the heparin and start aspirin.
d   All of the above.

129   *Which of the following medications may be used to manage patients with heparin-induced thrombocytopenia?*

a   Aspirin
b   Clopidogrel (Plavix)
c   Lepirudin (Refludan)
d   Enoxaparin (Lovenox)

130   *A 30-year-old athlete is abusing anabolic steroids. Which of the following psychiatric disorders would you expect?*

a   Depression
b   Schizophrenia
c   Delirium
d   Mania

131   *A patient is receiving lepirudin (Refludan). How do you monitor its efficacy?*

a   Follow bleeding times.
b   Follow aPTT.
c   Follow PT/INR.
d   Follow platelet counts.

132   *A 65-year-old man is seen in the emergency department after splattering a drain cleaner in his eyes.*

He rinsed his eyes vigorously at home and is complaining of bilateral eye pain. Which of the following interventions should be done immediately?

a   Irrigate the eye again.
b   Consult ophthalmology.
c   Assess visual acuity.
d   Give analgesia.

133   *Which of the following symptoms may be associated with iron toxicity?*

a   Seizures and tremors
b   Abdominal pain and vomiting
c   Headaches
d   Fever and chills

134   *A patient is brought to the emergency department with methadone overdose. What is the antidote for methadone?*

a   Acetylcysteine (Mucomyst)
b   Naloxone (Narcan)
c   Diazepam (Valium)
d   Oxazepam (Serax)

135   *A tension pneumothorax may lead to hemodynamic compromise by:*

a   causing arrhythmias.
b   causing hyperinflation of both lungs.
c   creating crepitus.
d   compressing the heart and great structures.

136   *A 45-year-old man is 2 days postoperative from a lung resection and has a chest tube in place. The nurse notifies you that there is no respiratory variation in the chest tube system. This finding may indicate that the:*

a   patient has a pneumothorax.
b   chest tube is not functioning and may be clotted.
c   chest tube is not placed properly.
d   chest tube drainage system may need to be changed.

137   *Visual disturbances associated with migraine headache include:*

a   intense eye pain.
b   burning and pruritus of the eye.
c   photophobia.
d   delayed pupillary response.

138   *A patient with a closed head injury has hyponatremia and low urine output. These findings suggest:*

a   Addisonian crisis.
b   diabetes mellitus.
c   syndrome of inappropriate antidiuretic hormone (SIADH).
d   increased intracranial pressure.

139 *You examine a 60-year-old woman with sudden onset of slurred speech and generalized weakness. Past medication history is significant for type 2 diabetes mellitus. She is taking metformin (Glucophage). What should be done in the initial evaluation of this patient?*

a Computed tomography (CT) scan of the head
b Lumbar puncture
c Serum glucose and electrolytes levels
d Magnetic resonance imaging (MRI) scan of the head

140 *Which of the following findings may indicate meningococcal meningitis?*

a Headache
b Petechiae
c Fever over 101°F
d Anorexia

141 *Which of the following laboratory values would you expect in a patient with hyperglycemic hyperosmolar nonketotic coma?*

a Positive urine ketones, ph of 7.2, and serum osmolarity of 300 mOsm/L
b Negative urine ketones, pH of 7.3, and serum osmolarity of 275 mOsm/L
c Positive urine ketones, pH of 7.45, and serum osmolarity of 300 mOsm/L
d Negative urine ketones, pH of 7.15, and serum osmolarity of 250 mOsm/L

142 *The main reason(s) for multiple drug resistance and treatment failures in patients with tuberculosis is(are):*

a patient noncompliance.
b human immunodeficiency virus infection.
c drug tolerance.
d all of the above.

143 *Which of the following medications may be used to treat the catecholamine effects associated with hyperthyroidism and thyroid storm?*

a Dopamine (Inotropin)
b Metoprolol (Lopressor)
c Epinephrine
d Clonidine (Catapres)

144 *Bloody penile discharge may be associated with:*

a penile ulcerations.
b urethritis.
c cancer of the penis.
d all of the above.

145 *The most common cause of male infertility is:*

a abstinence.
b variocele.
c hydrocele.
d undescended testes.

146 *Which of the following findings on urinalysis indicates an allergic reaction?*

a hyaline cast.
b elevated white blood cell count.
c eosinophils.
d presence of leukoesterase.

147 *The joint most likely to be affected by degenerative joint disease is the:*

a wrist.
b shoulder.
c knee.
d hip.

148 *The most common cause of degenerative joint disease is:*

a trauma.
b infection.
c obesity.
d immobility.

149 *Which of the following intravenous fluids should be used initially in patients with diabetic ketoacidosis?*

a Lactated Ringer's injection
b 0.9% sodium chloride solution
c Dextrose 5% in 0.45% sodium chloride solution
d Dextrose 10%

150 *Aminocaproic acid (Amicar) is used to:*

a inhibit plasminogen activators.
b increase platelet counts.
c stop bleeding in post-surgical patients.
d inhibit red blood cell breakdown.

Answers

1 Answer b
Content area: Chapter 24, Infections

2 Answer b
Content area: Chapter 3, Cardiovascular Problems

3 Answer a
Content area: Chapter 3, Cardiovascular Problems

4 Answer d
Content area: Chapter 3, Cardiovascular Problems

5 Answer d
Content area: Chapter 3, Cardiovascular Problems

6 Answer d
Content area: Chapter 3, Cardiovascular Problems

7 Answer a
Content area: Chapter 3, Cardiovascular Problems

8 Answer b
Content area: Chapter 3, Cardiovascular Problems

9 Answer c
Content area: Chapter 3, Cardiovascular Problems

10 Answer c
Content area: Chapter 3, Cardiovascular Problems

11 Answer c
Content area: Chapter 3, Cardiovascular Problems

12 Answer a
Content area: Chapter 3, Cardiovascular Problems

13 Answer b
Content area: Chapter 17, Shock

14 Answer b
Content area: Chapter 24, Infection

15 Answer b
Content area: Chapter 18, Nutritional Imbalances

16 Answer c
Content area: Chapter 17, Shock

17 Answer b
Content area: Chapter 8, Gastrointestinal Problems

18 Answer d
Content area: Chapter 8, Gastrointestinal Problems

19 Answer a
Content area: Chapter 24, Infections

20 Answer c
Content area: Chapter 5, Endocrine Problems

21 Answer b
Content area: Chapter 28, Management of Rapidly Changing Situations

22 Answer c
Content area: Chapter 31, Health Promotion and Risk Assessment

23 Answer a
Content area: Chapter 20, Poisoning and Drug Toxicities

24 Answer d
Content area: Chapter 20, Poisoning and Drug Toxicities

25 Answer c
Content area: Chapter 12, Head, Ear, Nose, and Throat Problems

26 Answer b
Content area: Chapter 8, Gastrointestinal Problems

27 Answer c
Content area: Chapter 8, Gastrointestinal Problems

28 Answer a
Content area: Chapter 4, Pulmonary Problems

29 Answer d
Content area: Chapter 9, Hematology and Oncology Problems

30 Answer b
Content area: Chapter 9, Hematology and Oncology Problems

31 Answer b
Content area: Chapter 9, Hematology and Oncology Problems

32 Answer d
Content area: Chapter 8, Gastrointestinal Problems

33 Answer b
Content area: Chapter 11, Musculoskeletal Problems

34 Answer c
Content area: Chapter 11, Musculoskeletal Problems

35 Answer c
Content area: Chapter 15, Psychosocial Issues

36 Answer a
Content area: Chapter 15, Psychosocial Issues

37 Answer c
Content area: Chapter 10, Immunology Problems

38 Answer b
Content area: Chapter 28, Age- and Culture-Related Considerations

39 Answer c
Content area: Chapter 19, Fluid, Electrolyte, and Acid-Base Imbalances

40 Answer b
Content area: Chapter 19, Fluid, Electrolyte, and Acid-Base Imbalances.

41 Answer b
Content area: Chapter 20, Poisoning and Drug Toxicities

42 Answer c
Content area: Chapter 27, Management of Rapidly Changing Situations

43 Answer b
Content area: Chapter 7, Renal, Genitourinary, and Gynecologic Problems

44 Answer a
Content area: Chapter 3, Cardiovascular Problems

45 Answer b
Content area: Chapter 27, Management of Rapidly Changing Situations

46 Answer d
Content area: Chapter 8, Gastrointestinal Problems

47 Answer b
Content area: Chapter 19, Fluid, Electrolyte, and Acid-Base Imbalances.

48 Answer c
Content area: Chapter 22, Comorbidities

49 Answer d
Content area: Chapter 9, Hematology and Oncology Problems

50 Answer b
Content area: Chapter 9, Hematology and Oncology Problems

51 Answer a
Content area: Chapter 27, Management of Rapidly Changing Situations

52 Answer c
Content area: Chapter 5, Endocrine Problems

53 Answer a
Content area: Chapter 5, Endocrine Problems

54 Answer b
Content area: Chapter 5, Endocrine Problems

55 Answer b
Content area: Chapter 10, Immunology Problems

56 Answer c
Content area: Chapter 3, Cardiovascular Problems

57 Answer b
Content area: Chapter 18, Nutritional Imbalances

58 Answer a
Content area: Chapter 18, Nutritional Imbalances

59 Answer b
Content area: Chapter 27, Management of Rapidly Changing Situations

60 Answer b
Content area: Chapter 27, Management of Rapidly Changing Situations

61 Answer c
Content area: Chapter 27, Management of Rapidly Changing Situations

62 Answer c
Content area: Chapter 8, Gastrointestinal Problems

63 Answer a
Content area: Chapter 9, Hematology and Oncology Problems

64 Answer b
Content area: Chapter 9, Hematology and Oncology Problems

65 Answer c
Content area: Chapter 4, Pulmonary Problems

66 Answer b
Content area: Chapter 4, Pulmonary Problems

67 Answer d
Content area: Chapter 31, Health Promotion and Risk Assessment

68 Answer b
Content area: Chapter 9, Hematology and Oncology Problems

69 Answer c
Content area: Chapter 9, Hematology and Oncology Problems

70 Answer a
Content area: Chapter 9, Hematology and Oncology Problems

71 Answer a
Content area: Chapter 9, Hematology and Oncology Problems

72 Answer d
Content area: Chapter 9, Hematology and Oncology Problems

73 Answer d
Content area: Chapter 10, Immunology Problems

74 Answer a
Content area: Chapter 7, Renal, Genitourinary, and Gynecologic Problems

75 Answer c
Content area: Chapter 27, Management of Rapidly Changing Situations

76 Answer d
Content area: Chapter 22, Comorbidities

77 Answer d
Content area: Chapter 8, Gastrointestinal Problems

78 Answer b
Content area: Chapter 31, Health Promotion and Risk Assessment

79 Answer d
Content area: Chapter 7, Renal, Genitourinary, and Gynecologic Problems

80 Answer a
Content area: Chapter 7, Renal, Genitourinary, and Gynecologic Problems

81 Answer b
Content area: Chapter 7, Renal, Genitourinary, and Gynecologic Problems

82 Answer c
Content area: Chapter 7, Renal, Genitourinary, and Gynecologic Problems

83 Answer d
Content area: Chapter 9, Hematology and Oncology Problems

84 Answer d
Content area: Chapter 26, Palliative Care

85 Answer a
Content area: Chapter 35, Endocrine Problems

86 Answer a
Content area: Chapter 9, Hematology and Oncology Problems

87 Answer d
Content area: Chapter 8, Gastrointestinal Problems

88 Answer c
Content area: Chapter 8, Gastrointestinal Problems

89 Answer c
Content area: Chapter 8, Gastrointestinal Problems

90 Answer d
Content area: Chapter 8, Gastrointestinal Problems

91 Answer c
Content area: Chapter 4, Pulmonary Problems

92 Answer a
Content area: Chapter 4, Pulmonary Problems

93 Answer c
Content area: Chapter 22, Comorbidities

94 Answer d
Content area: Chapter 19, Fluid, Electrolyte, and Acid-Base Imbalances

95 Answer d
Content area: Chapter 19, Fluid, Electrolyte, and Acid-Base Imbalances

96 Answer a
Content area: Chapter 19, Fluid, Electrolyte, and Acid-Base Imbalances

97 Answer a
Content area: Chapter 19, Fluid, Electrolyte, and Acid-Base Imbalances

98 Answer b
Content area: Chapter 19, Fluid, Electrolyte, and Acid-Base Imbalances

99 Answer a
Content area: Chapter 19, Fluid, Electrolyte, and Acid-Base Imbalances

100 Answer c
Content area: Chapter 27, Management of Rapidly Changing Situations

101 Answer d
Content area: Chapter 4, Pulmonary Problems

102 Answer b
Content area: Chapter 18, Nutritional Imbalances

103 Answer c
Content area: Chapter 9, Hematology and Oncology Problems

104 Answer d
Content area: Chapter 10, Immunology Problems

105 Answer c
Content area: Chapter 6, Neurologic Problems

106 Answer b
Content area: Chapter 22, Comorbidities

107 Answer d
Content area: Chapter 22, Comorbidities

108 Answer a
Content area: Chapter 27, Management of Rapidly Changing Situations

109 Answer b
Content area: Chapter 6, Neurologic Problems

110 Answer a
Content area: Chapter 15, Psychosocial Issues

111 Answer c
Content area: Chapter 15, Psychosocial Issues

112 Answer b
Content area: Chapter 15, Psychosocial Issues

113 Answer a
Content area: Chapter 15, Psychosocial Issues

114 Answer a
Content area: Chapter 15, Psychosocial Issues

115 Answer c
Content area: Chapter 24, Infections

116 Answer b
Content area: Chapter 8, Gastrointestinal Problems

117 Answer b
Content area: Chapter 8, Gastrointestinal Problems

118 Answer c
Content area: Chapter 7, Renal, Genitourinary, and Gynecologic Problems

119 Answer a
Content area: Chapter 31, Health Promotion and Risk Assessment

120 Answer c
Content area: Chapter 8, Gastrointestinal Problems

121 Answer a
Content area: Chapter 8, Gastrointestinal Problems

122 Answer d
Content area: Chapter 8, Gastrointestinal Problems

123 Answer b
Content area: Chapter 27, Management of Rapidly Changing Situations

124 Answer c
Content area: Chapter 27, Management of Rapidly Changing Situations

125 Answer b
Content area: Chapter 9, Hematology and Oncology Problems

126 Answer a
Content area: Chapter 9, Hematology and Oncology Problems

127 Answer c
Content area: Chapter 9, Hematology and Oncology Problems

128 Answer a
Content area: Chapter 27, Management of Rapidly Changing Situations

129 Answer c
Content area: Chapter 27, Management of Rapidly Changing Situations

130 Answer d
Content area: Chapter 15, Psychosocial Issues

131 Answer b
Content area: Chapter 9, Hematology and Oncology Problems

132 Answer c
Content area: Chapter 20, Poisoning and Drug Toxicities

133 Answer b
Content area: Chapter 20, Poisoning and Drug Toxicities

134 Answer b
Content area: Chapter 20, Poisoning and Drug Toxicities

135 Answer d
Content area: Chapter 4, Pulmonary Problems

136 Answer b
Content area: Chapter 4, Pulmonary Problems

137 Answer c
Content area: Chapter 6, Neurologic Problems

138 Answer c
Content area: Chapter 19, Fluid, Electrolyte, and Acid-Base Imbalances

139 Answer c
Content area: Chapter 22, Comorbidities

140 Answer b
Content area: Chapter 24, Infections

141 Answer a
Content area: Chapter 5, Endocrine Problems

142 Answer a
Content area: Chapter 24, Infections

143 Answer b
Content area: Chapter 5, Endocrine Problems

144 Answer d
Content area: Chapter 7, Renal, Genitourinary, and Gynecologic Problems

145 Answer b
Content area: Chapter 7, Renal, Genitourinary, and Gynecologic Problems

146 Answer c
Content area: Chapter 7, Renal, Genitourinary, and Gynecologic Problems

147 Answer d
Content area: Chapter 11, Musculoskeletal Problems

148 Answer c
Content area: Chapter 11, Musculoskeletal Problems

149 Answer b
Content area: Chapter 19, Fluid, Electrolyte, and Acid-Base Imbalances

150 Answer a
Content area: Chapter 9, Hematology and Oncology Problems